Public Health 101
Healthy People– Healthy Populations

Richard Riegelman, MD, MPH, PhD

Professor and Founding Dean
The George Washington University
School of Public Health and Health Services
Washington, DC

JONES AND BARTLETT PUBLISHERS
Sudbury, Massachusetts
BOSTON   TORONTO   LONDON   SINGAPORE

World Headquarters
Jones and Bartlett Publishers
40 Tall Pine Drive
Sudbury, MA 01776
978-443-5000
info@jbpub.com
www.jbpub.com

Jones and Bartlett Publishers Canada
6339 Ormindale Way
Mississauga, Ontario L5V 1J2
Canada

Jones and Bartlett Publishers International
Barb House, Barb Mews
London W6 7PA
United Kingdom

Jones and Bartlett's books and products are available through most bookstores and online booksellers. To contact Jones and Bartlett Publishers directly, call 800-832-0034, fax 978-443-8000, or visit our website, www.jbpub.com.

Substantial discounts on bulk quantities of Jones and Bartlett's publications are available to corporations, professional associations, and other qualified organizations. For details and specific discount information, contact the special sales department at Jones and Bartlett via the above contact information or send an email to specialsales@jbpub.com.

This publication is designed to provide accurate and authoritative information in regard to the Subject Matter covered. It is sold with the understanding that the publisher is not engaged in rendering legal, accounting, or other professional service. If legal advice or other expert assistance is required, the service of a competent professional person should be sought.

Production Credits
Publisher: Michael Brown
Editorial Assistant: Catie Heverling
Editorial Assistant: Teresa Reilly
Senior Production Editor: Tracey Chapman
Senior Marketing Manager: Sophie Fleck
Manufacturing and Inventory Control Supervisor: Amy Bacus
Composition: Auburn Associates, Inc.
Cover Design: Kristin E. Parker
Cover Image: (left to right, top to bottom) © Temelko Temelkov/ShutterStock, Inc.; © sergel telegin/ShutterStock, Inc.;
    © Muriel Lasure/ShutterStock, Inc.; © Bill Jonscher/Dreamstime.com
Printing and Binding: Courier Stoughton
Cover Printing: John Pow Company

Library of Congress Cataloging-in-Publication Data
Riegelman, Richard K.
    Public health 101 : healthy people - healthy populations / Richard Riegelman.
        p.   ; cm.
    Includes bibliographical references and index.
    ISBN-13: 978-0-7637-6044-1 (pbk.)
    ISBN-10: 0-7637-6044-7 (pbk.)
    1. Public health—Textbooks.   I. Title.
    [DNLM: 1. Public Health. WA 100 R554p 2009]
    RA425.R36 2009
    362.1—dc22
                                                2009004511

6048
Printed in the United States of America
13 12 11 10 09   10 9 8 7 6 5 4 3 2 1

Contents

Section II   Tools of Population Health   39

Chapter 3   Health Informatics and Health Communications   41

Chapter 4   Social and Behavioral Sciences and Public Health   55

Section IV Health Professionals, Healthcare Institutions, and Healthcare Systems 127

The Essential Public Health Series

CURRENT AND FORTHCOMING TITLES IN THE *ESSENTIAL PUBLIC HEALTH SERIES*:

ABOUT THE EDITOR:

Richard K. Riegelman, MD, MPH, PhD, is Professor of Epidemiology-Biostatistics, Medicine, and Health Policy, and founding dean of The George Washington University School of Public Health and Health Services in Washington,

DC. He has taken a lead role in developing the Educated Citizen and Public Health initiative which has brought together arts and sciences and public health education associations to implement the Institute of Medicine of the National Academies' recommendation that ". . .all undergraduates should have access to education in public health." Dr. Riegelman also led the development of George Washington's undergraduate public health major and minor and currently teaches "Public Health 101" and "Epidemiology 101" to undergraduates.

Dedication

To Nancy Alfred Persily, whose enthusiasm for teaching public health to undergraduates inspired *Public Health 101: Healthy People–Healthy Populations.*

Acknowledgments

Public Health 101: Healthy People–Healthy Populations is the culmination of a decade of effort aimed at introducing public health to undergraduates. The effort began with the teaching of an introductory course in public health in 1998 at the then newly created George Washington University School of Public Health and Health Services. The new course organized by Nancy Alfred Persily inspired my own efforts to teach and to learn from a new generation. The approach was designed as part of a liberal arts education stimulating the movement which came to be called The Educated Citizen and Public Health.

Efforts to think through the content of an introductory course in public health has involved a large number of people throughout the United States. Public health, arts and sciences, and clinical educators all participated in the 2006 Consensus Conference on Public Health Education which put forward the framework for "Public Health 101" upon which this book is based. Among those who led and continue to lead this effort is Susan Albertine whose insights into the relationship between public health and liberal education has formed the basis for much of The Educated Citizen and Public Health movement.

I have taught "Public Health 101" since 2002, providing an opportunity to teach and to learn from over 300 undergraduate students at The George Washington University. Their feedback and input has been central to writing and rewriting this book. Madison Hardee and Katie Harter deserve special recognition for their extensive feedback on many chapters of the book. Laura Olsen provided extremely valuable editing assistance. Paul Marantz from Albert Einstein School of Medicine utilized a draft of the book in teaching an introductory undergraduate course. His students also provided helpful feedback. I'd also like to thank Alan Greenberg and Dante Verme, the chair and vice chair of the Department of Epidemiology and Biostatistics at The George Washington University School of Public Health and Health Services, for their support of my efforts to expand the audience for undergraduate public health.

The draft of the text went through extensive review and feedback. I am grateful to all those who read chapters and provided constructive input. These include Doug Anderson, Constance Battle, Amanda Castel, James Cawley, Ellen Dawson, Diane Dewar, Mark Edberg, Leonard Friedman, Jaime Gofin, Michael Gough, Marc Hiller, Rebecca Katz, Ruth Long, Manya Magnus, David Michaels, Marjorie Rubenson, Richard Skolnik, Joel Teitelbaum, and Sara Wilensky.

Mike Brown, Publisher of public health books for Jones and Bartlett, has made an extraordinary contribution to this book and the series as a whole. His vision has helped craft the series and his publishing expertise made it happen. Catie Heverling, Tracey Chapman, Sophie Fleck, and Jessica Cormier of the editorial, production, and marketing staff of Jones and Bartlett deserve special recognition. Their commitment to this book and the entire *Essential Public Health* series has gone well beyond the expectations of their job. They have watched over this project to ensure that it meets the highest publishing standards and finds its role in the education of an entire generation of students new to public health. Sarah Hajduk's copyediting helped improve the clarity and consistency of this text.

Last, but by no means least, is my wife, Linda Riegelman, who encouraged this book and the *Essential Public Health* series from the beginning. She saw the need to reach out to students and make real the roles that public health plays in their everyday lives. Linda went the extra mile by reading and rereading every word I wrote. She deserves the credit for what works but the blame for what fails is all mine.

Confronting the challenge of putting together *Public Health 101* has been one of the great joys of my professional life. I hope that it will bring both joy and a challenge to you as enter into the important and engaging world of public health.

Richard Riegelman, MD, MPH, PhD
April 2009
Washington, DC

Preface: What Is *Public Health 101* All About?

Health care is vital to all of us some of the time, but public health is vital to all of us all of the time.
—C. Everett Koop[1]

Public health is about what makes us sick, what keeps us healthy, and what we can do TOGETHER about it. When we think about health, what often comes to mind first is individual health and wellness. In public health, what should come to mind first is the health of communities and society as a whole. Thus, in public health the focus shifts from the individual to the population, from me to us. Whether the issue is influenza, AIDS, climate change, or the cost of health care, we need to look at the impact on individuals and groups at risk as well as the population as a whole.

Public Health 101: Healthy People–Healthy Populations will introduce you to the population health approach to public health. Population health asks basic questions about what determines health and disease. It puts on the table the full range of options for intervention to promote health and prevent disease. These options can range from individualized medical care, to community-wide efforts to protect health and detect disease, to society-wide interventions ranging from laws to taxes.

Public Health 101 is divided into five sections:

- Section I—Principles of Population Health
- Section II—Tools of Population Health
- Section III—Preventing Disease, Disability, and Death
- Section IV—Health Professionals, Healthcare Institutions, and Healthcare Systems
- Section V—Public Health Institutions and Systems

Section I provides an overview of the principles of population health. We outline what determines disease and disability. We see how we can use evidence to come up with strategies for protecting health and reducing disease, disability, and death. In Chapter 1, we see how public health affects our daily life in ways that we often take for granted. We see how public health focuses on the needs of society as a whole, as well as the needs of populations with special vulnerabilities to disease and disability. We also explore the full range of potential interventions for protecting health and preventing disease, disability, and death. Chapter 2 demonstrates how population health places special emphasis on using evidence to define health problems; to understand the etiology or cause of disease; to develop recommendations for addressing health problems; and to implement and evaluate the benefits and harms of these interventions.

Section II examines the tools of population health designed to reach large numbers of people. These tools include: health information and communications; social and behavioral sciences; and health policy, law, and ethics. In Chapter 3, called Health

Informatics and Health Communications, we look at how health data is obtained and compiled and how it can be conveyed or communicated and used to make decisions. In Chapter 4, we look at the contributions of social sciences to our understanding of the sources of health and disease and the tools available to reduce disease, disability, and death. To do this, we examine how social, economic, and cultural factors affect health. We also examine how individual and group behavior can be changed to improve health. In Chapter 5, we take a look at how health policies and laws can be used to improve health. We also examine the legal, policy, and ethical limitations on their use.

Section III looks at the types of conditions that produce disability and death which include: non-communicable disease, communicable diseases, and environmental disease and injury. We explore the types of interventions that are available to protect health, and prevent disease, disability, and death for each of these types of conditions. Chapter 6 looks at a wide range of non-communicable diseases, including most cancers and diseases of the heart and blood vessels, as well as diseases that affect our mental health, from depression to Alzheimer's. We look at a range of options for intervention including: screening for risk factors and for early detection; genetic modification; and use of cost-effective treatments. Chapter 7 examines communicable diseases or diseases that can be transmitted from person-to-person or from other species to humans. It reviews the options for eliminating or controlling the impacts of these conditions. Options for intervention include: barriers to prevent spread of disease ranging from hand washing to quarantine; immunizations designed to protect individuals, as well as populations; and screening, case finding, and preventive treatment designed to cure and control disease. Chapter 8 explores the impact of the physical environment. We look at the health impacts of the unaltered or natural environment; the human-impacted or altered environment; and the impact of the physical environment built for human use including issues of injuries or safety. We explore the multiple ways that we interact with the physical environment and the resulting potential for disease and injury. We also explore approaches to reducing risk.

In Section IV, we step back and take a look from the population health perspective at health care and healthcare systems focused on the care of individuals one at a time. The healthcare system is such a large enterprise that it has consequences far beyond the individuals it directly serves. In Chapter 9, we examine the range of health professionals, including physicians, nurses, and public health professionals. We ask what we mean by a health professional and look at the roles that education and training play in that process. We also look at how society regulates and compensates health professionals. Chapter 10 examines the types of healthcare institutions in the United States, from hospitals to hospice. It examines how these organizations fit together to address issues of coordination and quality of health care. It asks what we can do to connect the components to ensure coordination and quality of care. In Chapter 11, we build upon what we have learned about healthcare professionals and healthcare institutions and examine the healthcare system as a whole. To do this, we need a basic understanding of how the healthcare system is financed and we look at the issue of access to care and the cost of health care. We examine choices you may need to make when selecting health insurance, as well as choices society as a whole needs to make to provide health care to everyone.

Finally, in Section V we look at the public health system, including the governmental structures that make public health *public*. We also ask basic questions about where we go from here as we explore the future of public health. Chapter 12 examines public health agencies at the local, state, federal, and global levels, and explores the roles that public health agencies are expected to play. It recognizes that even with close collaboration among agencies, the job of population health requires involvement of many other groups. We examine approaches to cooperation with other governmental agencies, nongovernmental organizations, and healthcare professionals. Chapter 13 concludes the book by asking you to think about the future of public health. We examine the emerging emphasis on protection of health through disaster preparation and response. We also see how we can plan for the future by learning lessons from the past and understanding current trends that are likely to continue.

How will we go about accomplishing all this? *Public Health 101: Healthy People–Healthy Populations* will not try to overload your mind with facts. It is about providing you with frameworks for thinking, and applying these frameworks to real situations and thought-provoking scenarios.

Each chapter begins and ends with scenarios designed to show you the types of situations you may confront. After each section, there are cases that relate to one or more chapters in the section. They provide realistic case studies and open-ended questions to help you think through the application of the key concepts presented in each section.

Public Health 101: Healthy People–Healthy Populations has been designed to fulfill the recommendations for "Public Health 101" developed as part of the faculty development program sponsored by the Association for Prevention Teaching and Research (APTR) and the Association of American Colleges and Universities (AAC&U) and funded by the Centers for Disease Control and Prevention (CDC).[2] These recommendations include learning outcomes, as well as enduring understandings, designed to identify key concepts and frameworks that students should take away from "Public Health 101" and integrate into their thinking, their work, and their lifelong learning.

Public Health 101 is designed as a gateway to the world of public health. You should take advantage of the Public Health 101 Web site at www.publichealth101.org.

Hopefully, you will come away from reading *Public Health 101* with an appreciation of how the health of the public is influenced by and can be improved by efforts directed at the population, as well as at the individual level. Let us begin in Chapter 1 by exploring the ways that public health affects everyone's daily life.

REFERENCES

1. C. Everett Koop. What is Public Health? Available at: http://sphcm.washington.edu/about/whatis.asp. Accessed April 2, 2009.
2. Association for Prevention Teaching and Research and Association of American Colleges and Universities. Recommendations for Undergraduate Public Health Education. Available at: http://www.aptrweb.org/resources/pdfs/Recommendations.pdf. Accessed April 2, 2009.

About the Author

Richard Riegelman, MD, MPH, PhD, is Professor of Epidemiology–Biostatistics, Medicine, and Health Policy, and founding dean of The George Washington University School of Public Health and Health Services. His education includes an MD from the University of Wisconsin, plus a MPH and PhD in Epidemiology from The Johns Hopkins University. Dr. Riegelman practiced primary care internal medicine for over 20 years.

Dr. Riegelman has over 70 publications, including six books for students and practitioners of medicine and public health. He is currently editor of the Jones and Bartlett book series *Essential Public Health*. The series provides books and ancillary materials for the full spectrum of curricula for undergraduate public health education, as well as the core and crosscutting competencies covered by the Certification in Public Health examination of the National Board of Public Health Examiners.

Dr. Riegelman has spearheaded efforts to fulfill the Institute of Medicine's recommendation that "…all undergraduates should have access to education in public health." His work with national public health and arts and sciences organizations has developed into The Educated Citizen and Public Health Movement. This movement now includes efforts by the Association of Schools of Public Health (ASPH), the Association for Prevention Teaching and Research (APTR), the Association of American Colleges and Universities (AAC&U), and the American Public Health Association (APHA), to implement undergraduate public health education. Richard Riegelman teaches medical school, graduate, and undergraduate public health courses, which include "Public Health 101" and "Epidemiology 101."

SECTION I

Principles of
Population Health

Introduction Section I

Section I of Public Health 101: Healthy People—Healthy Populations introduces you to the ways that public health affects your every waking moment from the food you eat, to the water you drink, to the car you drive. Even sleep matters. In public health we use bed nets to prevent malaria as well as beds that prevent back pain and encourage a good night's sleep.

In Section I we will examine a range of approaches to public health that have been used over the centuries. Then we will focus on a 21st century approach known as population health. Population health includes the full range of options for intervention to address health problems from healthcare systems to community control of communicable disease and environmental health to public policies such as taxation and laws designed to reduce cigarette smoking.

In this section we will also examine an evidence-based approach to population health that focuses on defining the problem, establishing the etiology, making evidence-based recommendations, and evaluating the impacts of interventions. The population health and evidence-based approaches introduced in section I provide an underpinning for all that follows.

At the end of Section I, as with each section, there are cases with discussion questions that draw on chapters from the section. Each case is designed as a realistic description of the types of problems we face as we seek to achieve healthy people and healthy populations.

So with no further ado, let's take a look at how public health can and does affect your daily lives.

Public Health: The Population Health Approach

I woke up this morning, got out of bed, and went to the bathroom where I used the toilet, washed my hands, brushed and flossed my teeth, drank a glass of water, and took my blood pressure medicine, cholesterol medication, and an aspirin. Then, I did my exercises and took a shower.

On the way to the kitchen, I didn't even notice the smoke detector I passed or the old ashtrays in the closet. I took a low fat yogurt out of the refrigerator and prepared hot cereal in the microwave oven for my breakfast.

Then, I walked out my door into the crisp clean air and got in my car. I put on my seat belt, saw the light go on for the air bag, and safely drove to work. I got to my office where I paid little attention to the new defibrillator at the entrance, the "no smoking" signs, or the absence of asbestos. I arrived safely in my well-ventilated office and got ready to teach Public Health 101.

It wasn't a very eventful morning, but then it's all in a morning's work when it comes to public health.

This rather mundane morning is made possible by a long list of achievements that reflect the often-ignored history of public health.[1] We take for granted the fact that water chlorination, hand washing, and indoor plumbing largely eliminated the transmission of common bacterial disease, which so often killed the young and not-so-young for centuries. Don't overlook the impact of prevention on our teeth and gums. Teeth brushing, flossing, and fluoridation of water have made a dramatic impact on dental health of children and adults.

The more recent advances in the prevention of heart disease have been a major public health achievement. Preventive successes include: the reduction of blood pressure and cholesterol, cigarette cessation efforts, use of low-dose aspirin, an understanding of the role of exercise, and the widespread availability of defibrillators. These can be credited with at least half the dramatic reductions in heart disease that have reduced the death rate from coronary artery disease by approximately 50 percent in the United States and most other developed countries in the last half century.

The refrigerator was one of the most important advances in food safety which illustrates the impact of social change and innovation not necessarily intended to improve health. Food and product safety are public health achievements that require continued attention. It was public pressure for food safety that in large part brought about the creation of the U.S. Food and Drug Administration. The work of this public health agency continues to affect all of our lives from the safety of the foods we eat to the drugs and cosmetics we use.

Radiation safety, like radiation itself, usually goes unnoticed from the regulation of microwave ovens to the reduction of radon in buildings. We rarely notice when disease does not occur.

public health interventions

Highway safety illustrates the wide scope of activities required to protect the public's health. From seat belts, child restraints, and air bags to safer cars, highways, designated driver programs and enforcement of drunk driving laws, public health efforts require collaboration with professionals not usually thought of as having a health focus.

The physical environment too has been made safer by the efforts of public health. Improvement in the quality of the air we breathe both outdoors and indoors has been an ongoing accomplishment of what we will call "population health." Our lives are safer today because of interventions ranging from installation of smoke detectors to removal of asbestos from buildings. However, the challenges continue. Globalization increases the potential for the spread of existing and emerging diseases and raises concerns about the safety of the products we use. Climate change and ongoing environmental deterioration continue to produce new territory for "old" diseases, such as malaria. Overuse of technologies, such as antibiotics, have encouraged the emergence of resistant bacteria.

The 20th century saw an increase in life expectancy of almost 30 years in most developed countries, much of it due to the successes of public health initiatives.[2] We cannot assume that these trends will continue indefinitely. The epidemic of obesity already threatens to slow down or reverse the progress we have been making. The challenges of 21st century public health include protection of health and continued improvement in its quality, not just its quantity. Chapter (5)

To understand the role of public health in these achievements and ongoing challenges, let us start at the beginning and ask: what do we mean by public health?

WHAT DO WE MEAN BY PUBLIC HEALTH?

Ask your parents what public health means and they might say "health care for the poor." Well, they are right that public health has always been about providing services for those with special vulnerabilities either directly or through the healthcare system. But that is only one of the ways that public health serves the most needy and vulnerable in our population. Public health efforts often focus on the most vulnerable populations from reducing exposure to lead paint in deteriorating buildings to food supplementation to prevent birth defects and goiters. Addressing the needs of vulnerable populations has always been a cornerstone of public health. As we will see, however, the definition of vulnerable populations continues to change as do the challenges of addressing their needs.

Ask your grandparents what public health means and they might say "washing your hands." Well, they are right too—public health has always been about determining risks to health and providing successful interventions that are applicable to

everyone. But hand washing is only the tip of the iceberg. The types of interventions that apply to everyone and benefit everyone span an enormous range: from food and drug safety to controlling air pollution; from measures to prevent the spread of tuberculosis to vaccinating against childhood diseases; from prevention and response to disasters to detection of contaminants in our water.

The concerns of society as a whole are always in the forefront of public health. These concerns keep changing and the methods for addressing them keep expanding. New technologies and global, local, and national interventions are becoming a necessary part of public health. To understand what public health has been and what it is becoming, let us look at some definitions of public health. The following are two definitions of public health—one from the early 20th century and one from more recent years.

Public health is ". . . the science and art of preventing disease, prolonging life and promoting health . . . through organized community effort. . . ."[3]

The substance of public health is the "organized community efforts aimed at the prevention of disease and the promotion of health."[4]

These definitions show how little the concept of public health changed in the 20th century, however the concept of public health in the 21st century is beginning to undergo important changes in a number of ways including:

- The goal of prolonging life is being complemented by an emphasis on the quality of life.
- Protection of health when it already exists is becoming a focus along with promoting health when it is at risk.
- Use of new technologies, such as the Internet, are redefining "community," as well as offering us new ways to communicate.
- The enormous expansion in the options for intervention, as well as the increasing awareness of potential harms and costs of intervention programs, require a new science of "evidence-based" public health.
- Public health and clinical care, as well as public and private partnerships, are coming together in new ways to produce collaborative efforts rarely seen in the 20th century.

Thus, a new 21st century definition of public health is needed. One such definition might read as follows:

The totality of all evidence-based public and private efforts that preserve and promote health and prevent disease, disability, and death.

This broad definition recognizes public health as the umbrella for a range of approaches which need to be viewed as a part of a big picture or population perspective. Specifically, this definition enlarges the traditional scope of public health to include:

[handwritten: what factors led to the disease]

- An examination of the full range of environmental, social, and economic determinants of health—not just those traditionally addressed by the public health and clinical health care
- An examination of the full range of interventions to address health issues, including the structure and function of healthcare delivery systems, plus the role of public policies that affect health even when health is not their intended effect

If you are asked by your children what is public health, you might respond: *"It is about the big picture issues that affect our own health and the health of our community every day of our lives. It is about protecting health in the face of disasters; preventing disease from addictions such as cigarettes; controlling infections such as the human immunodeficiency virus (HIV); and developing systems to ensure the safety of the food we eat and the water we drink."*

A variety of terms have been used to describe this big picture perspective that takes into account the full range of factors that affect health and considers their interactions.[5] A variation of this approach has been called the social-ecological model, systems thinking, or the **population health approach**. We will use the latter term. Before exploring what we mean by the population health approach, let us examine how the approaches to public health have changed over time.[a]

HOW HAS THE APPROACH OF PUBLIC HEALTH CHANGED OVER TIME?

Organized community efforts to promote health and prevent disease go back to ancient times.[6, 7] The earliest human civilizations integrated concepts of prevention into their culture, their religion, and their laws. Prohibitions against specific foods—including pork, beef, and seafood—plus customs for food preparation, including officially-designated methods of killing cattle and methods of cooking, were part of the earliest practices of ancient societies. Prohibitions against alcohol or its limited use for religious ceremony have long been part of societies' efforts to control behavior, as well as prevent disease. Prohibition of cannibalism, the most

universal of food taboos, has strong grounding in the protection of health.[b]

Sexual practices have been viewed as having health consequences from the earliest civilizations. Male circumcision, premarital abstinence, and marital fidelity have all been shown to have impacts on health.

Quarantine or isolation of individuals with disease or exposed to disease has likewise been practiced for thousands of years. The intuitive notion that isolating individuals with disease could protect individuals and societies led to some of the earliest organized efforts to prevent the spread of disease. At times they were successful, but without a solid scientific basis. Efforts to separate individuals and communities from epidemics sometimes led to misguided efforts, such as the unsuccessful attempts to control the black plague by barring outsiders from walled towns and not recognizing that it was the rats and fleas that transmitted the disease.

During the 18th and first half of the 19th century individuals occasionally produced important insights into the prevention of disease. In the 1740s, British naval commander James Lind demonstrated that lemons and other citrus fruit could prevent and treat scurvy, a then-common disease of sailors whose daily nourishment was devoid of citrus fruit, the best source of vitamin C.

In the last years of the 18th century, English physician Edward Jenner recognized that cowpox, a common mild ailment of those who milked cows, protected those who developed it against life-threatening smallpox. He developed what came to be called a vaccine—derived from the Latin *"vacs,"* meaning cows. He placed fluid from cowpox sores under the skin of recipients, including his son, and exposed them to smallpox. Despite the success of these smallpox prevention efforts, widespread use of vaccinations was slow to develop partially because at that time there was not an adequate scientific basis to explain the reason for its success.

All of these approaches to disease prevention were known before organized public health existed. Public health awareness began to emerge in Europe and America in the mid-19th century. The American public health movement had its origins in Europe where concepts of disease as the consequence of social conditions took root in the 1830s and 1840s. This movement, which put forth the idea that disease emerges from social conditions of inequality, produced the concept of

---

[a] Turnock[2] has described several meanings of public health. These include the system and social enterprise, the profession, the methods, the government services, and the health of the public. The population health approach used in this book may be thought of as subsuming all of these different perspectives on public health.

---

[b] In recent years, this prohibition has been indirectly violated by feeding beef products containing bones and brain matter to other cattle. The development of "mad cow" disease and its transmission to humans has been traced to this practice, which can be viewed as analogous to human cannibalism.

social justice. Many attribute public health's focus on vulnerable populations to this tradition.

While early organized public health efforts paid special attention to vulnerable members of society, they also focused on the hazards that affected everyone: contamination of the environment. This focus on sanitation and public health was often called the hygiene movement, which began even before the development of the germ theory of disease. Despite the absence of an adequate scientific foundation, the hygiene movement made major strides in controlling infectious diseases, such as tuberculosis, cholera, and waterborne diseases largely through alteration of the physical environment.

The fundamental concepts of epidemiology also developed during this era. In the 1850s, John Snow, often called the father of epidemiology, helped establish the importance of careful data collection and documentation of rates of disease before and after an intervention to evaluate effectiveness. He is known for his efforts to close down the Broad Street pump, which supplied water contaminated by cholera to a district of London. His actions quickly terminated that epidemic of cholera. John Snow's approach has become a symbol of the earliest epidemiological thinking.

Semmelweis, an Austrian physician, used much the same approach in the mid-19th century to control puerperal fever—or fever of childbirth—then a major cause of maternal mortality. Noting that physicians frequently went from autopsy room to delivery room without washing their hands, he instituted a hand washing procedure and was able to document a dramatic reduction in the frequency of puerperal fever. Unfortunately, he was unable to convince many of his contemporaries to accept this intervention without a clear mechanism of action. Until the acceptance of the germ theory of disease, puerperal fever continued to be the major cause of maternal deaths in Europe and North America.

The mid-19th century in England also saw the development of birth and death records, or vital statistics, which formed the basis of population-wide assessment of health status. From the beginning, there was controversy over how to define the cause of death. Two key figures in the early history of organized public health took opposing positions that reflect this continuing controversy. Edwin Chadwick argued that specific pathological conditions or diseases should be the basis for the cause of death. William Farr argued that underlying factors, including what we would today call risk factors and social conditions, should be seen as the actual causes of death.

Thus, the methods of public health were already being established before the development of the germ theory of disease by Louis Pasteur and his European colleagues in the mid-1800s. The revolutions in biology that they ignited ushered in a new era in public health. American physicians and public health leaders often went to Europe to study new techniques and approaches and brought them back to America to use at home.

After the Civil War, American public health began to produce its own advances and organizations. In 1872, the American Public Health Association (APHA) was formed. According to its own historical account, "the APHA's founders recognized that two of the association's most important functions were advocacy for adoption by the government of the most current scientific advances relevant to public health, and public education on how to improve community health."[8]

The biological revolution of the late 19th and early 20th centuries that resulted from the germ theory of disease laid the groundwork for the modern era of public health. An understanding of the contributions of bacteria and other organisms to disease produced novel diagnostic testing capabilities. For example, scientists could now identify tuberculosis cases through skin testing, bacterial culture, and the newly discovered chest X-ray. Concepts of vaccination advanced with the development of new vaccines against toxins produced by tetanus- and diphtheria-causing bacteria. Without antibiotics or other effective cures, much of public health in this era relied on prevention, isolation of those with disease, and case-finding methods to prevent further exposure.

In the early years of the 20th century, epidemiology methods continued to contribute to the understanding of disease. The investigations of pellagra by Goldberger and the United States Public Health Service overthrew the assumption of the day that pellagra was an infectious disease and established that it was a nutritional deficiency that could be prevented or easily cured with vitamin B-6 (niacin) or a balanced diet. Understanding of the role of nutrition was central to public health's emerging focus on prenatal care and childhood growth and development. Incorporating key scientific advances, these efforts matured in the 1920s and 1930s and introduced a growing alphabet of vitamins and nutrients to the American vocabulary.

A new public health era of effective intervention against active disease began in force after World War II. The discovery of penicillin and its often miraculous early successes convinced scientists, public health practitioners, and the general public that a new era in medicine and public health had arrived.

During this era, public health's focus was on filling the holes in the healthcare system. In this period, the role of public health was often seen as assisting clinicians to effectively deliver clinical services to those without the benefits of private medical care and helping to integrate preventive efforts into the practice of medicine. Thus, the great public health success of organized campaigns for the eradication of polio was mistakenly seen solely as a victory for medicine. Likewise, the successful passage of Medicaid and Medicare, outgrowths of public health's commitment to social justice, was simply viewed as efforts to expand the private practice of medicine.

This period, however, did lay the foundations for the emergence of a new era in public health. Epidemiological methods designed for the study of noncommunicable diseases demonstrated the major role that cigarette smoking plays in lung cancer and a variety of other diseases. The emergence of the randomized clinical trial and the regulation of drugs, vaccines, and other interventions by the Food and Drug Administration developed the foundations for what we now call evidence-based public health and evidence-based medicine.

The 1980s and much of the 1990s were characterized by a focus on individual responsibility for health and interventions at the individual level. Often referred to as health promotion and disease prevention, these interventions targeted individuals to effect behavioral change and combat the risk factors for diseases. As an example, to help prevent coronary artery disease, efforts were made to help individuals address high blood pressure and cholesterol, cigarette smoking, and obesity. Behavioral change strategies were also used to help prevent the spread of the newly emerging HIV/AIDS epidemic. Efforts aimed at individual prevention and early detection as part of medical practice began to bear some fruit with the widespread introduction of mammography for detection of breast cancer and the worldwide use of Pap smears for the detection of cervical cancer. Newborn screening for genetic disease became a widespread and often legally-mandated program, combining individual and community components.

Major public health advances during this era resulted from the environmental movement, which brought public awareness to the health dangers of lead in gasoline and paint. The environmental movement also focused on reducing cancer by controlling radiation exposure from a range of sources including sunlight and radon, both naturally-occurring radiation sources. In a triumph of global cooperation, governments worked together to address the newly-discovered hole in the ozone layer. In the United States, reductions in air pollution levels and smoking rates during this era had an impact on the frequency of chronic lung disease, asthma, and most likely coronary artery disease.

The heavy reliance on individual interventions that characterized much of the last half of the 20th century changed rapidly in the beginning of the 21st century. A new era in public health that is often called "population health" has begun to transform professional and public thought about health. From the potential for bioterrorism to the high costs of health care to the control of pandemic influenza and AIDS, the need for community-wide or population-wide, public health efforts have become increasingly evident. This new era is characterized by a global perspective and the need to address international health issues. It includes a focus on the potential impacts of climate change, emerging and reemerging infectious diseases, and the consequences of trade in potentially contaminated or dangerous products, ranging from food to toys.

Table 1-1 outlines these eras of public health, identifies their key defining elements, and highlights important events that symbolize each era.[9]

Thus, today we have entered an era in which a focus on the individual is increasingly coupled with a focus on what needs to be done at the community and population level. This era of public health can be viewed as "the era of population health."

WHAT IS MEANT BY POPULATION HEALTH?

The concept of population health has emerged in recent years as a broader concept of public health that includes all the ways that society as a whole or communities within society are affected by health issues and how they respond to these issues. Population health provides an intellectual umbrella for thinking about the wide spectrum of factors that can and do affect the health of individuals and the population as a whole. Figure 1-1 provides an overview of what falls under the umbrella of population health.

Population health also provides strategies for considering the broad range of potential **interventions** to address these issues. By intervention we mean the full range of strategies designed to protect health, and prevent disease, disability, and death. Interventions include: preventive efforts, such as nutrition and vaccination; curative efforts, such as antibiotics and cancer surgery; and efforts to prevent complications and restore function—from chemotherapy to physical therapy. Thus, population health is about *healthy people and healthy populations*.

The concept of population health can be seen as a comprehensive way of thinking about the modern scope of public health. It utilizes an evidence-based approach to analyze the determinants of health and disease and the options for intervention to preserve and improve health. Population health requires us to define what we mean by **health issues** and what we mean by **population(s)**. It also requires us to define what we mean by **society's shared health concerns**, as well as **society's vulnerable groups**.

To understand population health, we therefore need to define what we mean by each of these four components:

- Health issues
- Population(s)
- Society's shared health concerns
- Society's vulnerable groups

TABLE 1-1 Eras of Public Health

Eras of public health	Focus of attention/ Paradigm	Action framework	Notable events and movements in public health and epidemiology
Health protection (Antiquity–1830s)	Authority-based control of individual and community behaviors	Religious and cultural practices and prohibited behaviors	Quarantine for epidemics; sexual prohibitions to reduce disease transmission; dietary restrictions to reduce food-borne disease
Hygiene movement (1840–1870s)	Sanitary conditions as basis for improved health	Environmental action on a community-wide basis distinct from health care	Snow on Cholera; Semmelweis and puerperal fever; collection of vital statistics as empirical foundation for public health and epidemiology
Contagion control (1880–1940s)	Germ theory: demonstration of infectious origins of disease	Communicable disease control through environmental control, vaccination, sanatoriums, and outbreak investigation in general population	Linkage of epidemiology, bacteriology, and immunology to form TB sanatoriums; outbreak investigation, e.g., Goldberger and pellagra
Filling holes in the medical care system (1950s–mid-1980s)	Integration of control of communicable diseases; modification of risk factors; and care of high-risk population as part of medical care	Public system for care of and control of specific infectious diseases and vulnerable populations distinct from general health care system; Integrated health maintenance organizations with integration of preventive services into general health care system	Antibiotics; randomized clinical trials; concept of risk factors; Surgeon General reports on cigarette smoking; Framingham study on cardiovascular risks; health maintenance organizations and community health centers with integration of preventive services into general healthcare system
Health promotion/ Disease prevention (Mid-1980–2000)	Focus on individual behavior and disease detection in vulnerable and general populations	Clinical and population-oriented prevention with focus on individual control of decision making and multiple interventions	AIDS epidemic and need for multiple interventions to reduce risk; reductions in coronary heart disease through multiple interventions
Population health (21st century)	Coordination of public health and health care delivery based upon shared evidence-based systems thinking	Evidence-based recommendations and information management; focus on harms and costs as well as benefits of interventions; globalization	Evidence-based medicine and public health; information technology; medical errors; antibiotic resistance; global collaboration, e.g., SARS, tobacco control, climate change

Source: Awofeso N. What's new about the "New Public Health"? *American Journal of Public Health.* 2004;94(5):705–709.

FIGURE 1-1 The full spectrum of population health

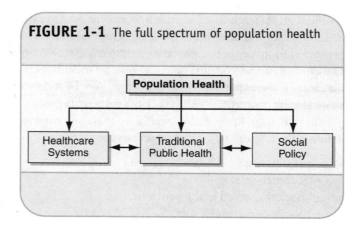

What Are the Implications of Each of the Four Components of Population Health?

All four of the key components of public health have changed in recent years. Let us take a look at the historical, current, and emerging scopes of each component and consider their implications.

For most of the history of public health, the term "health" focused solely on physical health. Mental health has now been recognized as an important part of the definition; conditions such as depression and substance abuse make enormous contributions to disability in populations throughout the world. The boundaries of what we mean by health continue to expand and the limits of health are not clear. Many novel medical interventions, including modification of genes and treatments to increase height, improve cosmetic appearance, and improve sexual performance, confront us with the question: are these health issues?

The definition of a population, likewise, is undergoing fundamental change. For most of recorded history, a population was defined geographically. Geographic communities, such as cities, states, and countries, defined the structure and functions of public health. The current definition of population has expanded to include the idea of a global community, recognizing the increasingly interconnected issues of global health. The definition of population is also focusing more on nongeographic communities. Universities now include the distance-learning community; health care is delivered to members of a health plan; and the Internet is creating new social communities. All of these new definitions of a population are affecting the thinking and approaches needed to address public health issues.

What about the meaning of society-wide concerns—have they changed as well? Historically, public health and communicable disease were nearly synonymous, as symbolized by the field of epidemiology which actually derives its name from the study of communicable disease epidemics. In recent decades, the focus of society-wide concerns has greatly expanded to include toxic exposures from the physical environment, transportation safety, and the costs of health care. However, communicable disease never went away as a focus of public health and the 21st century is seeing a resurgence in concern over emerging infectious diseases, including HIV/AIDS, pandemic flu, and newly drug-resistant diseases, such as staph infections and tuberculosis. Additional concerns, ranging from the impact of climate change to the harms and benefits of new technologies, are altering the meaning of society-wide concerns.

Finally, the meaning of vulnerable populations continues to transform. For most of the 20th century, public health focused on maternal and child health and high risk occupations as the operational definition of vulnerable populations. While these groups remain important to public health, additional groups now receive more attention, including the disabled, the frail elderly, and those without health insurance. Attention is also beginning to focus on the immune-suppressed among those living with HIV/AIDS, who are at higher risk of infection and illness, and those whose genetic code documents their special vulnerability to disease.

Public health has always been about our shared health concerns as a society and our concerns about vulnerable populations. These concerns have changed over time, and new concerns continue to emerge. Table 1-2 outlines historical, current, and emerging components of the population health approach to public health. As is illustrated by communicable diseases, past concerns cannot be relegated to history.

SHOULD WE FOCUS ON EVERYONE OR ON VULNERABLE GROUPS?

Public health is often confronted with the potential conflict of focusing on everyone and addressing society-wide concerns

TABLE 1-2 Components of Population Health

	Health	Population	Examples of society-wide concerns	Examples of vulnerable groups
Historical	Physical	Geographically limited	Communicable disease	High risk maternal and child, high risk occupations
Current	Physical and mental	Local, state, national, global, governmentally-defined	Toxic substances, product and transportation safety, communicable diseases, costs of health care	Disabled, frail elderly, uninsured
Emerging	Cosmetic, genetic, social functioning	Defined by local, national, and global communications	Disasters, climate change, technology hazards, emerging infectious diseases	Immune-suppressed, genetic vulnerability

versus focusing on the needs of vulnerable populations.[10] This conflict is reflected in the two different approaches to addressing public health problems. We will call them the **high-risk approach** and the **improving-the-average approach**.

The high-risk approach focuses on those with the highest probability of developing the disease and aims to bring their risk close to the levels experienced by the rest of the population. Figure 1-2A illustrates the high risk approach.

The success of the high-risk approach, as shown in Figure 1-2B, assumes that those with a high probability of developing disease are heavily concentrated among those with exposure to what we call **risk factors**. Risk factors include a wide range of exposures from cigarette smoke and other toxic substances to high risk sexual behaviors.

The improving-the-average approach focuses on the entire population and aims to reduce the risk for everyone. Figure 1-3 illustrates this approach.

The improving-the-average approach assumes that everyone is at some degree of risk and the risk increases with the extent of exposure. In this situation, most of the disease occurs

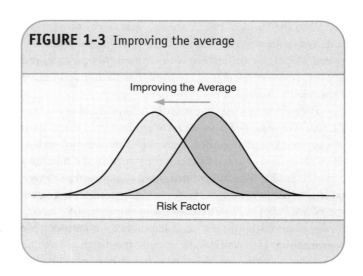

FIGURE 1-3 Improving the average

FIGURE 1-2A High risk

FIGURE 1-2B Reducing high risk

among the large number of people who have only modestly increased exposure. The successful reduction in average cholesterol levels through changes in the American diet and the anticipated reduction in diabetes via a focus on weight reduction among children illustrate this approach.

One approach may work better than the other in specific circumstances, but in general both approaches are needed if we are going to successfully address today's and tomorrow's health issues. These two approaches parallel public health's longstanding focus on both the health of vulnerable populations and society-wide health concerns.[c]

Now that we understand what is meant by population health, let us take a look at the range of approaches that may be used to promote and protect health.

WHAT ARE THE APPROACHES AVAILABLE TO PROTECT AND PROMOTE HEALTH?

The wide range of strategies that have been, are being, and will be used to address health issues can be divided into three general categories: health care, traditional public health, and social interventions.

Health care includes the delivery of services to individuals on a one-on-one basis. It includes services for those who are sick or disabled with illness or diseases, as well as for those who are asymptomatic. Services delivered as part of clinical prevention have been categorized as vaccinations, behav-

[c] An additional approach includes reducing disparities by narrowing the curve. For instance, this might be accomplished by transferring financial and/or health services from the low risk to the high risk category through taxation or other methods. Depending on the distribution of the factors affecting health, this approach may or may not reduce the overall frequency of disease more than the other approaches. The distribution of risk in Figures 1-1 and 1-2 assumes a bell-shaped or normal distribution. The actual distribution of factors affecting health may not follow this distribution.

ioral counseling, screening for disease, and preventive medications.[11]

Traditional public health efforts have a population-based preventive perspective utilizing interventions targeting communities or populations, as well as defined high risk or vulnerable groups. Communicable disease control, reduction of environmental hazards, food and drug safety, and nutritional and behavioral risk factors have been key areas of focus of traditional public health approaches.

Both health care and traditional public health approaches share a goal to directly affect the health of those they reach. In contrast, social interventions are primarily aimed at achieving other nonhealth goals, such as increasing convenience, pleasure, economic growth, and social justice. Social interventions range from improving housing, improving education and services for the poor, to increased global trade. These interventions may have dramatic and sometimes unanticipated positive or negative health consequences. Social interventions, like increased availability of food, may improve health, while the availability of high-fat or high-calorie foods may pose a risk to health.

Table 1-3 describes the characteristics of health care, traditional public health, and social approaches to population health and provides examples of each approach.

None of these approaches is new. However, they have traditionally been separated or put into silos in our thinking process with the connections between them often ignored. As we will see in subsequent chapters, connecting the pieces is an important part of the 21st century challenge of defining public health.

Now that we have explained what we mean by public health and seen the scope and methods that we call population health, let us continue our big-picture approach by taking a look at what we mean by the determinants of health and disease.

WHAT FACTORS DETERMINE THE OCCURRENCE OF DISEASE, DISABILITY, AND DEATH?

To complete our look at the big picture issues in public health, we need to gain an understanding of the forces that determine disease and the outcome of disease including what in public health has been called morbidity (disability) and mortality (death).[d]

As we will see in Chapter 2, we need to establish what are called contributory causes based on evidence. **Contributory causes** can be thought of as causes of disease. For instance, the HIV virus and cigarette smoking are two well-established contributory causes of disease, disability, and death. They produce disease, as well as disability and death. However, knowing these contributory causes of disease is often not enough. We need to ask: what determines whether people will smoke or come in contact with the HIV virus? What determines their course once exposed to cigarettes or HIV? In public health we use the term **determinants** to identify these underlying factors that ultimately bring about disease.

Determinants look beyond the known contributory causes of disease to factors that are at work often years before a dis-

---

[d] We will use the term "disease" as shorthand for the broad range of outcomes that includes injuries and exposures that result in death and disability.

TABLE 1-3 Approaches to Population Health

	Characteristics	Examples
Health care	Systems for delivering one-on-one individual health services including those aimed at prevention, cure, palliation, and rehabilitation	Clinical preventive services including: vaccinations, behavioral counseling, screening for disease, and preventive medications
Traditional public health	Group- and community-based interventions directed at health promotion and disease prevention	Communicable disease control, control of environmental hazards, food and drug safety, reduction in risk factors for disease
Social	Interventions with another nonhealth-related purpose, which have secondary impacts on health	Interventions that improve the built environment, increase education, alter nutrition, or address socioeconomic disparities through changes in tax laws; globalization and mobility of goods and populations

ease develops.[12,13] These underlying factors may be thought of as "upstream" forces. Like great storms, we know the water will flow downstream, often producing flooding and destruction along the way. We just don't know exactly when and where the destruction will occur.

There is no official list or agreed-upon definition of what is included in determinants of disease.[e] Nonetheless, there is wide agreement that the following factors are among those that can be described as determinants in that they increase or at times decrease the chances of developing conditions that threaten the quantity and/or quality of life.

Behavior
Infections
Genetics

Geography
Environment
Medical care
Socio-economic-cultural

BIG GEMS provides a convenient device for remembering these determinants of disease. Let's see what we mean by each of the determinants.

Behavior—Behavior implies actions that increase exposure to the factors that produce disease or protect individuals from disease. Actions such as cigarette smoking, exercise, diet, alcohol consumption, unprotected intercourse, and seat belt use are all examples of the ways that behaviors help determine the development of disease.

Infection—Infections are often the direct cause of disease. In addition, we are increasingly recognizing that early or long-standing exposures to infections may contribute to the development of disease or even protection against disease. Diseases as diverse as gastric and duodenal ulcers, gallstones, and hepatoma or cancer originating in the liver, are increasingly suspected to have infection as an important determinant of the disease. Early exposure to infections may actually reduce diseases ranging from polio to asthma.

Genetics—The revolution in genetics has focused our attention on roles that genetic factors play in the development

and outcome of disease. Even when contributory causes, such as cigarettes, have been clearly established as producing lung cancer, genetic factors also play a role in the development and progression of the disease. While genetic factors play a role in many diseases, they are only occasionally the most important determinant of disease.

Geography—Geographic location influences the frequency and even the presence of disease. Infectious diseases such as malaria, Chagas disease, schistosomiasis, and Lyme disease occur only in defined geographic areas. Geography may also imply local geological conditions, such as those that produce high levels of radon—a naturally-occurring radiation that contributes to the development of lung cancer.

Environment—Environmental factors determine disease and the course of disease in a number of ways. The unaltered or "natural" physical world around us may produce disability and death from sudden natural disasters, such as earthquakes and volcanic eruptions, to iodine deficiencies due to low iodine content in the food-producing soil. The altered physical environment produced by human intervention includes exposures to toxic substances in occupational or nonoccupational settings. The physical environment built for use by humans— the **built environment**—produces determinants ranging from indoor air pollution, to "infant-proofed" homes, to hazards on the highway.

Medical care—Access to and the quality of medical care can be a determinant of disease. When a high percentage of individuals are protected by vaccination, nonvaccinated individuals in the population may be protected as well. Cigarette smoking cessation efforts may help smokers to quit, and treatment of infectious disease may reduce the spread to others. Medical care, however, often has its major impact on the course of disease by attempting to prevent or minimize the disability and death once disease develops.

Social-economic-cultural—In the United States, socioeconomic factors have been defined as education, income, and occupational status. These measures have all been shown to be determinants of diseases as varied as breast cancer, tuberculosis, and occupational injuries. Cultural and religious factors are increasingly being recognized as determinants of diseases because beliefs sometimes influence decisions about treatments, in turn affecting the outcome of the disease. While most diseases are more frequent in lower socioeconomic groups, others such as breast cancer are often more common in higher socioeconomic groups.

We will return to determinants again and again as we explore the work of population health. Historically, understanding determinants has often allowed us to prevent diseases and their consequences even when we did not fully understand the

---

[e] Health Canada[12] has identified 12 determinants of health that are: 1) income and social status; 2) employment; 3) education; 4) social environments; 5) physical environments; 6) healthy child development; 7) personal health practices and coping skills; 8) health services; 9) social support networks; 10) biology and genetic endowment; 11) gender; and 12) culture. Many of these are subsumed under socio-economic-cultural determinants in the BIG GEMS framework. The World Health Organization's Commission on Social Determinants of Health has also produced a list of determinants that is consistent with the BIG GEMS framework.[13]

mechanism by which the determinants produced their impact. For instance:

- Scurvy was controlled by citrus fruits well before vitamin C was identified.
- Malaria was partially controlled by clearing swamps before the relationship to mosquito transmission was appreciated.
- Hepatitis B and HIV infections were partially controlled even before the organisms were identified through reduction in use of contaminated needles and blood transfusions.
- Tuberculosis death rates were greatly reduced through less crowded housing, the use of TB sanitariums, and better nutrition.

Using asthma as an example, Box 1-1 illustrates the many ways that determinants can affect the development and course of a disease.

Thus, population health focuses on the big picture issues and the determinants of disease. Increasingly, public health also emphasizes a focus on the research evidence as a basis for understanding the cause or etiology of disease and the intervention that can improve the outcome. Let us now turn our attention to Chapter 2 which explores what we mean by evidence-based public health.

BOX 1-1 Asthma and the Determinants of Disease.

Jennifer, a teenager living in an urban rundown apartment in a city with high levels of air pollution, develops severe asthma. Her mother also has severe asthma, yet both of them smoke cigarettes. Her clinician prescribed medications to prevent asthma attacks, but she takes them only when she experiences severe symptoms. Jennifer is hospitalized twice with pneumonia due to common bacterial infections. She then develops an antibiotic-resistant infection. During this hospitalization, she requires intensive care on a respirator. After several weeks of intensive care and every known treatment to save her life, she dies suddenly.

Asthma is an inflammatory disease of the lung coupled with an increased reactivity of the airways, which together produce a narrowing of the airways of the lungs. When the airways become swollen and inflamed, they become narrower, allowing less air through to the lung tissue and causing symptoms such as wheezing, coughing, chest tightness, breathing difficulty, and predisposition to infection. Once considered a minor ailment, asthma is now the most common chronic disorder of childhood. It affects over six million children under the age of 18 in the United States alone.

Jennifer's tragic history illustrates how a wide range of determinants of disease may affect the occurrence, severity, and development of complications of a disease. Let's walk through the BIG GEMS framework and see how each determinant impacts in Jennifer's story.

Behavior—Behavioral factors play an important role in the development of asthma attacks and in their complications. Cigarette smoking makes asthma attacks more frequent and more severe. It also predisposes individuals to developing infections such as pneumonia. Treatment for severe asthma requires regular treatments along with more intensive treatment when an attack occurs. It is difficult for many people, especially teenagers, to take medication regularly, yet failure to adhere to treatment greatly complicates the disease.

Infection—Infection is a frequent precipitant of asthma and asthma increases the frequency and severity of infections. Infectious diseases, especially pneumonia, can be life-threatening in asthmatics requiring prompt and high quality medical care. The increasing development of antibiotic-resistant infections pose special risks to those with asthma.

Genetics—Genetic factors predispose people to childhood asthma. However, many children and adults without a family history develop asthma.

Geography—Asthma is more common in geographic areas with high levels of naturally occurring allergens due to flowering plants. However, today even populations in desert climates in the United States are often affected by asthma, as irrigation results in the planting of allergen-producing trees and other plants.

Environment—The physical environment, including that built for use by humans, has increasingly been recognized as a major factor affecting the development of asthma and asthma attacks. Indoor air pollution is the most common form of air pollution in many developing countries. Along with cigarette smoke, air pollution inflames the lungs acutely and chronically. Cockroaches often found in rundown buildings have been found to be highly allergenic and predisposing to asthma. Other factors in the built environment, including mold and exposure to pet dander, can also trigger wheezing in susceptible individuals.

(continues)

BOX 1-1 continued.

Medical care—The course of asthma can be greatly affected by medical care. Management of the acute and chronic effects of asthma can be positively affected by efforts to understand an individual's exposures, reducing the chronic inflammation with medications, managing the acute symptoms, and avoiding life-threatening complications.

Socio-economic-cultural—Disease and disease progression are often influenced by an individual's socioeconomic status. Air pollution is often greater in lower socioeconomic neighborhoods of urban areas. Mold and cockroach infestations may be greater in poor neighborhoods. Access to and quality of medical care may be affected by social, economic, and cultural factors.

Thus, asthma is a condition which demonstrates the contributions made by the full range of determinants included in the BIG GEMS framework. No one determinant alone explains the bulk of the disease. The large number of determinants and their interactions provide opportunities for a range of health care, traditional public health, and social interventions.

Key Words

- Population health approach
- Social justice
- Interventions
- Health issues
- Population(s)
- Society's shared health concerns
- Society's vulnerable groups
- High-risk approach
- Improving-the-average approach

- Risk factor
- Contributory causes
- Determinants
- Built environment
- Behavior
- Infections
- Genetics
- Geography
- Environment
- Medical care
- Socio-economic-cultural

Discussion Question

1. Think about a typical day in your life and identify ways that public health affects it.

REFERENCES

1. Pfizer Global Pharmaceuticals. *Milestones in Public Health: Accomplishments in Public Health over the Last 100 Years.* New York: Pfizer Global Pharmaceuticals; 2006.

2. Turnock BJ. *Public Health: What It Is and How It Works,* 4th ed. Sudbury, MA: Jones and Bartlett Publishers; 2009.

3. Winslow CEA. The untilled field of public health. *Mod. Med.* 1920; 920;2:183–191.

4. Institute of Medicine. *The Future of Public Health.* Washington, DC: National Academy Press; 1988:41.

5. Young TK. *Population Health: Concepts and Methods.* New York: Oxford University Press; 1998.

6. Rosen G. *A History of Public Health.* Baltimore: Johns Hopkins University Press; 1993.

7. Porter D. *Health, Civilization, and the State: A History of Public Health from Ancient to Modern Times.* Oxford: Rutledge; 1999.

8. American Public Health Association. APHA History and Timeline. Available at: http://www.apha.org/about/news/presskit/aphahistory.htm? NRMODE=Published&NRNODEGUID=%7b8AF0A3FE-8B29-4952-87EF-2757B9B2668F%7d&NRORIGINALURL=%2fabout%2fnews%2fpresskit% 2faphahistory.htm&NRCACHEHINT=NoModifyGuest&PF=true. Accessed March 12, 2009.

9. Awofeso N. What's new about the "New Public Health"? *American Journal of Public Health.* 2004;94(5):705–709.

10. Rose G, Khaw KT, Marmot M. *Rose's Strategy of Preventive Medicine.* New York: Oxford University Press; 2008.

11. Agency for Healthcare Research and Quality. Preventive Services. Available at: http://www.ahrq.gov/. Accessed March 12, 2009.

12. Public Health Agency of Canada. Population Health Approach— What Determines Health? Available at: http://www.phac-aspc.gc.ca/ph-sp/ determinants/index-eng.php. Accessed March 12, 2009.

13. Commission on Social Determinants of Health. *Closing the gap in a generation: health equity through action on the social determinants of health. Final Report of the Commission on Social Determinants of Health.* Geneva: World Health Organization; 2008.

Evidence-based Public Health

Tobacco was introduced to Europe as a new world crop in the early 1600s. Despite the availability of pipe tobacco and later, cigars, the mass production and consumption of tobacco through cigarette smoking did not begin until the development of the cigarette rolling machine by James Duke in the 1880s. This invention allowed mass production and distribution of cigarettes for the first time. Men were the first mass consumers of cigarettes. During World War I, cigarettes were widely distributed free of charge to American soldiers.

Cigarette smoking first became popular among women in the 1920s—an era noted for changes in the role and attitudes of women—and at this time advertising of cigarettes began to focus on women. The mass consumption of cigarettes by women, however, trailed that of men by at least two decades. By the 1950s, over 50 percent of adult males and approximately 25 percent of adult females were regular cigarette smokers.

The health problems of cigarette smoking were not fully recognized until decades after the habit became widespread. As late as the 1940s, R.J. Reynolds advertised that "more doctors smoke Camels than any other cigarette."

Epidemiologists observed that lung cancer deaths were increasing in frequency in the 1930s and 1940s. The increase in cases did not appear to be due to changes in efforts to recognize the disease, ability to recognize the disease, or the definition of the disease. Even after the increasing average life span and aging of the population was taken into account, it was evident that the rate of death from lung cancer was increasing—and more rapidly for men than women. In addition, it was noted that residents of states with higher rates of smoking had higher rates of lung cancer. In the 1950s, the number of lung cancer deaths in females also began to increase and by the 1960s, the disease had become the most common cause of cancer-related deaths in males and was still rising among women.[1, 2]

This type of information was the basis for describing the problems of cigarette smoking and lung cancer and developing ideas or hypotheses about its etiology, or cause. Let us take a look at how the evidence-based public health approach has been used to address the problem of cigarette smoking. There are four basic questions that we need to ask that together make up what we will call the evidence-based public health approach.[3]

1. **Problem:** What is the health problem?
2. **Etiology:** What is/are the contributory cause(s)?
3. **Recommendations:** What works to reduce the health impacts?
4. **Implementation:** How can we get the job done?

These four questions provide a framework for defining, analyzing, and addressing a wide range of public health issues and can be applied to cigarette smoking for the purposes of this chapter.[4] We will call this framework the **P.E.R.I. process**. This process is really circular as illustrated in Figure 2-1. If the evaluation suggests that more needs to be done, the cycle can and should be repeated. Thus, it is an ongoing process.

Using cigarette smoking as an example, we will illustrate the steps needed to apply the evidence-based public health approach.

HOW CAN WE DESCRIBE A HEALTH PROBLEM?

The first step in addressing a health problem is to describe its impact. That is, we need to begin by understanding the occurrence of disability and death due to a disease, which we call the **burden of disease**. In public heath, disability is often called **morbidity** and death is called **mortality**. We also need to determine whether there has been a recent change in the impact of the disease. Thus, the first question we ask in describing a health problem is: what is the burden of disease in terms of morbidity and mortality and has it changed over time?

The second question we need to ask is: are there differences in the distribution of disease and can these differences generate ideas or hypotheses about the disease's etiology (cause)? That is, we need to examine how the disease is spread out or distributed in a population. We call this the **distribution of disease**. Public health professionals called **epidemiologists** investigate factors known as "person" and "place" to see if they can find patterns or associations in the frequency of a disease. We call these **group associations**. Group associations may suggest ideas or hypotheses about the cause, or etiology of a disease.

"Person" includes demographic characteristics which describe people, such as age, gender, race, and socioeconomic factors. It also includes behaviors or exposures, such as cigarette smoking, exercise, radiation exposure, and use of medications. "Place" implies geographic location, such as a city or state, but it also includes connections between people, such as a university community or a shared Internet site. When these types of factors occur more frequently among groups with the disease than among groups without the disease we call them **risk indicators** or **risk markers**.[a]

Finally, epidemiologists take a scientific approach to addressing public health problems. They are often skeptical of initial answers to a question and ask: could there be another explanation for the differences or changes in the distribution of disease? They often ask: are the differences or changes real or are they artifactual? **Artifactual** implies that the apparent association is actually the result of the data collection process.

When trying to determine whether an association is artifactual or real, epidemiologists ask whether, the observed changes or differences may be due to comparing apples to oranges—for example comparing groups of subjects of different average ages. Age is especially important to epidemiologists because it is very strongly related to the occurrence of disease. Thus, the third question that we need to ask in describing a problem is: are the differences or changes used to suggest group associations artifactual or real?

Before we can answer these three questions we need to understand more about the measurements that epidemiologists use to describe a health problem. We need to look carefully at how we measure the changes or differences in disease, disability, and death. In public health, we use **rates** to summarize our measurement. Let us begin by looking at what we mean by rates and then we will return to the three questions that need to be addressed when describing a health problem.

WHAT DO WE NEED TO KNOW ABOUT RATES IN ORDER TO DESCRIBE A HEALTH PROBLEM?

The term "rate" will be used to describe the types of measurements that have a numerator and a denominator where the numerator is a subset of the denominator—that is, the numerator includes only individuals who are also included in the denominator. In a rate, the numerator measures the number of times an event, such as the diagnosis of lung cancer, occurs. The denominator measures the number of times the event

FIGURE 2-1 Evidence-based public health: The P.E.R.I. approach

Source: Adopted from Riegelman RK. Evidence-Based Public Health: The Population Health Approach—Cigarettes and Health. Available at: http://www.aptrweb.org/undergraduatepublichealth/Evidence-Based%20Public%20Health.doc. Accessed December 18, 2008.

---

[a] The term risk indicator or risk marker needs to be distinguished from the term risk factor. A risk factor is a candidate for being a contributory cause and implies that at least an association at the individual level has been established as we will discuss later in this chapter. We will also add "time" to "person" and "place" as a basic characteristic for generating hypotheses.

could occur. We often use the entire population in the denominator, but at times we may only use the **at-risk population**. For instance, when measuring the rate of cervical cancer we would only use the population of women in the denominator and when measuring rates of prostate cancer we would only use the population of men in the denominator.[b]

There are two basic types of rates that are key to describing a disease.[5, 6] These are called **incidence** rates and **prevalence**. Incidence rates measure the chances of developing a disease over a period of time—usually one year. That is, incidence rates are the number of new cases of a disease that develop during a year divided by the number of people in the at-risk population, as in the following equation:

$$Incidence\ rate = \frac{\#\ of\ new\ cases\ of\ a\ disease\ in\ a\ year}{\#\ of\ people\ in\ the\ at\text{-}risk\ population}$$

We often express incidence rates as the number of events per 100,000 population in the denominator. For instance, the incidence rate of lung cancer might be 100 per 100,000 per year. In evidence-based public health, comparing incidence rates is often a useful starting point when trying to establish the cause of a problem.

Mortality rates are a special type of incidence rate that measure the incidence of death due to a disease during a particular year. When most people who develop a disease die from the disease, as is the situation with lung cancer, the mortality rate and the incidence rates are very similar. Thus, if the incidence rate of lung cancer is 100 per 100,000 per year, the mortality rate might be 95 per 100,000 per year. When mortality rates and incidence rates are similar and mortality rates are more easily or more reliably obtained, epidemiologists may substitute mortality rates for incidence rates.[c]

The relationship between the incidence rate and the mortality rate is important since it estimates the chances of dying from the disease once it is diagnosed. We call this the **case-fatality**. In our example, the chances of dying from lung cancer—the morality rate divided by the incidence rate—is 95 percent, which indicates that lung cancer results in a very poor prognosis once it is diagnosed.

Prevalence is the number of individuals who have a disease at a particular time divided by the number of individuals who could potentially have the disease. It can be represented by the following equation:

$$Prevalence = \frac{\#\ living\ with\ a\ particular\ disease}{\#\ in\ the\ at\text{-}risk\cdot population}$$

Thus, prevalence tells us the proportion or percentage of individuals who have the disease.[5, 6]

Despite the fact that lung cancer has become the most common cancer, the prevalence will be low—perhaps one-tenth of one percent or less—because those who develop lung cancer do not generally live for a long period of time. Therefore, you will rarely see people with lung cancer. The prevalence of chronic diseases of prolonged duration, such as asthma or chronic obstructive pulmonary disease (COPD), is often relatively high, hence you will often see people with these diseases.[d]

Prevalence is often useful when trying to assess the total impact or burden of a health problem in a population and can help identify the need for services. For example, knowledge that there is a high prevalence of lung cancer in a certain region may indicate that there is a need for healthcare services in that area. Prevalence is also very useful in clinical medicine as the starting point for screening and diagnosis, as we will discuss in Chapter 6. Now that we have addressed rates, we can return to the three questions for describing a health problem.

WHAT IS THE BURDEN OF DISEASE IN TERMS OF MORBIDITY AND MORTALITY AND HAS IT CHANGED OVER TIME?

As we have seen, lung cancer is a disease with a very poor prognosis; therefore, the burden of disease is high as measured by its high mortality rate. This was the situation in the past and to a large extent continues to be the situation.

Mortality rates have been obtained from death certificates for many years. The cause of death on death certificates is classified using a standardized coding system known as the International Classification of Diseases (ICD). No equally complete or accurate system has been available for collecting data on the incidence rate of lung cancer. However, as we learned in

---

[b] When talking about the term "rate," many epidemiologists also include a unit of time, such as a day or a year, over which the number of events in the numerator is measured. This may also be called a **true rate**. The term "rate," as used in this book includes true rates, as well as proportions. A **proportion** is a fraction in which the numerator is a subset of the denominator. A time period is not required for a proportion, however, it often reflects the situation at one point in time.

[c] This is an example of the pragmatic approach that is often taken by epidemiologists when they are limited by the available data. The question facing epidemiologists is frequently: is the data good enough to address the question? Thus, epidemiology can be thought of as an approximation science.

---

[d] The relationship between incidence and prevalence rates is approximately: the incidence rate × average duration of the disease = the prevalence rate. Both the incidence rate and the average duration affect the prevalence of the disease. Together, the incidence, prevalence, and case-fatality rates provide a population-based summary of the course of a disease. Incidence reflects the chance of developing the disease, prevalence indicates the chances of having the disease, and case-fatality indicates the prognosis or chance of dying from the disease.

our discussion of rates, the incidence rates and mortality rates for lung cancer are very similar. Therefore, we can use mortality data as a substitute for incidence data when evaluating the overall burden of lung cancer in a population.

By the 1930s, epidemiologists had concluded from the study of death certificates that lung cancer deaths were rapidly increasing. This increase continued through the 1950s—with cancer occurring two decades or more after the growth in consumption of cigarettes. Therefore, it was not immediately obvious that the two were related. In order to hypothesize that cigarettes were a cause of lung cancer, one needed to conclude that there was a long delay and/or a need for long-term exposure to cigarettes before lung cancer developed. There was a need for more evidence linking cigarettes and lung cancer. Let us turn our attention to the second question to see where this evidence came from.

ARE THERE DIFFERENCES IN THE DISTRIBUTION OF DISEASE AND CAN THESE DIFFERENCES GENERATE IDEAS OR HYPOTHESES ABOUT THEIR ETIOLOGY OR CAUSE?

In looking at the distribution of disease and the potential risk factors, epidemiologists found some important relationships.

In terms of "person," the increases in lung cancer mortality observed in the 1930s through 1950s were far more dramatic among men than among women, though by the 1950s the mortality rate among women had begun to increase as well. It was noted that cigarette use had increased first in men and later among women. There appeared to be a delay of several decades between the increase in cigarette smoking and the increase in lung cancer mortality among both men and women. This illustrates that "time" along with "person" and "place" is important in generating hypotheses.

In terms of "place," it was found that the relationship between cigarette smoking and lung cancer mortality was present throughout the United States, but was strongest in those states where cigarette smoking was most common. Therefore, changes over time and the distribution of disease using "person" and "place" led epidemiologists to the conclusion that there was an association between groups of people who smoked more frequently and the group's mortality rates due to lung cancer. These relationships generated the idea that cigarettes might be a cause of lung cancer. Box 2-1 illustrates some other examples of how distributions of disease by "person", "place," and "time" can generate hypotheses about their cause.

BOX 2-1 Generating Hypotheses from Distributions of Person and Place.

An increased frequency of disease based upon occupation has often provided the initial evidence of a group association based upon a combination of "person" and "place." The first recognized occupational disease was found among chimney sweeps often exposed for long periods of time to large quantities of coal dust who were found to have a high incidence of testicular cancer.

The Mad Hatter described in *Alice's Adventures in Wonderland* by Lewis Carroll made infamous the 19th century recognition that exposure to mercury fumes was associated with mental changes. Mercury fumes were created when making the felt used for hats, hence the term "mad as a hatter."

The high frequency of asbestosis among those who worked in shipyards suggested a relationship decades before the dangers of asbestos were fully recognized and addressed. A lung disease known as silicosis among those who worked in the mining industry likewise suggested a relationship that led to in-depth investigation and greater control of the risks.

More recently, a rare tumor called angiosarcoma was found to occur among those exposed over long periods to polyvinyl chloride (PVC), a plastic widely used in construction. The initial report of four cases of this unusual cancer among workers in one PVC plant was enough to strongly suggest a cause-and-effect relationship based upon "place" alone.

An important example of the impact that "place" can have on generating ideas or hypotheses about causation is the history of fluoride and cavities. In the early years of the 20th century, children in the town of Colorado Springs, Colorado, were found to have a very high incidence of brown discoloration of the teeth. It was soon recognized that this condition was limited to those who obtained their water from a common source. Ironically, those with brown teeth were also protected from cavities. This clear relationship to "place" was followed by over two decades of research that led to the understanding that fluoride in the water reduces the risk of cavities, while very high levels of the compound also lead to brown teeth. Examination of the levels of fluoride in other water systems eventually led to the establishment of levels of fluoride that could protect against cavities without producing brown teeth.

Such strong and clear-cut relationships are important, but relatively unusual. Often, examinations of the characteristics of "person," "place," and "time" in populations suggests hypotheses that can be followed-up among individuals to establish cause and effect relationships.[5, 6]

It is important to realize that these mortality rates are group rates. This data did not include any information about whether those who died from lung cancer were smokers. It merely indicated that groups who smoked more, such as males, also had higher mortality rates from lung cancer. The most that we can hope to achieve from this data is to generate hypotheses based on associations between groups or group associations. When we try to establish causation or etiology, we will need to go beyond group association and focus on associations at the individual level. However, before addressing etiology, we need to ask our third question:

ARE THE DIFFERENCES OR CHANGES USED TO SUGGEST GROUP ASSOCIATIONS ARTIFACTUAL OR REAL?

As we have seen from the 1930s through the 1950s, a large number of studies established that lung cancer deaths were increasing among men, but not among women. That is, there was a change over time and a difference between groups. When epidemiologists observe these types of changes and differences in rates, they ask: are the changes or differences in rates real or could they be artificial or artifactual? There are three basic reasons that changes in rates may be artifactual rather than real:

- Changes in the interest in identifying the disease
- Changes in the ability to identify the disease
- Changes in the definition of the disease

For some conditions, such as HIV/AIDS, these changes have all occurred. New and effective treatments have increased the interest in detecting the infection. Improved technology has increased the ability to detect HIV infections at an earlier point in time. In addition, there have been a number of modifications of the definition of AIDS based on new opportunistic infections and newly recognized complications. Therefore, with HIV/AIDS we need to be especially attentive to the possibility that artifactual changes have occurred.

With lung cancer, on the other hand, the diagnosis at the time of death has been of great interest for many years. The ability to diagnose the disease has not changed substantially. In addition, the use of ICD codes on death certificates has helped standardize the definition of the disease. Epidemiologists concluded that it was unlikely that changes in interest, ability, or definition explained the changes in the rates of lung cancer observed in males, thus they concluded that the changes were not artifactual, but real.[e]

However, it was still possible that the increased mortality rates from lung cancer were due to the increasing life span that was occurring between 1930 and 1960, along with the subsequent aging of the population. Perhaps older people are more likely to develop lung cancer and the aging of the population itself explains the real increase in the rates. To address this issue, epidemiologists use what is called **age adjustment**. To conduct age adjustment, epidemiologists look at the rates of the disease in each age group and also the **age distribution** or the number of people in each age group in the population. Then, they combine the rates for each age group taking into account or adjusting for the age distribution of a population.[f]

Taking into account the age distribution of the population in 1930 and 1960 did have a modest impact on the changes in the mortality rates from lung cancer, but large differences remained. As a result, epidemiologists concluded that lung cancer mortality rates changed over this period especially among men; the changes in rates were real; and the changes could not be explained simply by the aging of the population. Thus, epidemiologists had established the existence of a group association between groups that smoked more cigarettes and groups that developed lung cancer.

WHAT IS THE IMPLICATION OF A GROUP ASSOCIATION?

Group associations are established by investigations that use information on groups or a population without having information on the specific individuals within the group. These studies have been called **population comparisons** or **ecological studies**. Having established the existence of a group association, we still don't know if the individuals who smoke cigarettes are the same ones who develop lung cancer. We can think of a group association as a hypothesis that requires investigation at the individual level. The group association between cigarettes and lung cancer was the beginning of a long road to establish that cigarettes are a cause of lung cancer.

Not all group associations are also individual associations. Imagine the following situation: the mortality rates from drowning are higher in southern states than northern states. The per capita consumption of ice cream is also higher in southern states than northern states. Thus, a group association was established between ice cream consumption and drowning. In thinking about this relationship, you will soon realize that there is another difference between southern and northern states. The average temperature is higher in southern states and higher temperatures are most likely associated with

---

[e] There are actually several types of lung cancer defined by the ICD codes. Most, but not all, types of lung cancer are strongly associated with cigarette smoking.

[f] Adjustment for age is often performed by combining the rates in each age group using the age distribution of what is called a standard population. The age distribution of the U.S. population in 2000 is currently used as the standard population. Adjustment is not limited to age and may at times be conducted using other characteristics that may differ among the groups, such as gender or race, which may affect the probability of developing a disease.

more swimming and also more ice cream consumption. Ice cream consumption is therefore related both to swimming and to drowning. We call this type of factor a **confounding variable**. In this situation, there is no evidence that those who drown actually consumed ice cream. That is, there is no evidence of an association at the individual level. Thus group associations can be misleading if they suggest relationships that do not exist at the individual level.

Epidemiology research studies that look at associations at the individual level are key to establishing etiology, or cause. Etiology is the second component of the P.E.R.I. approach. Let us turn our attention to how to establish etiology.

ETIOLOGY: HOW DO WE ESTABLISH CONTRIBUTORY CAUSE?

Understanding the reasons for disease is fundamental to the prevention of disability and death. We call these reasons etiology or causation. In evidence-based public health, we use a very specific definition of causation—**contributory cause**. The evidence-based public health approach relies on epidemiological research studies to establish a contributory cause. This requires that we go beyond group association and establish three definitive requirements.[7]

1. The "cause" is associated with the "effect" at the individual level. That is, the potential "cause" and the potential "effect" occur more frequently in the same individual than would be expected by chance. Therefore, we need to establish that individuals with lung cancer are more frequently smokers than individuals without lung cancer.

2. The "cause" precedes the "effect" in time. That is, the potential "cause" is present at an earlier time than the potential "effect." Therefore, we need to establish that cigarette smoking comes before the development of lung cancer.

3. Altering the "cause" alters the "effect." That is, when the potential "cause" is reduced or eliminated, the potential "effect" is also reduced or eliminated. Therefore, we need to establish that reducing cigarette smoking reduces lung cancer rates.

Box 2-2 illustrates the logic behind using these three criteria to establish a cause-and-effect relationship, as well as what the implications of a contributory cause are.

These three definitive requirements are ideally established using three different types of studies, all of which relate potential "causes" to potential "effects" at the individual level. That is, they investigate whether individuals who smoke cigarettes are the same individuals that develop lung cancer.[6] The three basic types of investigations are called **case-control** or **retrospective studies**, **cohort studies** or **prospective studies**, and **randomized clinical trials** or **experimental studies**.

Case-control studies are most useful for establishing requirement #1 previously, i.e., the "cause" is associated with the "effect" at the individual level. Case-control studies can demonstrate that cigarettes and lung cancer occur together more

---

BOX 2-2   Lightning, Thunder, and Contributory Cause.

The requirements for establishing the type of cause-and-effect relationship known as contributory cause used in evidence-based public health can be illustrated by the cause-and-effect relationship between lightning and thunder that human beings have recognized from the earliest times of civilization.

First, lightning is generally associated with thunder, that is, the two occur together far more often than one would expect if there were no relationship. Second, with careful observation it can be concluded that the lightning is seen a short time before the thunder is heard. That is, the potential "cause" (the lightning) precedes in time the "effect" (the thunder). Finally, when the lightning stops, so does the thunder—thus, altering the "cause" alters the "effect."

Notice that lightning is not always associated with thunder. "Heat lightning" may not produce audible thunder or the lightning may be too far away for the thunder to be heard. Lightning is not sufficient in and of itself to guarantee that our ears will subsequently always hear thunder. Conversely, in recent years it has been found that the sound of thunder does not always require lightning. Other reasons for rapidly expansion of air, such as an explosion, can also create a sound similar or identical to thunder.

The recognition of lightning as a cause of thunder came many centuries before human beings had any understanding of electricity or today's appreciation for the science of light and sounds. Similarly, cause-and-effect relationships established by epidemiological investigations do not always depend on understanding the science behind the relationships.

frequently than would be expected by chance alone. To accomplish this, cases with the disease (lung cancer) are compared to controls without the disease to determine whether the cases and the controls previously were exposed to the potential "cause" (cigarette smoking).

When a factor such as cigarettes has been demonstrated to be associated on an individual basis with an outcome such as lung cancer, we often refer to that factor as a **risk factor**.[g]

During the 1940s and early 1950s, a number of case-control studies established that individuals who developed lung cancer were far more likely to be regular smokers compared to similar individuals who did not smoke cigarettes. These case-control studies established requirement #1—the "cause" is associated with the "effect" at the individual level. They established that cigarettes are a risk factor for lung cancer.

Cohort studies are most useful for establishing requirement #2 previously—the "cause" precedes the "effect." Those with the potential "cause" or risk factor (cigarette smoking) and those without the potential "cause" are followed over time to determine who develops the "effect" (lung cancer).[h]

Several large scale cohort studies were conducted in the late 1950s and early 1960s. One conducted by the American Cancer Society followed nearly 200,000 individuals over three or more years to determine the chances that smokers and nonsmokers would develop lung cancer. Those who smoked regularly at the beginning of the study had a greatly increased chance of developing lung cancer over the course of the study, thus establishing requirement #2, the "cause" precedes the "effect" in time.

Randomized clinical trials are most useful for establishing requirement #3—altering the "cause" alters the "effect." Using a chance process known as **randomization**, individuals are assigned to be exposed or not exposed to the potential "cause" (cigarette smoking). Individuals with and without the potential "cause" are then followed over time to determine who develops the "effect." Conducting a randomized clinical trial of cigarettes and lung cancer would require investigators to randomize individuals to smoke cigarettes or not smoke cigarettes

and follow them over many years. This illustrates the obstacles that can occur in seeking to definitively establish contributory cause. Once there was a strong suspicion that cigarettes might cause lung cancer, randomized clinical trials were not practical or ethical as a method for establishing cigarette smoking as a contributory cause of lung cancer. Therefore, we need to look at additional criteria that we can use to help us establish the existence of contributory cause.[i]

Figure 2-2 illustrates the requirements for definitively establishing contributory cause and the types of studies that may be used to satisfy each of the requirements. Notice that the requirements for establishing contributory cause are the same as the requirements for establishing **efficacy**. Efficacy implies that an intervention works, that is, it increases positive outcomes or benefits in the population being investigated.

WHAT CAN WE DO IF WE CANNOT DEMONSTRATE ALL THREE REQUIREMENTS TO DEFINITIVELY ESTABLISH CONTRIBUTORY CAUSE?

When we cannot definitively establish a contributory cause, we often need to look for additional supportive evidence.[7] In evidence-based public health, we often utilize what have been called **supportive** or **ancillary criteria** to make scientific judgments about cause and effect. A large number of these criteria have been used and debated. However, four of them are widely used and pose little controversy. They are:

- Strength of the relationship
- Dose-response relationship
- Consistency of the relationship
- Biological plausibility

Let us examine what we mean by each of these criteria. The **strength of the relationship** implies that we are interested in knowing how closely related the risk factor (cigarette smoking) is to the disease (lung cancer). In other words, we want to know the probability of lung cancer among those who smoke cigarettes compared to the probability of lung cancer among those who do not smoke cigarettes. To measure the strength of the relationship we calculate what we call the **relative risk**. The

---

[g] A risk factor, as we just discussed, usually implies that the factor is associated with the disease at the individual level. At times it may be used to imply that the factor not only is associated with the disease at the individual level, but that it precedes the disease in time. Despite the multiple uses of the term, a risk factor does not in and of itself imply that a cause-and-effect relationship is present, though it may be considered a possible cause.

[h] It may seem obvious that cigarette smoking precedes the development of lung cancer. However, the sequence of events is not always so clear. For instance, those who have recently quit smoking cigarettes have an increased chance of being diagnosed with lung cancer. This may lead to the erroneous conclusion that stopping cigarette smoking is a cause of lung cancer. It is more likely that early symptoms of lung cancer lead individuals to quit smoking. The conclusion that stopping cigarette smoking causes lung cancer is called **reverse causality**. Thus, it was important that cohort studies followed smokers and nonsmokers for several years to establish that the cigarette smoking came first.

[i] At times, a special form of a cohort study called a **natural experiment** can help establish that altering the cause alters the effect. A natural experiment implies that an investigator studies the results of a change in one group, but not in another similar group that was produced by forces outside the investigator's control. For instance, after the Surgeon General's *1964 Report on Smoking and Health* was released, approximately 100,000 physicians stopped smoking. This did not happen among other professionals. Over the next decade, the rates of lung cancer among physicians dropped dramatically, but not among other professionals. Despite the fact that natural experiments can be very useful, they are not considered as reliable as randomized clinical trials. Randomization, especially in large studies, eliminates differences between groups or potential confounding differences, even when these differences in characteristics are not recognized by the investigators.

FIGURE 2-2 Fulfilling requirements for establishing contributory cause or efficacy

ask whether smoking more cigarettes is associated with a greater chance of developing lung cancer. If it is, then we say there is a **dose-response relationship**. For instance, smoking one pack of cigarettes per day over many years increases the chances of developing lung cancer compared to smoking half a pack per day. Similarly, smoking two packs per day increases the chances of developing the disease compared to smoking one pack per day. These examples show that a dose-response relationship is present.[k]

Consistency implies that studies in different geographic areas and among a wide range of groups produce similar results. A very large number of studies of cigarettes and lung cancer in many countries and among those of nearly every race and socioeconomic group have consistently demonstrated a strong individual association between cigarette smoking and lung cancer.

The final support criterion is **biological plausibility**. This term implies that we can explain the occurrence of disease based upon known and accepted biological mechanisms. We can explain the occurrence of lung cancer by the fact that cigarette smoke contains a wide range of potentially toxic chemicals which reach the locations in the body where lung cancer occurs.

Thus, the ancillary criteria add support to the argument that cigarette smoking is a contributory cause of lung cancer. Table 2-1 summarizes the use of ancillary or support criteria in making scientific judgments about contributory cause and illustrates these principles using the cigarette smoking and lung cancer scenario. It also cautions to use these criteria carefully because a cause-and-effect relationship may be present even when some or all of these criteria are not fulfilled.[7]

We have now summarized the approach used in evidence-based public health to establish a contributory cause. We

relative risk is the probability of developing the disease if the risk factor is present compared to the probability of the disease if the risk factor is not present. Therefore, the relative risk for cigarette smoking is calculated as:

$$Relative\ risk = \frac{probability\ of\ lung\ cancer\ for\ cigarette\ smokers}{probability\ of\ lung\ cancer\ for\ nonsmokers}$$

The relative risk for cigarette smoking and lung cancer is approximately ten. A relative risk of ten is very large. It tells us that the chances or probability of developing lung cancer are ten times as great for the average smoker compared to the average nonsmoker.[j]

In addition to looking at the strength of the overall relationship between smoking cigarettes and lung cancer, we can

---

[j] A relative risk of ten does not tell us the **absolute risk**. The absolute risk is the actual chance or probability of developing the disease (lung cancer) in the presence of the risk factor (cigarette smoking), expressed numerically—for example, as 0.03 or 3%. A relative risk of ten might imply an increase from 1 in 1000 individuals to 1 in 100 individuals. Alternatively it might imply an increase from 1 in 100 individuals to 1 in 10 individuals. A relative risk can be calculated whenever we have follow-up data on groups of individuals; therefore, it does not in and of itself imply that a contributory cause is present. We need to be careful not to imply that the risk factor will increase the chances of developing the disease or that reducing or eliminating the risk factor will reduce or eliminate the disease unless we have evidence of contributory cause. For case-control studies, a measure known as the **odds ratio** can be calculated and is often used as an approximation of relative risk.

---

[k] A dose-response relationship may also imply that greater exposure to a factor is associated with reduced probability of developing the disease, such as with exercise and coronary artery disease. In this case, the factor may be called a **protective factor** rather than a risk factor.

TABLE 2-1 Ancillary or Supportive Criteria—Cigarettes and Lung Cancer

Criteria	Meaning of the criteria	Evidence for cigarettes and lung cancer	Cautions in using criteria
Strength of the relationship	The relative risk for those with the risk factor is greatly increased compared to those without the risk factor	The relative risk is large or substantial. The relative risk is greater than 10 for the average smoker implying that the average smoker has more than 10 times the probability of developing lung cancer compared to nonsmokers	Even relatively modest relative risks may make important contributions to disease when the risk factor is frequently present. A relative risk of 2 for instance implies a doubling of the probability of developing a disease.
Dose-response relationship	Higher levels of exposure and/or longer duration of exposure to the "cause" is associated with increased probability of the "effect"	Studies of cigarette and lung cancer establish that smoking half a pack a day over an extended period of time increases the risk compared to no smoking. Smoking one pack per day and two packs per day further increases the risk	No dose-response relationship may be evident between no smoking and smoking one cigarette a day or between smoking three and four packs per day
Consistency of the relationship	Studies at the individual level produce similar results in multiple locations among populations of varying socioeconomic and cultural backgrounds	Hundreds of studies in multiple locations and populations consistently establish an individual association between cigarettes and lung cancer	Consistency requires the availability of numerous studies that may not have been conducted
Biological plausibility	Known biological mechanisms can convincingly explain a cause-and-effect relationship	Cigarette smoke directly reaches the areas where lung cancer appears	Exactly which component(s) of cigarette smoking produce lung cancer are just beginning to be understood

started with the development of group associations that generate hypotheses and moved on to look at the definitive requirements for establishing contributory cause. We also looked at the ancillary or supportive criteria that are often needed to make scientific judgments about contributory cause. Table 2-2 summarizes this process and applies it to cigarette smoking and lung cancer.

WHAT DOES CONTRIBUTORY CAUSE IMPLY?

Establishing a contributory cause on the basis of evidence is a complicated, and often a time, consuming job. In practice, our minds often too quickly jump to the conclusion that a cause-

and-effect relationship exists. Our language has a large number of words which may subtly imply a cause-and-effect relationship, even in the absence of evidence. Box 2-3 illustrates how we often rapidly draw conclusions about cause and effect.

It is important to understand what the existence of a contributory cause implies and what it does not imply. Despite the convincing evidence that cigarette smoking is a contributory cause of lung cancer, some individuals never smoke and still develop lung cancer. Therefore, cigarettes are not what we call a **necessary cause** of lung cancer. Others smoke cigarettes all their lives and do not develop lung cancer. Thus, cigarettes are not what we call a **sufficient cause** of lung cancer.

TABLE 2-2 Cigarettes and Lung Cancer—Establishing Cause and Effect

Requirements for contributory cause	Meaning of the requirements	Types of studies that can establish the requirement	Evidence for cigarette smoking and lung cancer
Associated at a population level (Group association)	A group relationship between a "cause" and an "effect."	Ecological study or population comparison study: a comparison of population rates between an exposure and a disease.	Men began mass consumption of cigarettes decades before women and their rates of lung cancer increased decades before those of women.
Individual association: "Requirement #1"	Individuals with a disease ("effect") also have an increased chance of having a potential risk factor ("cause").	Case-control studies: cases with the disease are compared to similar controls without the disease to see who had the exposure.	Lung cancer patients were found to have 10 times or greater chance of smoking cigarettes regularly compared to those without lung cancer.
Prior association: "Requirement #2"	The potential risk factor precedes—in time—the outcome.	Cohort studies: exposed and similar nonexposed individuals are followed over time to determine who develops the disease.	Large cohort studies found that those who smoke cigarettes regularly have a 10 times or greater chance of subsequently developing lung cancer.
Altering the "cause" alters the "effect": "Requirement #3"	Active intervention to expose one group to the risk factor results in a greater chance of the outcome.	Randomized clinical trials allocating individuals by chance to be exposed or not exposed are needed to definitively establish contributory cause. Note: these studies are not always ethical or practical.	Alternatives to randomized clinical trials, such as "natural experiments" established that those who quit smoking have greatly reduced chances of developing lung cancer. In addition, the four supportive criteria also suggest contributory cause.

The fact that not every smoker develops lung cancer implies that there must be factors that protect some individuals from lung cancer. The fact that some nonsmokers develop lung cancer implies that there must be additional contributory causes of lung cancer. Thus, the existence of a contributory cause implies that the "cause" increases the chances that the "effect" will develop. Its presence does not guarantee that the disease will develop. In addition the absence of cigarette smoking does not guarantee that the disease will not develop.

Despite the fact that cigarettes have been established as a contributory cause of lung cancer, they are not a necessary or a sufficient cause of lung cancer. In fact, the use of the concepts of necessary and sufficient cause is not considered useful in the evidence-based public health approach because so few, if any, diseases fulfill the definitions of necessary and sufficient

cause. These criteria are too demanding to be used as standards of proof in public health or medicine.

By 1964, the evidence that cigarette smoking was a contributory cause of lung cancer was persuasive enough for the Surgeon General of the United States to produce the first Surgeon General's *Report on Smoking and Health*. The report concluded that cigarettes are an important cause of lung cancer. Over the following decades, the Surgeon General's reports documented the evidence that cigarette smoking not only caused lung cancer, but other cancers—including cancer of the throat and larynx. Cigarette smoking is also a contributory cause of chronic obstructive pulmonary disease (COPD) and coronary artery disease. Smoking during pregnancy poses risks to the unborn child and passive or second-hand smoke creates increased risks to those exposed—especially children.[8] Based on the Surgeon

---

BOX 2-3   Words that Imply Causation.

Often when reading the newspaper or other media you will find that conclusions about cause and effect are made based upon far less rigorous examination of the data than we have indicated are needed to definitively establish cause and effect. In fact, we often draw conclusions about cause and effect without even consciously recognizing we have done so. Our language has a large number of words that imply a cause-and-effect relationship, some of which we use rather casually.

Let's take a look at the many ways that a hypothetical newspaper article might imply the existence of a cause-and-effect relationship or a contributory cause even when the evidence is based only upon a group association or upon speculation about the possible relationships.

*Over several decades the mortality rates from breast cancer in the United States were observed to increase each year. This trend was **due to** and can be **blamed on** a variety of factors including the increased use of estrogens and exposure to estrogens in food. The recent reduction in breast cancer **resulted from** and can be **attributed to** the declining use of estrogens for menopausal and postmenopausal women. The declining mortality rate was also **produced by** the increased use of screening tests for breast cancer that were **responsible for** early detection and treatment. These trends **demonstrate that** reduced use of estrogens and increased use of screening tests have **contributed to** and **explain** the reduction in breast cancer.*

While these conclusions sound reasonable and may well be cause-and-effect relationships, note that they rely heavily on assertions for which there is no direct evidence provided. For instance, the following words are often used to imply a cause-and-effect relationship when evidence is not or cannot be presented to support the relationship:

- due to
- blamed on
- result from
- attributable to
- produced by
- responsible for
- contributed to
- explained by

It is important to be aware of conscious or unconscious efforts to imply cause-and-effect relationships when the data suggest only group associations and do not meet our more stringent criteria establishing cause and effect.

General's findings, there is clearly overwhelming evidence that cigarette smoking is a contributory cause of lung cancer and a growing list of other diseases. Thus, let us turn our attention to the third component of the P.E.R.I. process: recommendations.

RECOMMENDATIONS: WHAT WORKS TO REDUCE THE HEALTH IMPACT?

The evidence for cigarette smoking as a cause of lung cancer, as well as other diseases, was so strong that it cried out for action. In evidence-based public health, however, action should be grounded in **recommendations** that incorporate evidence. That is, evidence serves not only to establish contributory cause, but is central to determining whether or not specific interventions work.[9, 10] Recommendations are built upon the evidence from studies of interventions. Thus, recommendations are summaries of the evidence of which interventions

work to reduce the health impacts and they indicate whether actions should be taken. These studies utilize the same types of investigations we discussed for contributory cause. In fact, the requirements of contributory cause are the same as those for establishing that an intervention works or has efficacy on the particular population that was studied.

In the decades since the Surgeon General's initial report, a long list of interventions have been implemented and evaluated. As we have discussed, the term intervention is a very broad term in public health. Interventions range from individual counseling and prescription of pharmaceutical drugs which aid smoking cessation; to group efforts, such as peer support groups; to social interventions, such as cigarette taxes and legal restriction on smoking in restaurants.

Recommendations for action have been part of public health and medicine for many years. Evidence-based recommendations, however, are relatively new. They have been contrasted with the traditional *eminence-based* recommendation, which uses the opinion of a respected authority as its foundation. Evidence-based recommendations ask about the research evidence supporting the benefits and harms of potential interventions. In evidence-based recommendations the opinions of experts are most important when research evidence does not or cannot provide answers.

Before looking at the evidence-based recommendations on cigarette smoking made by the Centers for Disease Control and Prevention (CDC), let us look at how they are often made and can be graded. Evidence-based recommendations are based upon two types of criteria—the quality of the evidence and the magnitude of the impact. Each of these criteria is given what is called a **score**.[9, 10] The quality of the evidence is scored based in large part upon the types of investigations and how well the investigation was conducted. Well-conducted randomized clinical trials that fully address the health problem are considered the highest quality evidence. Often, however, cohort and case control studies are needed and are used as part of the recommendation.

Expert opinion, though lowest on the hierarchy of evidence, is often essential to fill in the holes in the research evidence.[9, 10] The quality of the evidence also determines whether the data collected during an intervention is relevant to its use in a particular population or setting. Data from young adults may not be relevant to children or the elderly. Data from severely ill patients may not be relevant to mildly ill patients. Thus, high quality evidence needs to be based not only on the research which can establish efficacy in one particular population, but on the **effectiveness** of the intervention in the specific population in which it will be used.

In evidence-based public health the quality of the evidence is often scored as good, fair, or poor. Good quality implies that the evidence fulfills all the criteria for quality. Poor quality evidence implies that there are fatal flaws in the evidence and recommendations cannot be made. Fair quality lies in between having no fatal flaws.[l]

In addition to looking at the quality of the evidence, it is also important to look at the magnitude of the impact of the intervention. The magnitude of the impact asks the question: how much of the disability and/or death due to the disease can be potentially removed by the intervention? In measuring the magnitude of the impact, evidence-based recommendations take into account the potential benefits of an intervention, as well as the

potential harms. Therefore, we can regard the magnitude of the impact as the benefits minus the harms, or the "net benefits."[m]

The magnitude of the impact, like the quality of the evidence, is scored based upon a limited number of potential categories. In one commonly-used system, the magnitude of the impact is scored as substantial, moderate, small, and zero/negative.[9] A substantial impact may imply that the intervention works extremely well for a small number of people, such as a drug treatment for cigarette cessation. These are the types of interventions that are often the focus of individual clinical care. A substantial impact may also imply that the intervention has a modest net benefit for any one individual, but can be applied to large numbers of people, such as in the form of media advertising or taxes on cigarettes. These are the types of interventions that are most often the focus of traditional public health and social policy.

Evidence-based recommendations combine the score for the quality of the evidence with the score for the impact of the intervention.[9] Table 2-3 summarizes how these aspects can be combined to produce a classification of the strength of the recommendation—graded as A, B, C, D, and I.

It may be useful to think of these grades as indicating the following:

A = Must—A strong recommendation
B = Should—In general, the intervention should be used unless there are good reasons or contraindications for not doing so.
C = May—The use of judgment is often needed on an individual-by-individual basis. Individual recommendations depend on the specifics of an individual's situation, risk-taking attitudes, and values.
D = Don't—There is enough evidence to recommend against using the intervention.
I = Indeterminant, insufficient or I don't know—The evidence is inadequate to make a recommendation for or against the use of the intervention at the present time.

Notice that evidence-based public health and medicine rely primarily on considerations of benefits and harms.

---

[l] To fulfill the criteria for good quality data, evidence is also needed to show that the outcome being measured is a clinically important outcome. Short-term outcomes called **surrogate outcomes**, such as changes in laboratory tests, may not reliably indicate longer term or clinically important outcomes.

[m] The magnitude of the impact can be measured using the relative risk calculation. When dealing with interventions, the people who receive the intervention are often placed in the numerator. Thus, an intervention that reduces the bad outcomes by half would have a relative risk of 0.5. The smaller the relative risk is, the greater the measured impact of the intervention. If the relative risk is 0.20, then those with the intervention have only 20 percent of the risk remaining. Their risk of a bad outcome has been reduced by 80 percent. The reduction in bad outcome is called the **attributable risk percentage** or the **percent efficacy**. The intervention can only be expected to accomplish this potential reduction in risk when a contributory cause is present and the impact of the "cause" can be immediately and completely eliminated.

TABLE 2-3 Classification of Recommendations

	Magnitude of the impact			
	Net benefit: substantial	Net benefit: moderate	Net benefit: small	Net benefit: zero/negative
Quality of the evidence				
Good	A	B	C	D
Fair	B	B	C	D
Poor (insufficient evidence)	I	I	I	I

Source: Agency for Healthcare Research and Quality, U.S. Preventive Services Task Force Guide to Clinical Preventive Services Vol 1, AHRQ Pub. No.02-500.

portant to appreciate the source of the recommendations, as well as the methods used to develop them.[7]

Let us take a look at some examples of how interventions to prevent smoking, detect lung cancer early, or cure lung cancer have been graded. The CDC publishes *The Guide to Community Prevention Services*.[10] This guide indicates that the following interventions are recommended, implying a grade of A or B:

However, recently issues of financial cost have begun to be integrated into evidence-based recommendations. At this point, however, cost considerations are generally only taken into account for "close calls." Close calls are often situations where the net benefits are small to moderate and the costs are large.

The evidence-based public health approach increasingly relies on the use of evidence-based recommendations that are graded based on the quality of the evidence and the expected impact of the intervention. The recommendations are made by a wide array of organizations as discussed in Box 2-4. It is im-

- Clean indoor air legislation prohibiting tobacco use in indoor public and private workplaces
- Federal, state, and local efforts to increase taxes on tobacco products as an effective public health intervention to promote tobacco use cessation and to reduce the initiation of tobacco use among youths
- The funding and implementation of long-term, high-intensity mass media campaigns using paid broadcast times and media messages developed through formative research

BOX 2-4 Who Develops Evidence-Based Recommendations?

Evidence-based recommendations may be developed by a range of groups including government, practitioner-oriented organizations, consumer-oriented organizations, organized health care systems, and even for-profit organizations. Organizations developing evidence-based recommendations, however, are expected to acknowledge their authorship and identify the individuals who participated in the process, as well as their potential conflicts of interest. In addition, regardless of the organization, the evidence-based recommendations should include a description of the process used to collect the data and make the recommendations.

For-profit organizations may make evidence-based recommendations. However, their obvious conflicts of interest often lead them to fund other groups to make recommendations. Thus, the funding source(s) supporting the development of evidence-based recommendations should also be acknowledged as part of the report.

One well-regarded model for development of evidence-based recommendations is the task force model used by the United States Preventive Services Task Force of the Agency for Healthcare Research and Quality (AHRQ), as well as by the Task Force on Community Preventive Services of the Centers for Disease Control and Prevention (CDC).[9, 10] The task force model aims to balance potential conflicts of interest and ensures a range of expertise by selecting a variety of experts, as well as community participants based upon a public nomination process. Once the task force members are appointed, their recommendations are made by a vote of the task force and do not require approval by the government agency.

Thus, as a reader of evidence-based recommendations, it is important that you begin by looking at which group developed the recommendations, whether they have disclosed their membership including potential conflicts of interest, and the groups' procedures for developing the recommendations.

- Proactive telephone cessation support services (quit lines)
- Reduced or eliminated copayments for effective cessation therapies
- Reminder systems for healthcare providers (encouraging them to reinforce the importance of cigarette cessation)
- Efforts to mobilize communities to identify and reduce the commercial availability of tobacco products to youths

Additional recommendations encourage clinicians to specifically counsel patients against smoking, prescribe medications for adults, encourage support groups for smoking cessation, and treat lung cancer with the best available treatments when detected.

Of interest is the grade of D for recommending against screening for early detection of lung cancer using traditional chest X-rays. The evidence strongly suggests that screening using this method may detect cancer at a slightly earlier stage, but not early enough to alter the course of the disease. Therefore early detection does not alter the outcome of the diseases. Research continues to find better screening methods to detect lung cancer in time to make a difference.

Recommendations are not the end of the process. There may be a large number of recommendations among which we may need to choose. In addition, we need to decide the best way(s) to put the recommendations into practice. Thus, implementation is not an automatic process. Issue of ethics, culture, politics, and risk-taking attitudes can and should have major impacts on implementation. A fourth step in the evidence-base public health approach requires us to look at the options for implementation and to develop a strategy for getting the job done.

IMPLEMENTATION: HOW DO WE GET THE JOB DONE?

Strong recommendations based upon the evidence are ideally the basis of implementation. At times, however, it may not be practical or ethical to obtain the evidence needed to establish contributory cause and develop evidence-based recommendations. Naturally-occurring implementation itself may be part of the process of establishing causation, as it was for cigarette smoking in the 1960s when 100,000 physicians stopped smoking and their rates of lung cancer declined rapidly, as compared to other similar professionals who did not stop smoking.

Today, there are often a large number of interventions with adequate data to consider implementation. Many of the interventions have potential harms, as well as potential bene-

fits. The large and growing array of possible interventions means that health decisions require a systematic method for deciding which interventions to use and how to combine them in the most effective and efficient ways. One method for examining the options for implementation uses a structure we will call the "When-Who-How" approach.

"When" asks about the timing in the course of disease in which an intervention occurs. This timing allows us to categorize interventions as **primary**, **secondary**, and **tertiary**. Primary interventions take place before the onset of the disease. They aim to prevent the disease from occurring. Secondary interventions occur after the development of a disease or risk factor, but before symptoms appear. They are aimed at early detection of disease or reducing risk factors while the patient is asymptomatic. Tertiary interventions occur after the initial occurrence of symptoms, but before irreversible disability. They aim to prevent irreversible consequences of the disease. In the cigarette smoking and lung cancer scenario, primary interventions aim to prevent cigarette smoking. Secondary interventions aim to reverse the course of disease by smoking cessation efforts or screening to detect early disease. Tertiary interventions diagnose and treat diseases caused by smoking in order to prevent permanent disability and death.

"Who" asks: at whom should we direct the intervention? Should it be directed at individuals one at a time as part of clinical care? Alternatively, should it be directed at groups of people, such as vulnerable populations, or should it be directed at everyone in a community or population?[n]

Finally, we need to ask: how should we implement interventions? There are three basic types of interventions when addressing the need for behavioral change. These interventions can be classified as: information (education), motivation (incentives), and obligation (requirements).[o]

---

[n] The CDC defines four levels of intervention: the individual, the relationship (e.g., the family), the community, and society or the population as a whole. This framework has the advantage of separating immediate family interventions from community interventions. The group or at-risk group relationship used here may at times refer to the family unit or geographic communities. It may also refer to institutions or at-risk vulnerable groups within the community. The use of group or at-risk group relationship provides greater flexibility allowing application to a wider range of situations. In addition, the three levels used here correlate with the measurements of relative risk, attributable risk percentage, and population attributable percentage, which are the fundamental epidemiological measurements applied to the magnitude of the impact of an intervention.[7]

[o] An additional option is innovation. Innovation implies a technical or engineering solution. The development of a safer cigarette might be an innovation. A distinct advantage of technical or engineering solutions is that they often require far less behavior change. Changing human behavior is frequently difficult. Nonetheless, it is an essential component of most, if not all, successful public health interventions. Certainly, that is the case with cigarette smoking.

TABLE 2-4 Framework of Options for Implementation

	When	Who	How
Levels	1) Primary—Prior to disease or condition 2) Secondary—Prior to symptoms 3) Tertiary—Prior to irreversible complications	1) Individual 2) At-risk group 3) General population/ community	1) Information (education) 2) Motivation (incentives) 3) Obligation (requirement)
Meaning of levels	1) Primary—Remove underlying cause, increase resistance, or reduce exposure 2) Secondary—Post-exposure intervention, identify and treat risk factors or screen for asymptomatic disease 3) Tertiary—Reverse the course of disease (cure), prevent complications, restore function	1) Individual often equals patient care 2) At-risk implies groups with common risk factors 3) General population includes defined populations with and without the risk factor	1) Information—Efforts to communicate information and change behavior on basis of information 2) Motivation—Rewards to encourage or discourage without legal requirement 3) Obligation—Required by law or institutional sanction
Cigarette smoking example	1) Primary—Prevention of smoking, reduction in second-hand exposure 2) Secondary—Assistance in quitting, screening for cancer if recommended 3) Tertiary—Health care to minimize disease impact	1) Individual smoker 2) At-risk—Groups at risk of smoking or disease caused by smoking, e.g., adolescents as well as current and ex-smokers 3) Population—Entire population including those who never have or never will smoke	1) Information—Stop smoking campaigns, advertising, warning on package, clinician advice 2) Motivation—Taxes on cigarettes, increased cost of insurance 3) Obligation—Prohibition on sales to minors, exclusion from athletic eligibility, legal restrictions on indoor public smoking

An information or education strategy aims to change behavior through individual encounters, group interactions, or the mass media. Motivation implies use of incentives for changing or maintaining behavior. It implies more than strong or enthusiastic encouragement, it implies tangible reward. Obligation relies on law and regulations requiring specific behaviors. Table 2-4 illustrates how options for intervention for cigarettes might be organized using the "When-Who-How" approach. To better understand the "who" and "how" of the options for intervention when behavior change is needed, refer to Table 2-5, which outlines nine different options.

Deciding when, who, and how to intervene depends in large part upon the available options and the evidence that they work. They also depend in part on our attitudes toward different types of interventions. In American society, we prefer to rely on information or educational strategies. These approaches preserve freedom of choice which we value in public, as well as private, decisions. Use of mass media informational strategies may be quite economically efficient relative to the large number of individuals they reach though messages often need to be tailored to different audiences. However, information is often ineffective in accomplishing behavioral change—at least on its own.

Strategies based upon motivation, such as taxation and other incentives, may at times be more effective than information alone, though educational strategies are still critical to justify and rein-

TABLE 2-5 Examples of "Who" and "How" Related to Cigarette Smoking

	Information	Motivation	Obligation
Individual	Clinician provides patient with information explaining reasons for changing behavior	Clinician encourages patient to change behavior in order to qualify for a service or gain a benefit, e.g., status or financial	Clinician denies patient a service unless patient changes behavior
	Example: Clinician distributes educational packet to a smoker and discusses his or her own smoking habit	*Example: Clinician suggests that the financial savings from not buying cigarettes be used to buy a luxury item*	*Example: Clinician implements recommendation to refuse birth control pills to women over 35 who smoke cigarettes*
High-risk group	Information is made available to all those who engage in a behavior	Those who engage in a behavior are required to pay a higher price	Those who engage in a behavior are barred from an activity or job
	Example: Warning labels on cigarette packages	*Examples: Taxes on cigarettes*	*Example: Smokers banned from jobs that will expose them to fumes that may damage their lungs*
Population	Information is made available to the entire population, including those who do not engage in the behavior	Incentives are provided for those not at risk to discourage the behavior in those at risk	An activity is required or prohibited for those at risk and also for those not at risk of the condition
	Example: Media information on the dangers of smoking	*Example: Lower health care costs for everyone results from reduced percentage of smokers*	*Example: Cigarettes sales banned for those under 18*

force motivational interventions. Motivational interventions should be carefully constructed and judiciously used or they may result in what has been called **victim blaming**. For example, victim blaming in the case of cigarette smoking implies that we regard the consequences of smoking as the smokers' own fault.

The use of obligation or legally-required action can be quite effective if clear-cut behavior and relatively simple enforcement, such as restrictions on indoor public smoking, are used. These types of efforts may be regarded by some as a last resort, but others may see them as a key to effective use of other strategies. Obligation inevitably removes freedom of choice and if not effectively implemented with regard for individual rights, the strategy may undermine respect for the law. Enforcement may become invasive and expensive, thus obligation requires careful consideration before use as a strategy.

Understanding the advantages and disadvantages of each type of approach is key to deciphering many of the controversies we face in deciding how to implement programs to address public health problems; however, implementation is not the end of the evidence-based public health process.

WHAT HAPPENS AFTER IMPLEMENTATION?

Public health problems are rarely completely eliminated with one intervention—there are few magic bullets in this field. Therefore, it is important to evaluate whether an intervention or combination of interventions has been successful in reducing the problem. It is also critical to measure how much of the problem has been eliminated by the intervention(s).

For instance, studies of cigarette smoking between the mid-1960s and the late 1990s demonstrated that there was nearly a 50 percent reduction in cigarette smoking in the United States and that the rates of lung cancer were beginning to fall—at least among males. However, much of the problem still existed because the rates among adolescent males and females remained high and smoking among adults was preceded by smoking as adolescents nearly 90 percent of the time. Thus, an evaluation of the success of cigarette smoking interventions led to a new cycle of the P.E.R.I. process. It focused on how to address the issue of adolescent smoking and nicotine addiction among adults. Many of the interventions being used today grew out of this effort to cycle once again through the evidence-based public health process and look for a new understanding of the problem, its etiology, evidence-based recommendations, and options for implementation as illustrated in Figure 2-3.

Deciding the best combination of approaches to address a public health problem remains an important part of the judgment needed for the practice of public health. In general, multiple approaches are often needed to effectively address a complex problem like cigarette smoking. Population and high risk group approaches, often used by public health professionals, and individual approaches, often used in as part of health care, should be seen as complementary. Often using both types of interventions is more effective than either approach alone. Social interventions, such as cigarette taxes and restrictions on public smoking are also important interventions to consider when asking how to intervene.

The scope of public health problems and the options for intervention are expanding rapidly and now include global, as well as local and national efforts. In China, for instance, 75 percent of adult males are reported to be smokers making China—with its large population—number one in terms of the number of smokers, as well as the number of deaths caused by smoking. An important example of a social intervention is global collaboration to address smoking and health. World Health Organization's (WHO) efforts have led to what the WHO calls the Framework Convention on Tobacco Control (WHO FCTC).[11]

Today, an enormous body of evidence exists on the relationship between tobacco and health. Understanding the nature of the problems, the etiology or cause-and-effect relationships, the evidence-based recommendations, and the approaches for implementing and evaluating the options for interventions, remain key to the public health approach to smoking and health.[4] Figure 2-3 diagrams the full P.E.R.I approach. Table 2-6 summarizes the questions to ask in the evidence-based public health approach.

The P.E.R.I. process summarizes as a mneumonic the steps in evidence-based public health. It emphasizes the need to understand the nature of the problem and its underlying causes. It also helps structure the use of evidence to make recommendations and decide on which options to put into practice. Finally the circular nature of the P.E.R.I. process reminds us that the job of improving health goes on often requiring multiple efforts to understand and address the problem.[12]

Now that we have an understanding of the basic approach of evidence-based public health let us turn our attention in Section II to the fundamental tools at our disposal for addressing public health problems.

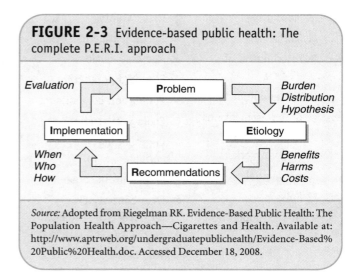

FIGURE 2-3 Evidence-based public health: The complete P.E.R.I. approach

Source: Adopted from Riegelman RK. Evidence-Based Public Health: The Population Health Approach—Cigarettes and Health. Available at: http://www.aptrweb.org/undergraduatepublichealth/Evidence-Based%20Public%20Health.doc. Accessed December 18, 2008.

TABLE 2-6 Questions to Ask—Evidence-Based Public Health Approach

1. **Problem**—What is the health problem?
   • What is the burden of disease and has it changed over time?
   • Are there differences in the distribution of disease and can these differences generate ideas or hypotheses about their etiology?
   • Are the differences or changes used to suggest group associations artifactual or real?
2. **Etiology**—What are the contributory cause(s)?
   • Has an association been established at the individual level?
   • Does the "cause" precede the "effect"?
   • Has altering the "cause" been shown to alter the "effect" (if not use ancillary criteria)?
3. **Recommendations**—What works to reduce the health impacts?
   • What is the quality of the evidence for the intervention?
   • What is the impact of the intervention in terms of benefits and harms?
   • What grade should be given indicating the strength of the recommendation?
4. **Implementations**—How can we get the job done?
   • When should the implementation occur?
   • At whom should the implementation be directed?
   • How should the intervention(s) be implemented?

Source: Adapted from Riegelman RK. Evidence-Based Public Health: The Population Health Approach—Cigarettes and Health. Available at: http://www.aptrweb.org/undergraduatepublichealth/Evidence-Based%20Public%20Health.doc. Accessed December 18, 2008.

Key Words

- P.E.R.I. process
- Burden of disease
- Morbidity
- Mortality
- Distribution of disease
- Epidemiologists
- Group associations
- Risk indicators (or risk markers)
- Artifactual
- Rate
- At-risk population
- True rate

- Incidence rate
- Prevalence rate
- Case-fatality
- Age adjustment
- Age distribution
- Standard population
- Population comparisons
- Ecological studies
- Confounding variable
- Contributory cause
- Case-control or retrospective studies
- Cohort or prospective studies

- Randomized clinical trials or experimental studies
- Risk factor
- Reverse causality
- Randomization
- Natural experiment
- Efficacy
- Supportive criteria
- Ancillary criteria
- Relative risk
- Absolute risk
- Odds ratio
- Dose-response relationship
- Protective factor

- Biological plausibility
- Necessary cause
- Sufficient cause
- Effectiveness
- Surrogate outcomes
- Attributable risk percentage (or the percent efficacy)
- Primary, secondary, and tertiary interventions
- Victim blaming
- Proportion
- Consistency
- Recommendation
- Evidence

Discussion Questions

1. Use the P.E.R.I. framework and the list of questions to outline how each step in the P.E.R.I. process was accomplished for cigarette smoking.

2. How would you use the P.E.R.I. process to address the remaining issues of cigarette smoking?

REFERENCES

1. Cable News Network. Focus: Tobacco Under Attack. Available at: http://www.cnn.com/US/9705/tobacco/history/#cigars.htm. Accessed December 20, 2008.

2. Johnson, Dr. G. A Long Trail of Evidence Links Cigarette Smoking to Lung Cancer. ON SCIENCE column. Available at: http://www.txtwriter.com/Onscience/Articles/smokingcancer2.html. Accessed March 12, 2009.

3. Centers for Disease Control and Prevention. The Public Health Approach to Violence Prevention. Available at: http://www.cdc.gov/ncipc/dvp/PublicHealthApproachTo_ViolencePrevention.htm. Accessed March 12, 2009.

4. Riegelman RK. The Population Health Approach—Cigarettes and Health. Available at: http://www.teachprevention.org/. Accessed March 12, 2009.

5. Gordis L. *Epidemiology*, 4th ed. Philadelphia: Elsevier Saunders; 2009.

6. Friis RH, Sellers TA. *Epidemiology for Public Health Practice*, 4th ed. Sudbury, MA: Jones and Bartlett Publishers; 2009.

7. Riegelman RK. *Studying a Study and Testing a Test: How to Read the Medical Evidence*, 5th ed. Philadelphia: Lippincott, Williams & Wilkins; 2005.

8. United States Department of Health and Human Services. Surgeon General's Reports on Smoking and Tobacco Use. Available at: http://www.cdc.gov/tobacco/data_statistics/sgr/index.htm. Accessed March 12, 2009.

9. Agency for Healthcare Research and Quality, *U.S. Preventive Services Task Force Guide to Clinical Preventive Services*. 2002; Vols. 1 and 2, AHRQ Pub. No. 02-500.

10. Centers for Disease Control and Prevention. The Community Guide. Available at: http://www.thecommunityguide.org/. Accessed March 12, 2009.

11. World Health Organization. Global tobacco treaty enters into force with 57 countries already committed. Available at: http://www.who.int/mediacentre/news/releases/2005/pr09/en/index.html. Accessed March 12, 2009.

12. Centers for Disease Control and Prevention. The Social-Ecological Model: A Framework for Prevention. Available at: http://www.cdc.gov/ncipc/dvp/social-ecological-model_dvp.htm. Accessed March 12, 2009.

Section I:
Cases and Discussion Questions

HIV/AIDS Determinants and Control of the Epidemic

A report appeared in the CDC's Morbidity and Morbidity Weekly Report (MMWR) on June 5, 1981 describing a previously unknown deadly disease in five young homosexual males all in Los Angeles. The disease was characterized by dramatically reduced immunity allowing otherwise innocuous organisms to become "opportunistic infections," rapidly producing fatal infections or cancer. Thus, acquired immune deficiency syndrome (AIDS) first became known to the public health and medical communities. It was soon traced to rectal intercourse, blood transfusions, and reuse of injection needles as methods of transmission. Reuse of needles was a common practice in poor nations. It was also widespread among intravenous drug abusers. Within several years the disease was traced to a previously unknown retrovirus which came to be called the human immunodeficiency virus (HIV).

A test was developed to detect the disease and was first used in testing blood for transfusion. Within a short period of time, the blood supply was protected by testing all donated blood and transmission of HIV by blood transfusion became a rare event. Diagnostic tests for HIV/AIDS soon became available for testing individuals. For many years, these were used by clinicians only for high risk individuals. More recently, the CDC has moved toward recommending universal testing as part of routine health care.

In subsequent years, much has been learned about HIV/AIDS. Today it is primarily a heterosexually-transmitted disease with greater risk of transmission from male to females than females to males. In the United States, African-Americans are at the greatest risk. Condoms have been demonstrated to reduce the risk of transmission. Abstinence and monogamous sexual relationship likewise eliminate or greatly reduce the risk. Even serial monogamy reduces the risk compared to multiple simultaneous partners. Male circumcision has been shown to reduce the potential to acquire HIV infection by approximately 50 percent.

In major U.S. cities, the frequency of HIV is often greater than 1 percent of the population fulfilling the CDC definition of high risk. In these geographic areas the risk of unprotected intercourse is substantially greater than in most suburban or rural areas. Nearly everyone is susceptible to HIV infection despite the fact that a small number of people have well documented protection on a genetic basis.

Maternal-to-child transmission is quite frequent and has been shown to be largely preventable by treatments during pregnancy and at the time of delivery. CDC recommendations for universal testing of pregnant women and intervention for all HIV-positive patients has been widely implemented by clinicians and hospitals and have resulted in greatly reduced frequency of maternal-to-child transmissions in the developed countries and in developing countries as well in recent years.

Medication is now available that greatly reduces the load of HIV present in the blood. These medications delay the progression of HIV, and also reduce the ease of spread of the disease. These treatments were rapidly applied to HIV/AIDS patients in developed countries, but it required about a decade before they were widely used in most developing countries. Inadequate funding from developed countries and controversies over patent protection for HIV/AIDS drugs delayed widespread use of these treatments in developing countries.

New and emerging approaches to HIV prevention include use of antiviral medications during breast feeding, postcoital treatments, and rapid diagnosis and follow-up to detect and treat those recently exposed.

Discussion Questions

1. Use the BIG GEMS framework to examine the factors in addition to infection that have affected the spread of HIV and control or failure to control the HIV/AIDS epidemic.
2. What roles has health care played in controlling or failing to control the HIV/AIDS epidemic?
3. What roles has traditional public health played in controlling or failing to control the HIV/AIDS epidemic?

4. What roles have social factors (beyond the sphere of health care or public health) played in controlling or failing to control the HIV/AIDS epidemic?

Smoking and Adolescents— The Continuing Problem

The rate of smoking in the United States has been reduced by approximately one-half since the 1960s. However, the rate of smoking among teenagers increased in the 1980s and 1990s, especially among teenage females. This raised concerns that young women would continue smoking during pregnancy. In addition, it was found that nearly 90 percent of those who smoked started before the age of 18, and in many cases at a considerably younger age.

In the 1980s and most of the 1990s, smoking was advertised to teenagers and even preteens or "tweens," through campaigns such as Joe Camel. In recent years, a series of interventions directed at teenagers and tweens were put into effect. These included elimination of cigarette vending machines, penalties for those who sell cigarettes to those under 18, and elimination of most cigarette advertising aimed at those under 18. In addition, the Truth® campaign aimed to convince adolescents that not smoking was a sign of independence from the tobacco companies who sought to control their behavior, rather than seeing smoking as a sign of independence from their parents. Evaluation studies concluded that these interventions have worked to reduce adolescent smoking by about one-third.

Despite the successes of the early years of the 21st century in lowering the rates of cigarette smoking among adolescents, the rates have now stabilized at over 20 percent. Evidence indicates that adolescents who smoke generally do not participate in athletics, more often live in rural areas, and more often white and less often African-American. Males and females smoke about the same amount overall, but white females smoke more and Asian females smoke less than their male counterparts.

New drugs have recently been shown to increase the rates of success in smoking cessation among adults with few side effects. Evidence that the benefits are greater than the harms in adolescents is insufficient to recommend them for widespread use because of increased potential for adverse effects including suicide. A series of interventions has been suggested for addressing the continuing problem of adolescent smoking. These include:

- Expulsion from school for cigarette smoking
- Focus on adolescents in tobacco warning labels
- Selective use of prescriptions for cigarette cessation drugs
- No smoking rules for sporting events, music concerts, and other adolescent-oriented events
- Fines for adolescents who falsify their age and purchase cigarettes
- Higher taxes on tobacco products
- Rewards to students in schools with the lowest smoking rates in a geographic area
- Higher auto insurance premiums for adolescents who smoke
- Application of technology to reduce the quantity of nicotine allowed in tobacco products to reduce the potential for addiction
- Testing of athletes for nicotine and exclusion from competition if they test positive
- Research to develop safer types of cigarettes
- Provision of tobacco counseling as part of medical care covered through insurance

As a recent high school graduate, you are asked to participate in a focus group to determine which of these interventions is likely to be most successful.

Discussion Questions

1. How does this case illustrate the P.E.R.I. process?
2. Which of these interventions do you think would be most successful? Explain.
3. How would you classify each of these potential interventions as education (information), motivation (incentives), obligation (required), or innovation (technological change)?
4. What other interventions can you suggest to reduce adolescent smoking?

Reye's Syndrome: A Public Health Success Story

Reye's Syndrome is a potentially fatal disease of childhood which typically occurs in the winter months at the end of an episode of influenza, chicken pox, or other acute viral infection. It is characterized by progressive stages of nausea and vomiting, liver dysfunction, and mental impairment that progress over hours to days and result in a range of symptoms from irritability to confusion to deepening stages of loss of consciousness. Reye's Syndrome is diagnosed by putting together a pattern of signs and symptoms. There is no definitive diagnostic test for the disease.

Reye's Syndrome was first defined as a distinct condition in the early 1960s. By the 1980s, over 500 cases per year were being diagnosed in the United States. When Reye's Syndrome was diagnosed there was over a 30 percent case-fatality rate. Early diagnosis and aggressive efforts to prevent brain damage were shown to reduce the deaths and limit the mental complications, but there is no cure for Reye's Syndrome.

In the late 1970s and early 1980s, a series of case-control studies compared Reye's Syndrome children with similar children who also had an acute viral infection, but did not develop the syndrome. These studies suggested that use of aspirin, then called "baby aspirin," was strongly associated with Reye's Syndrome with over 90 percent of those children afflicted with the syndrome having recently used aspirin.

Cohort studies were not practical because they would require observing very large numbers of children who might be given or not given aspirin by their caretakers. Randomized clinical trials were neither feasible nor ethical. Fortunately, it was considered safe and acceptable to reduce or eliminate aspirin use in children because there was a widely-used alternative—acetaminophen (often used as the brand name Tylenol)—that was not implicated in the studies of Reye's Syndrome.

As early as 1980, the CDC cautioned physicians and parents about the potential dangers of aspirin. In 1982, the U.S. Surgeon General issued an advisory on the danger of aspirin for use in children. By 1986, the U.S. Food and Drug Administration required a Reye's Syndrome warning be placed on all aspirin-containing medications. These efforts were coupled with public service announcements, informational brochures, and patient education by pediatricians and other health professionals who cared of children. The use of the term "baby aspirin" was strongly discouraged.

In the early 1980s, there were over 500 cases of Reye's Syndrome per year in the United States. In recent years, there have often been less than 5 per year. The success of the efforts to reduce or eliminate the use of "baby aspirin" and the subsequent dramatic reduction in the frequency of Reye's Syndrome provided convincing evidence that aspirin was a contributory cause of the condition and its removal from use was an effective intervention.

Discussion Questions

1. How does the Reye's Syndrome history illustrate the use of each of the steps in the P.E.R.I process?
2. What unique aspects of Reye's Syndrome made it necessary and feasible to rely on case-control studies to provide the evidence to help reduce the frequency of the syndrome?
3. What types of methods for implementation were utilized as part of the implementation process? Can you classify them in terms of when, who, and how?
4. How does the Reye's Syndrome history illustrate the use of evaluation to demonstrate whether the implementation process was successful?

SECTION II

Tools of Population Health

Introduction to Section II

In order to protect and promote health and prevent disease, disability, and death, public health uses an array of tools. In this section, we will examine three of the basic tools of public health: health informatics and health communications; social and behavioral sciences; and health policy, laws, and ethics. Figure 2-A provides a framework for thinking about the tools used in the population health approach and indicates where they are addressed in the book.

In Chapter 3, we will explore how health information is collected, compiled, and presented, as well as how it is perceived, combined, and used to make decisions in the arena of health informatics and health communications. Chapter 4 will examine the contributions of the social and behavioral sciences in helping us to understand the sources of health and disease and strategies available to reduce disease, disability, and death. To do this we will explore how social and economic factors affect health. We will also examine how individual and group behavior can be changed to improve health. Finally, in Chapter 5, we will learn how health policies and laws can be used to improve health, as well as how ethical and philosophical issues limit their use.

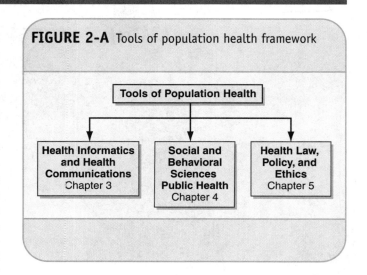

FIGURE 2-A Tools of population health framework

Health Informatics and Health Communications

By the end of this chapter the student will be able to:

- identify six basic types of public health data.
- explain the meaning, use, and limitations of the infant mortality rate and life expectancy measurements.
- explain the meanings and uses of HALEs and DALYs.
- identify criteria for evaluating the quality of information presented on a Web site.
- explain ways that perceptions affect how people interpret information.
- explain the roles of probabilities, utilities, and the timing of events in combining public health data.
- explain how attitudes, such as risk-taking attitudes, may affect decision making.
- identify three different approaches to clinical decision making and their advantages and disadvantages.

You read that the rate of use of cocaine among teenagers has fallen by 50 percent in the last decade. You wonder where that information might come from?

You hear that life expectancy in the United States is now approximately 80 years. You wonder what that implies about how long you will live and what that means for your grandmother who is 82 and in good health?

You hear on the news the gruesome description of a shark attack on a young boy from another state and decide to keep your son away from the beach. While playing at a friend's house your son nearly drowns after falling into the backyard pool. You ask why so many people think that drowning in a backyard pool is unusual when it is far more common than shark attacks?

Balancing the harms and benefits is essential to making decisions, your clinician says. The treatment you are considering

has an 80 percent chance of working but there is also a 20 percent chance of side effects. What do you need to consider when balancing the harms and the benefits, you ask?

You are faced with a decision to have a medical procedure, One physician tells you there's no other choice and you must undergo the procedure, another tells you about the harms and benefits and advises you to go ahead, and the third lays out the options and tells you it's your decision. Why are there such different approaches to making decisions these days?

These are the types of issues and questions that we will address as we look at health informatics and health communications.

WHAT ARE HEALTH INFORMATICS AND HEALTH COMMUNICATIONS?

The term "**health informatics**" deals with the methods for collecting, compiling, and presenting health information, while the term "**health communications**" deals with how we perceive information, combine information, and use information to make decisions. Thus, together these concepts are about information from its collection to its use. Figure 3-1 displays how these parts of the process fit into a continuous flow of information.

The fields of health informatics and health communications has been growing at the speed of the Internet. These fields have implications for most, if not all, aspects of public health, as well as health care. Therefore, we will focus on key issues in each of the above-mentioned components of this burgeoning field. We will look at the following aspects of health informat-

FIGURE 3-1 Health informatics and health communications and the flow of information

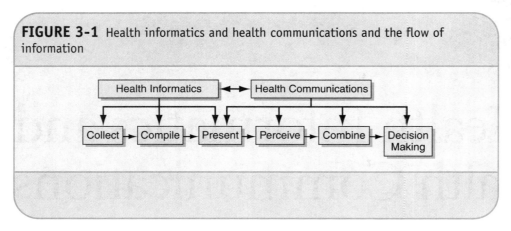

ics and health communications and ask the following questions:

- *Collecting data:* Where does public health data come from?
- *Compiling information:* How is public health information compiled or put together to measure the health of a population?
- *Presenting information:* How can we evaluate the quality of the presentation of public health information?
- *Perceiving information:* What factors affect how we perceive public health information?
- *Combing information:* What types of information need to be combined to make health decisions?
- *Decision making:* How do we utilize information to make health decisions?

We can only highlight key issues in this complex field of health informatics and health communications. To do this, we will use the above questions and provide frameworks and approaches to explore possible answers.

WHERE DOES PUBLIC HEALTH DATA COME FROM?

Public health **data** is collected in a wide variety of ways.[a]

These methods are often referred to as **public health surveillance**. Data of this type comes from a growing variety of sources. It is helpful, however, to classify these sources according to the way they are collected. Table 3-1 outlines the most common types of public health data, provides examples of each type, and indicates important uses, as well as the advantages and disadvantages of each type of data.

Data from different sources are increasingly being combined to create integrated health data systems or **databases**

[a] Data is usually defined as facts or representation of facts while **information** implies that the data is compiled and/or presented in a way designed for a range of uses. Thus the term data is used here only in the context of collection.

that can be rapidly and flexibly accessed by computers to address a wide range of questions. These systems have great potential to provide useful information to contribute to evidence-based public health. This information can help describe problems, examine etiology, assist with evidence-based recommendations, and examine the options for implementation, as well as help evaluate the outcomes. Despite their great potential, integrated databases also create the potential for abuse of the most intimate health information. Thus, protecting the privacy of data is now of great concern as part of the development of integrated databases.

Data can be used for a wide range of purposes in public health and health care. One particularly important use is the compilation of data to generate summary measurements of the health of a group or population. Let us take a look at how we compile this data.

HOW IS PUBLIC HEALTH INFORMATION COMPILED TO MEASURE THE HEALTH OF A POPULATION?

Measurements that summarize the health of populations are called **population health status measures**. For over a century, public health professionals have focused on how to summarize the health status of large populations, such as countries and large groups within countries—for example, males and females or large racial groups of a particular nation. In the 20th century, two measurements became standard for summarizing the health status of populations—the **infant mortality rate** and **life expectancy**. These measurements rely on death and birth certificate data, as well as census data. Toward the latter part of the 20th century, these sources of data became widely available and quite accurate in most parts of the world.

The infant mortality rate estimates the rate of death in the first year of life. For many years, it has been used as the primary measurement of child health. Life expectancy has been used to measure the overall health of the population using the probability of dying at each year of life.[1, 2] These measures were the mainstay of 20th century population health measurements. Let us look at each of these measures and see why additional health status measurements are needed for the 21st century.

At the turn of the 20th century, infant mortality rates were high even in today's developed countries. It was not usual for

TABLE 3-1 The 6 Ss of Sources of Public Health Data

Type	Examples	Uses	Advantages/Disadvantages
Single case or small series	Case reports of one or a small number of cases, such as SARS, anthrax, mad cow disease and new diseases (e.g., first report of AIDS)	Alert to new disease or resistant disease; alert to potential spread beyond initial area	Useful for dramatic, unusual, and new conditions; requires alert clinicians and rapid ability to disseminate information
Statistics ("Vital Statistics") and reportable diseases	Vital statistics: birth, death, marriage, divorce; reporting of key communicable and specially-selected noncommunicable diseases (e.g., elevated lead levels, child and spouse abuse, etc.)	Required by law—sometimes penalties imposed for noncompliance; births and deaths key to defining leading causes of disease; reportable disease may be helpful in identifying changes over time	Vital statistics very complete because of social and financial consequences; reportable disease often relies on institutional reporting rather than individual clinicians; frequent delays in reporting data
Surveys—sampling	National Health and Nutrition Examination Survey (NHANES); Behavioral Risk Factor Surveillance System (BRFSS)	Drawing conclusions about overall population and subgroups from representative samples	Well conducted surveys allow inference to be drawn about larger populations; frequent delays in reporting data
Self-reporting	Adverse effect monitoring of drugs and vaccines as reported by those affected	May help identify unrecognized or unusual events	Useful when unusual events closely follow initial use of drug or vaccine; tends to be incomplete; difficult to evaluate meaning because of selective process of reporting
Sentinel monitoring	Influenza monitoring to identify start of outbreak and changes in virus type	Early warnings or warning of previously unrecognized events	Can be used for "real-time" monitoring; requires considerable knowledge of patterns of disease and use of services to develop
Syndromic surveillance	Use of symptom patterns (e.g., headaches, cough/fever or gastrointestinal symptoms, plus increased sales of over-the-counter drugs) to raise alert of possible new or increased disease	May be able to detect unexpected and subtle changes, such as bioterrorism or new epidemic producing commonly occurring symptoms	May be used for early warning even when no disease is diagnosed; does not provide a diagnosis and may have false positives

over 100 of every 1000 newborns to die in the first year of life. In many parts of the world during this time, infant mortality far exceeded the death rate in any later years of childhood. For this reason, the infant mortality rate was often used as a surrogate or substitute measure for overall rates of childhood death. In the first half of the 20th century, however, great improvements in infant mortality occurred in what are today's developed countries. During the second half of the century, many developing countries also saw greatly reduced infant mortal-

ity rates. Today, many countries have achieved infant mortality rates below 10 per 1000 and a growing number of nations have achieved rates below 5 per 1000.[b]

---

[b] The infant mortality rate is measured using the number of deaths among those ages 0–1 in a particular year divided by the total number of live births in the same year. If the number of live births is stable from year to year, then the infant mortality rate is a measure of the rate of deaths. Health status measurements of child health have not sought to incorporate disability on the less-than-completely-accurate assumption that disability is not a major factor among children.

The degree of success in reducing mortality among children aged two to five has not been as great.[3] Malnutrition and old and new infectious diseases continue to kill young children. In addition, improvements in the care of severely ill newborns have extended the lives of many children—only to have them die after the first year of life. Children with HIV/AIDS often die not in the first year of life, but in the second, third or fourth year. Once a child survives to age five, they have a very high probability of surviving into adulthood in most countries. Thus, a new measurement known as under-5 mortality has now become the standard health status measure used by the World Health Organization (WHO) to summarize the health of children.

Let us take a look at the second traditional measure of population health status—life expectancy. Life expectancy is a snapshot of a population incorporating the probability of dying at each age of life in a particular year. Life expectancy tells us how well a country is doing in terms of deaths in a particular year. As an example, life expectancy at birth in a developed country might be 80 years. Perhaps in 1900, life expectancy at birth in that same country was only 50 years. In 2020, life expectancy might be 85 years. Thus, this metric allows us to make comparisons between countries and within a single country over time.

Despite its name, life expectancy cannot be used to accurately predict the future—that would require assuming that nothing will change. That is, it assumes that the death rates at all ages will remain the same in future years. We have seen increases in life expectancy in most countries over the last century, but declines occurred in Sub-Saharan Africa and countries of the former Soviet Union in the late 20th century.[c]

Life expectancy tells us only part of what we want to know. It reflects the impact of dying, but not the impact of disabilities. When considering the health status of a population in the 21st century, we need to consider disability, as well as death.

Today the World Health Organization (WHO) uses a measurement known as the health-adjusted life expectancy (HALE) to summarize the health of populations.[4] The HALE measurement starts with life expectancy and then incorporates measurements of the quality of health. The WHO utilizes survey data to obtain a country's overall measurement of

quality of health. This measurement incorporates key components including:[d]

- Mobility—the ability to walk without assistance
- Cognition—mental function including memory
- Self-care—activities of daily living including dressing, eating, bathing, and use of the toilet
- Pain—regular pain that limits function
- Mood—alteration in mood that limits function
- Sensory organ function—impairment in vision or hearing that impairs function

From these measurements, an overall quality of health score is obtained. In most countries, these range from 85 to 90 percent. We might consider a score of less than 85 percent as poor and greater than 90 percent as very good. A quality of health measurement of 90 percent indicates that the average person in the country loses 10 percent of their full health over their lifetime to one or more disabilities.

The quality of health measurement is multiplied by the life expectancy to obtain the HALE. Thus, a country which has achieved a life expectancy of 80 years and an overall quality of health score of 90 percent can claim a HALE of $80.00 \times 0.90 = 72.00$. Table 3-2 displays WHO data on life expectancy and HALEs at birth for a variety of large countries.[e]

Thus, today the under-5 mortality and HALEs are used by the WHO as the standard measures reflecting child health and the overall health of a population. An additional measure, known as the disability-adjusted life year (DALY) has been developed and used by the WHO to allow for comparisons and changes based on categories of diseases and conditions.[5] Box 3-1 describes DALYs and some of the data and conclusions that have come from using this measurement.

Table 3-3 displays DALYs according to these categories of diseases and conditions for the same large countries for which HALEs are displayed in Table 3-2.

---

[c] Life expectancy is greater than you might expect at older ages. For instance, in a country with a life expectancy of 80 years, a 60-year-old may still have a life expectancy of 25 years, not 20 years, because they escaped the risks of death during the early years of life. At age 80, the chances of death are very dependent on an individual's state of health because life expectancy combines the probability of death of those in good health and those in poor health. Healthy 80-year-olds have a very high probability of living to 90 and beyond.

[d] It can be argued that use of these measurements associate disability primarily with the elderly. Note that these qualities of health do not specifically include measures of the ability to work, engage in social interactions, or have satisfying sexual relationships, all of which may be especially important to younger populations.
[e] Not all countries accept the HALE as the method for expressing disabilities. A measurement known as the health-related quality of life (HRQOL) has been developed and used in the United States. The HRQOL incorporates a measure of unhealthy days. Unhealthy days are measured by asking a representative sample of individuals the number of days in the last 30 during which the status of either their mental or physical health kept them from their usual activities. It then calculates a measure of the quality of health by adding together the number of unhealthy days due to mental plus physical health. The quality of health is then obtained by dividing the number of healthy days by 30. This measurement is relatively easy to collect and calculate, but unlike the HALE, it does not reflect objective measures of disability and cannot be directly combined with life expectancy to produce an overall measure of health. That is, it does not include the impact of mortality.

TABLE 3-2 Life Expectancy and Health Adjusted Life Expectancy for a Range of Large Countries

Country	Life expectancy	Health-adjusted life expectancy (HALE)
Nigeria	48.8	41.5
India	62.8	53.5
Russian Federation	66.4	58.4
Brazil	71.7	59.8
China	73.4	64.1
United States	78.0	69.3
United Kingdom	79.2	70.6
Canada	80.6	72.0
Japan	82.6	75.0

Source: Data from World Health Organization. World Health Report 2004 Statistical Appendix 4; Geneva: World Health Organization; 2004.

The Global Burden of Disease (GBD) project has produced a number of important conclusions using DALYs including:

- Depression is a major contributor to most nation's DALY and may become the number one contributor in the next few decades in developing, as well as developed countries.
- Chronic disabling diseases, including hookworm, malaria, and HIV, affect the young and working-age population and are the greatest contributors to the burden of disease in many developing countries.
- Cancers—such as breast cancer, hepatomas (primary liver cancer), and colon cancer—which affect the working-age population and are common in many developing countries—have an important impact on the burden of disease as expressed in DALYs.
- Motor vehicle, occupational, and other forms of unintentional injuries have a disproportionate impact on the burden of disease compared to merely measuring deaths

BOX 3-1 DALYs.

Disability-adjusted life years (DALYs) are designed to examine the impacts that specific diseases and risk factors have on populations, as well as provide an overall measure of population health status. They allow comparisons between countries or within countries over time, based not only on overall summary numbers, such as life expectancy and HALEs, but based on specific diseases and risk factors. The DALY compares a country's performance to the country with the longest life expectancy, which is currently Japan. Japan has a life expectancy that is approximately 83 years. In a country with zero DALYs, the average person would live approximately 83 years without any disability and would then die suddenly. Of course, this does not occur even in Japan, so all countries have DALYs of greater than zero. The measurement is usually presented as DALYs per 1000 population in a particular country.[f]

Calculations of DALYs require much more data on specific diseases and disability than other measurements, such as life expectancy or HALEs. However, the WHO's Global Burden of Disease (GBD) project has made considerable progress in obtaining worldwide data collected using a consistent approach.[5] Data is often not available on the disability produced by a disease. The WHO then uses expert opinion to estimate the impact.

The GBD project presents data on DALYs divided into the following categories. Data is also available on specific diseases and risk factors.

- Communicable disease, maternal, neonatal and nutritional conditions
- Noncommunicable diseases
- Injuries

[f] The DALY is a complex and technical measurement. If, in a country with zero DALYs, 1000 newborns suddenly died, there would be a loss of as much as 83,000 DALYs from the death of these 1000 newborns. Thus, the total DALYs a country can lose in a particular year can range from zero to approximately 83,000 per 1000 persons. This somewhat overstates the possible loss due to the discounting and weighing that occurs in the calcualation of DALYs. Nonethe-less when interpreting a country's total DALYs, it may be useful to compare the number of DALYs to this maximum possible loss. It is also important to recognize that DALYs require a number of policy decisions that are hidden in the numbers. For instance, it was decided to emphasize the importance of death and disability among those of working age by giving them greater weight or importance in the calculation of this measurement. Working age was defined as age 16–60, which reflects a concept of working age more often used in developing countries. Death and disability at ages greater than the approximately 83 years of life expectancies of Japan do not add to the DALYs. In calculating DALYs, separate maximum life expectancies are used for males (~80 years) and females (>85 years), implying that loss of life among females is given slightly greater importance. These issues illustrate that in order to understand quantitative measures such as DALYs, you need to recognize that policy decisions are often subtly integrated into quantitative measurements. We need to appreciate the policy and sometimes the ethical decisions that are part of what appears to be objective measurements.

TABLE 3-3 DALYs Lost by Disease Categories and Total of All Categories Per 1,000 Population

Country	DALYs lost due to communicable diseases; maternal, neonatal, and nutritional conditions	DALYs lost due to noncommunicable diseases	DALYs lost due to injuries (unintentional + intentional)	Total DALYS lost
Nigeria	41,251	10,279	4,815	56,345
India	12,958	11,824	3,793	28,575
Russian Federation	2,189	18,752	6,411	27,352
Brazil	4,361	13,113	3,247	20,721
China	2,847	10,217	2,314	15,378
United States	941	11,939	1,387	14,267
United Kingdom	855	11,192	744	12,791
Canada	585	10,256	967	11,808
Japan	588	8,791	1,051	10,430

Source: Reprinted from World Health Organization. Global Burden of Disease Project 2004. Geneva: World Health Organization; 2004.

because these injuries produce long-term disabilities, as well as death at young ages.

- Obesity is rapidly overtaking malnutrition as a burden of disease in developing countries as early onset diabetes, heart disease, and strokes become major causes of death and disabilities among younger populations.

We have now looked at important sources of public health data and examined one key way that data is compiled to generate population health status measurements. Now, let us look at a third issue—the presentation of public health information.

HOW CAN WE EVALUATE THE QUALITY OF THE PRESENTATION OF HEALTH INFORMATION?

Having information is not enough. A key role and essential tool of public health is to effectively present the information in ways that serve as a basis for understanding and decision making. Issues of information presentation are increasingly important and increasingly complex. They require the study of a range of disciplines from mass media, to computer graphics, to statistics.[g] Public health information is often presented as graphics, Graphics create a picture in our mind of what is going on and a picture is truly worth a thousand words. Graphical presentations can accurately inform, but they can also mislead us in a wide variety of ways. The accurate presentation of visual information has become an art, as well as a science that deserves attention from all those who use information.[6]

Issues of quality are key to the presentation of information. The Internet is increasingly the primary source of public health information for the user. Thus, when we address issues of quality, we need to have a set of criteria for judging the quality of information presented on the Internet. Before relying on a Web site for health information, you should ask yourself key questions.[7] These questions are summarized in Table 3-4. Try these out the next time that you view a health information Web site.

The presentation of data may be viewed as the end of health informatics, but also the beginning of health communications. Even the most accurate data presentation does not tell us how the data will be perceived by the user. Let us take a look at the rapidly-growing component of health communications that deals with how we perceive information.

WHAT FACTORS AFFECT HOW WE PERCEIVE PUBLIC HEALTH INFORMATION?

Regardless of how accurately information is presented, communication also needs to consider how the information is perceived by the recipient. Therefore, we also need to look at factors known to affect the perception of information or the subjective interpretation of what the information means for an individual.

At least three types of effects can greatly influence our perceptions of potential harms and benefits.[8] We will call them

---

[g] The use of statistics is one approach to data presentation. It asks questions, such as: what are the strengths of the relationships between risk factors and diseases?. This is known as **estimation**. Statistical analysis also draws conclusions from data on small groups (**samples**) about larger groups or populations—this is called **inference** or **statistical significance testing**.

TABLE 3-4 Quality Standards for Health Information on the Internet

Criteria	Questions to Ask
Overall site quality	• Is the purpose of the site clear? • Is the site easy to navigate? • Are the site's sponsors clearly identified? • Are advertising and sales separated from health information?
Authors	• Are the authors of the information clearly identified? • Do the authors have health credentials? • Is contact information provided?
Information	• Does the site get its information from reliable sources? • Is the information useful and easy to understand? • Is it easy to tell the difference between fact and opinion?
Relevance	• Are there answers to your specific questions?
Timeliness	• Can you tell when the information was written? • Is it current?
Links	• Do the internal links work? • Are there links to related sites for more information?
Privacy	• Is your privacy protected? • Can you search for information without providing information about yourself?

Source: Data from American Public Health Association. Criteria for Assessing the Quality of Health Information on the Internet. Available at: http://www.apha.org/NR/rdonlyres/36630D3D-D50E-4215-8835-4B80298B0685/0/November152000.pdf. Accessed November 13, 2008.

the **dread effect**, the **unfamiliarity effect**, and the **uncontrollability effect**. The dread effect is present with hazards that easily produce very visualizable and feared consequences. It explains why we often fear shark attacks more than drowning in a swimming pool. The dread effect may also be elicited by the potential for catastrophic events, ranging from nuclear meltdowns to a poisoning of the water supply. Our degree of familiarity with a potential harm or a potential benefit can greatly influence how we perceive data and translate it for our own situation. Knowing a friend or relative who died of lung cancer may influence how we perceive the information on the hazards of smoking or the presence of radon. It also may explain why we often see the danger of sun exposure as low and food irradiation as high, despite the fact that the data indicates that the degree of harm is the other way around.

Finally, the uncontrollability effect may have a major impact on our perceptions and actions. We often consider hazards that we perceive as in our control as less threatening than ones that we perceive as out of our control. Automobile collisions, for instance, are often seen as less hazardous than airplane crashes, despite the fact that statistics show that commercial air travel is far safer than travel by automobile.

Perception of bad outcomes (or harms) and good outcomes (or benefits) needs to be considered along with the numbers if we are going to understand the ways information is used to make decisions. Not everyone perceives harms and benefits the same way. The selection of accurate and effective methods for conveying data is key to health communications.[h]

One approach to addressing differing perceptions of information is the use of a method known as **decision analysis**. Decision analysis relies on the vast information-processing ability of computers to formally combine information on benefits and harms to reach quantitative decisions. It provides us with insight into the types of information that need to be combined. Let us look at how we combine information—the next question in our flow of health information.

WHAT TYPE OF INFORMATION NEEDS TO BE COMBINED TO MAKE HEALTH DECISIONS?

Decision analysis focuses on three key types of information that need to be combined as the basis for making decisions. We can better understand these types of information by asking the following questions:

- *How likely?*—what is the probability or chance that the particular outcome will occur?
- *How important?*—what is the value or importance we place on a good or a bad outcome?
- *How soon?*—when, on average, will the particular outcome happen if it is going to happen?

When expressing the chances that an outcome will occur, we often express the results as a percentage from 0 to 100.

---

[h] For instance, we generally have difficulty distinguishing between small and very small numbers. The difference between 1 in 10,000 and 1 in 100,000 is difficult for most of us to grasp and incorporate into our decisions. When comparing these types of probabilities it is tempting to compare the outcomes to ones that are better known, such as those with similar emotional impacts. We might compare the chances of dying from a motorcycle accident with that of a truck or automobile accident. Comparison of different types of outcomes, such as between being struck by lightning compared to dying from a chronic exposure to chemicals or radiation, is far less informative.

Probabilities, on the other hand, range from 0 to 1. Percentages and probabilities are often used interchangeably—the probability of 0.10 can be converted to 10 percent and vice versa. When faced with a percentage or probability we need to ask: what period of time is being considered? For instance, if you hear that the chances of developing a blood clot while taking high-dose estrogen birth control pills is 5 percent, what does that mean? Does it mean 5 percent per cycle, 5 percent per year, or 5 percent over the time period that the average user is on the pill?

Outcomes vary from death to disabilities. Some outcomes greatly affect our function and limit our future, while we can learn to live with some outcomes despite the limitations they impose. When dealing with a quantitative approach, we are forced to place numbers on the value or importance of specific outcomes. A scale known as a **utility scale** is one method to measure and compare the value or importance that different people place on different outcomes.[9] This scale is intended to parallel the scale of probabilities, that is, it extends from 0 to 1 or from 0 to 100 percent. It defines 1 or 100 percent as the state of health in which there are no health-related limitations. Zero is defined as immediate death. On the utility scale there is nothing worse than immediate death. Figure 3-2 displays the utility scale.[i] Box 3-2 illustrates how we can use the utility scale to assign numbers to specific outcomes.

Utilities are important especially when we need to combine potential harms with potential benefits. Probabilities alone often do not give us the answers we need when addressing issues of hazards ranging from environmental toxins to unhealthy behaviors. Utilities are also critical when looking at particular interventions, such as prevention or treatment options that include positive benefits, but also involve side effects or harms. Thus, whenever we need to combine or balance benefits and harms, we need to consider the utility of the outcomes along with the chances or probabilities of the outcomes.

The expected timing of the occurrence of good and bad outcomes can also affect how we view the outcome. Most people view the occurrence of a bad outcome as worse if it occurs in the immediate future compared to its occurrence years from now. Conversely, we usually view a good outcome as more valuable if it occurs in the immediate future. Thus, whenever we consider harms and benefits and try to combine them, we need to ask: when are the outcomes expected to occur?[9] When both the good and the bad outcomes occur in the immediate future, the timing is not an issue. In public health and medi-

FIGURE 3-2 Scale used to measure utilities

cine, however, this is rarely the case. When dealing with many treatments the benefits come first while the harms may occur at a later time. When dealing with vaccines and surgery, the pain and side effects often precedes the potential gain. The timing of the benefits is rarely the same as the timing of the harms. Thus, we need to take this into account. This process is known as **discounting**. Discounting is a quantitative process in which we give greater emphasis or weight to events which are expected to occur in the immediate future compared to events which are expected to occur in the distant future.[k]

We have seen that probabilities, utilities, and timing are key components of health communications that need to be combined when making public health and healthcare decisions.[l] However, there are other factors that are characteristic not of the data itself, but of the **decision maker**. A decision maker may be an individual, a health professional, or it may be an organization like a nonprofit, a corporation, or a government agency. Let

---

[i] Many people consider prolonged incapacity or vegetative states as worse than death. The utility scale does not generally take this into account. This is a specific example of the more general limitation of quantitative decision making—that it focuses on the outcome and not on the process of getting there.

[k] The exact amount of discounting that should occur is controversial, but there is agreement that we should place less importance on outcomes that occur in the distant future than those which occur in the immediate future. There is also agreement that the rate of discounting for harms and for benefits should be the same. The concept of discounting comes from economics and can be most easily understood with a financial example. Let us imagine that we want to discount at 5 percent per year. A discount rate of 5 percent implies that I am willing to give you $95 today if you are willing to give me $100 one year from now.[9] Discounting is above and beyond inflation, so the actual return might be $100 plus the rate of inflation. Note that economists try to set the rate based on the average real return on money invested over a large number of years. In the past, this has been about 3 percent in most developed countries. When making decisions on a subjective basis, we often discount the future at a much higher rate. This is especially true of those who are very sick and are often focused heavily on the immediate future.

[l] Decision analysis is not the usual method used to combine information. Because the task of combining information is so complex and the ability of our minds to handle large quantities of information is so limited, we often use rules of thumb known as **heuristics**.[8] Heuristics allow us to make decisions more rapidly and often with less information. For instance, we often prefer to structure decisions to allow only one of two choices, rather than choosing from a large number of options presented to us at the same time. Thus, we often narrow the field of candidates in primary elections to allow side-by-side comparisons in the general elections. The one-on-one comparisons allow manipulation of the results by getting rid of candidates in the primaries who might have fared better in the general election.

> **BOX 3-2** Obtaining a Utility Score.
>
> Let us see how we can use the utility scale to put numbers on a specific outcome—complete and permanent blindness. Using the scale in Figure 3–2, place a number on the importance or value that you give to complete and permanent blindness.
>
> In large groups of individuals, the average utility placed on blindness is quite predictable—about 50 percent. However, the range of values among a group is generally quite wide ranging from 20 to 80 percent and sometimes even wider. Predicting an individual's utility is quite difficult since gender, socioeconomic group, and other predictors have little impact.[j]
>
> Individuals who place a high utility on complete and permanent blindness usually indicate that they can learn to live with blindness and it will not greatly affect their enjoyment of life. Those who place a low utility on blindness generally say just the opposite. Thus, we need to understand that a utility of 50 percent is an average including some with a much higher and some with a much lower utility. Therefore the best way to know the value or utility that an individual places on a particular outcome such as blindness is to ask them.
>
> ---
>
> [j] There are at least two predictors that are of some value. Those who have experienced an outcome usually find that they can adapt to it to a certain extent and usually rate its utility as somewhat higher than those who have not experienced the outcome. Second, age does have an impact on the scoring of utility. Younger people generally rate the utility of an outcome as somewhat worse or lower than older people, perhaps due to the longer-term impact the disability has on their future options. The average utility placed on blindness by college students, for instance, is often closer to 40 percent. Neither of these impacts is large on average, nor can they be used to successfully predict the utility of any one individual.

us turn our attention to decision makers and ask about how we can go about making decisions. To do this we need to address issues beyond probability, utility, and timing.

HOW DO WE UTILIZE INFORMATION TO MAKE HEALTH DECISIONS?

There are two key questions that we can ask to gain an understanding of how we use information to make health decisions:

- How do our risk-taking attitudes affect the way we make decisions?
- How do we incorporate information into our decisions?

There are a large number of attitudes that can affect the way we make decisions. One of the most important is known as our **risk-taking attitudes**.[m]

Let us examine what we mean by this term and see what type of risk-taking attitude you use in making decisions. Attitudes toward risk greatly influence the choices that we all make in the prevention and treatment of disease.[9] Box 3-3 illustrates how you can understand your own attitudes toward risk taking by making some choices. We will assume that you understand what we mean by utilities and that you have thought through what a wide range of utilities means to you personally.

Understanding attitudes toward risk is important for analyzing how individuals make decisions about their own lives. It is also key when trying to understand how group decisions are made that require society to balance harms and benefits. Perhaps the most common health decisions that you will make are the decisions related to your health care and that of your family. Therefore, let us complete our examination of health communications by looking at three different approaches that can be used to make clinical healthcare decisions.

There are three basic approaches to clinical decision making. We will call these approaches **inform of decision, informed consent**, and **shared decision making**. Preferences for these types of approaches have changed over time, yet all three are currently part of clinical practice.

The inform of decision approach implies that the clinician has all the essential information and can make decisions that are in the patient's best interest. The role of the clinician is then merely to inform the patient of what needs to be done, to prescribe the treatment, or write the orders. At one point in time, this type of decision-making approach was standard for practicing clinicians. In the not-too-distant past, clinicians rarely told patients that they had cancer—justifying their silence by arguments that the knowledge might make the patient depressed, which could interfere with their response to the disease and to the treatment. The decision to have many tests and receive a range of medications is still often done using the inform of decision approach.

A second type of decision-making approach is called informed consent. It rests on the principle that ultimately patients need to give their permission or consent before major

---

[m] In addition to a risk-taking attitude, there are other attitudes that affect our decision making. For instance, decision making may depend on whether we regard an error of omission as equal to an error of commission. Decision analysis and most ethicists regard them as equal, but many people see errors of omission as more acceptable than errors of commission. That is, most people consider a bad outcome resulting from inaction as more tolerable than a bad outcome resulting from their own actions.

BOX 3-3   Risk-Taking Attitudes.

Review the following situations and write down your decisions.

Situation A

Imagine that you have coronary artery disease and have a reduced quality of life with a utility of 0.80 compared to your previous state of full health with a utility of 1.00. You are offered the pair of options below. You can select only one option. Which of the following two options do you prefer?

OPTION #1: A treatment with the following possible outcomes:
  50% chance of raising the quality of your health (your utility) from 0.80 to 1.00
  50% chance of reducing the quality of your health (your utility) from 0.80 to 0.60
OPTION #2: Refuse the above treatment and accept a quality of your health (your utility) of 0.80

Situation B

Imagine that you have coronary artery disease and have a reduced quality of life that has a utility of 0.20 compared to your previous state of full health that had a utility of 1.00. You are offered the pair of options below. You can select only one option. Which of the following two options do you prefer?

OPTION #1: A treatment with the following possible outcomes:
  10% chance of raising the quality of your health (your utility) from 0.20 to 1.00
  90% chance of reducing the quality of your health (your utility) from 0.20 to 0.11
OPTION #2: Refuse the above treatment and accept a quality of your health (your utility) of 0.20

What was your answer in Situation A? Situation B? To understand the meaning of your answers you need to appreciate that in terms of the probabilities and utilities presented in each situation, these options are a "toss-up." That is, taking into account the probabilities and the utilities, there is no difference between these options.[n]

Thus, the information does not determine your choice; it must be your attitude toward taking chances, which is your attitude toward risk taking.

Did you choose Option #2 in Situation A and Option #1 in Situation B? Most, but not all, people make these choices. In Situation A, we begin with a utility of 0.80. For many people, this is a tolerable situation and they do not want to take any chances of being reduced to a lower, perhaps intolerable utility. Thus, they want to guarantee a tolerable level of health. We can call this the certainty effect. In Situation B, we begin with a utility of 0.20. For many people, this is an intolerable situation. Thus people are usually willing to take their chances of getting even worse in the hopes of a major improvement in their health. When the quality of life is bad enough, most, if not all, people are willing to take their chances or "go for it." This risk-taking behavior can be called the long-shot effect. Thus, risk-taking and risk-avoiding choices are both common, defensible, and reasonably predictable. Most of us are risk takers when conditions are intolerable and risk avoiders when conditions are tolerable.

A few people will choose Option #1 in both Situation A and B. These individuals are willing to take their chances in a range of situations in order to improve their outcome. We call them risk takers. Are you one of them? The only way to know is to ask yourself. Similarly, a few people will choose Option #2 in both situations. These individuals seek to avoid taking chances in a range of situations in order to preserve their current state of health. We call them risk avoiders. Are you one of them? Only you can answer that question.[o]

---

[n] Notice that the outcomes occur in the immediate future so there is no issue of timing or need to discount the benefits or the harms.

[o] There is a fourth option, which is to choose Option #2 in Situation A and Option #1 in Situation B. The small number of individuals who make this choice usually have a very different perception of what utilities mean to them. For instance, they might perceive little difference between a 0.80 and a 0.20 utility.

interventions, such as surgery, radiation, or chemotherapy, can be undertaken. Informed consent may be written, spoken, or implied. Clinically, informed consent implies that individuals have the right to know what will be done, why it will be done, and what the known benefits and harms are. Patients have the right to ask questions, including inquiring about the availability of other options. Informed consent does not mean that all possible options are presented to the patient, but it does imply that a clinician has made a recommendation for a specific intervention.

The third type of decision-making is called shared decision making. In this approach, the clinician's job is to provide information to the patient with which he or she can make a decision. This might include directly giving information to the patient, providing consultations, or referring patients to sources of information often on the Internet. Shared decision making places a far greater burden on the patient to seek out, understand, and use information. Using this approach, clinicians are not required to provide recommendations on specific interventions, though patients are free to ask for a clinician's opinion.

All three types of decision-making approaches are currently in use today. Table 3-5 outlines the process and roles implied by each of these approaches, as well as some of the potential advantages and disadvantages of each approach.

Health informatics and health communications are key tools for population health. We have taken a look at important issues related to each of them. We have asked questions about how public health data and information is collected, compiled, presented, perceived, combined, and used in decision making. Data and information are key public health tools for guiding our decision making. We will find ourselves coming back again and again to these principles as we study the population health approach. Now, let us turn our attention to Chapter 4, which discusses a second key tool—utilization of the social and behavioral sciences.

TABLE 3-5 Types of Individual Decision Making

Type of decision making	Process/Roles	Advantages	Disadvantages
Inform of decision	Clinician has all the essential information to make a decision that is in the patient's best interest Clinician aims to convey their decision as a clear and unambiguous action or order Patients accept the clinician's recommendation without necessarily understanding or agreeing with the underlying reasoning	May be efficient and effective when patients seek clear direction provided by an authoritative and trusted source Patient may favor if they do not seek out or feel they cannot handle independent decision-making responsibilities	Patient may not gain information and understanding of the nature of the problem or the nature of the treatment Patient may not be prepared to participate in the implementation of the decision Patient may not accept responsibility for the outcome of the treatment
Informed consent	Clinician has the responsibility to convey a recommendation to the patient Harms and benefits of treatment are weighed by the clinician in making a recommendation Clinician has a responsibility to provide information on the aim of the recommendation, the potential benefits, the known harms, and the process that will occur. The patient has the right to ask additional questions about the treatment and the availability of other alternatives	Patient gains information and understanding of the nature of the problem or the nature of the treatment Patient may be prepared to participate in the implementation of the decision Patient may accept responsibility for the outcome of the treatment	Time consuming compared to informing of the decision May require elaborate paperwork to implement formal informed consent process May increase emphasis on legal documents and malpractice law
Shared decision making	Clinicians serve as a source of information for patients including providing it directly or identifying means of obtaining information	May increase the control of the patients over their own lives May increase the types of information considered in decision making	May be time consuming for patients and clinicians May increase the costs of health care

continues

TABLE 3-5 Types of Individual Decision Making (continued)

Type of decision making	Process/Roles	Advantages	Disadvantages
	Patients can expect to be informed of the existence of a range of accepted options and be assisted in their efforts to obtain information	May reduce the adversarial nature of the relationship between clinicians and patients	May increase the stress/anxiety for patients
	Patients may seek information on experimental or alternative approaches and can discuss the advantages and disadvantages of these approaches with a clinician	May improve the outcome of care by increasing the patient's understanding and commitment to the chosen course of care	May shift the responsibility for bad outcomes from the clinician to the patient, i.e., takes the clinician off the hook/ clinician does not need to do the hard work of thinking through the decision and making a recommendation
	Considerations besides benefits and harms are part of the decision-making process, including such considerations as cost, risk-taking attitudes, and the distress/discomforts associated with the treatment		
	Patients are often directly involved in the implementation of care		

Key Words

- Health informatics
- Health communications
- Data
- Public health surveillance
- Databases
- Population health status measures
- Infant mortality rate
- Life expectancy
- Under-5 mortality
- Health-adjusted life expectancy (HALE)
- Disability-adjusted live year (DALY)
- Decision analysis
- Utility scale
- Discounting
- Decision maker
- Risk-taking attitude
- Dread effect
- Unfamiliarity effect
- Uncontrollability effect
- Inform of decision
- Informed consent
- Shared decision making
- Certainty effect
- Long-shot effect
- Risk takers
- Risk avoiders

Discussion Questions

Take a look at the questions posed in the following scenarios which were presented at the beginning of this chapter. See whether you can now answer these questions.

1. You read that the rate of use of cocaine among teenagers has fallen by 50 percent in the last decade. You wonder where that information might come from?

2. You hear that life expectancy in the United States is now approximately 80 years. You wonder what that implies about how long you will live and what that means for your grandmother who is 82 and in good health?

3. You hear on the news the gruesome description of a shark attack on a young boy from another state and decide to keep your son away from the beach. While playing at a friend's house your son nearly drowns after falling into the backyard pool. You ask why so many people think that drowning in a backyard pool is unusual when it is far more common than shark attacks?

4. Balancing the harms and benefits is essential to making decisions, your clinician says. The treatment you are considering has an 80 percent chance of working but there is also a 20 percent chance of side effects. What do you need to consider when balancing the harms and the benefits, you ask?

5. You are faced with a decision to have a medical procedure. One physician tells you there's no other choice and you must undergo the procedure, another tells you about the harms and benefits and advises you to go ahead, and the third lays out the options and tells you it's your decision. Why are there such different approaches to making decisions these days?

REFERENCES

1. Gordis L. *Epidemiology*, 4th ed. Philadelphia: Elsevier Saunders; 2009.
2. Friis RH Sellers TA. *Epidemiology for Public Health Practice*, 4th ed. Sudbury, MA; Jones and Bartlett Publishers; 2009.
3. Skolnik R. *Essentials of Global Health*. Sudbury, MA: Jones and Bartlett Publishers; 2008.
4. World Health Organization. Healthy life expectancy (HALE) at birth (years). Available at: http://www.who.int/whosis/indicators/compendium/2008/1hat/en/index.html. Accessed March 12, 2009.
5. World Health Organization. Global Burden of Disease. Available at: http://www.who.int/healthinfo/global_burden_disease/en/. Accessed March 12, 2009.
6. Tufte ER. *The Visual Display of Quantitative Information*, 2nd ed. Cheshire, CT: Graphics Press; 2001.
7. American Public Health Association. Criteria for Assessing the Quality of Health Information on the Internet. Available at: http://www.apha.org/NR/rdonlyres/36630D3D-D50E-4215–8835–4B80298B0685/0/November152000.pdf. Accessed March 12, 2009.
8. Dawes RM, Hastie R. *Rational Choice in an Uncertain World*. Thousand Oaks, CA: Sage Publications; 2001.
9. Riegelman RK. *Measures of Medicine: Benefits, Harms and Costs*. Cambridge, MA: Blackwell Science; 1995.

CHAPTER 4

Social and Behavioral Sciences and Public Health

LEARNING OBJECTIVES

By the end of this chapter the student will be able to:

- explain relationships between the social and behavioral sciences and public health.
- illustrate how socioeconomic status affects health.
- illustrate how culture and religion affects health.
- identify and illustrate the stages in behavioral change that constitute the Stages of Change model.
- identify ways that interventions at the individual level and at the social level can reinforce each other to influence behavioral change.
- explain the principles of social marketing.

You travel to a country in Asia and find that their culture affects most parts of life. From the food they eat and their method of cooking, to their attitudes toward medical care, to their beliefs about the cause of disease and the ability to alter it through public health and medical interventions, this country is profoundly different from the United States. You ask: how does culture affect health?

You are working in a country with strict Islamic practices and find that religion, like culture, can have major impacts on health. Religious practices differ widely—from beliefs about food and alcohol; to sexual practices, such as male circumcision and female sexual behavior; to acceptance or rejection of interventions aimed at women's health. You ask: how does religion affect health?

You're trying to help your spouse quit smoking cigarettes and your kids from starting. You know that gentle encouragement and support on a one-on-one basis are essential, but often are not enough because cigarettes are an addiction that produces withdrawal and long-term cravings. Like most addictions, it requires a combination of individual motivation, support from

family and friends, and sometimes the use of medications; but you wonder: do warning labels on cigarettes, taxes on cigarettes, and "no smoking" zones in public places make any difference?

Your efforts to convince your friends to avoid smoking (or at least stop smoking) focus on giving them the facts about how cigarettes cause lung cancer, throat cancer, and serious heart disease. You are frustrated by how little impact you have on your friends. You wonder, whether you would be more successful by focusing on the immediate negative impacts, such as stained teeth and bad breath, as well as the loss of control that goes along with addiction to nicotine?

As a new parent, you hear from your pediatrician, nurses in the hospital, and even from the makers of your brand of diapers, that babies should sleep on their backs. They call it "back-to-sleep." You're surprised to find that it's part of the class on babysitting given by the local community center and a required part of the training for those who work in registered day care centers. You find out that it's all part of a social marketing campaign that has reduced in half the number of deaths from sudden infant death syndrome. You ask: why has the "back-to-sleep" campaign been so successful?

Each of these cases illustrates ways that an understanding of social and behavioral sciences can contribute to an understanding of public health. Let us explore these connections.

HOW IS PUBLIC HEALTH RELATED TO THE SOCIAL AND BEHAVIORAL SCIENCES?

The development of social and behavioral sciences in the 19th and 20th centuries is closely connected with the

TABLE 4-1 Examples of Contributions of Social and Behavioral Sciences to Public Health

Social science discipline[a]	Examples of disciplinary contributions to public health
Psychology	Theories of the origins of behavior and risk taking tendencies and methods for altering individual and social behaviors
Sociology	Theories of social development, organizational behavior, and systems thinking. Social impacts on individual and group behaviors
Anthropology	Social and cultural influences on individual and population decision making for health with a global perspective
Political science/Public policy	Approaches to government and policy making related to public health. Structures for policy analysis and the impact of government on public health decision making
Economics	Understanding the micro- and macroeconomic impact on public health and health care systems
Communications	Theory and practice of mass and personalized communication and the role of media in communicating health information and health risks
Demography	Understanding demographic changes in populations globally due to aging, migration, and differences in birth rates, plus their impact on health and society
Geography	Understanding of the impacts of geography on disease and determinants of disease, as well as methods for displaying and tracking the location of disease occurrence

[a] A similar list of contributions of the humanities could be developed including the contributions of literature, the arts, history and philosophy, and ethics. These contributions of the social sciences are in addition to contributions of the sciences, mathematics, and humanities. Biology, chemistry, and statistics underpin much of epidemiology and environmental health. Languages and culture, history, and the arts provide key contributions to health communications and health policy. Thus, a broad arts and sciences education is often considered a key part of preparation for public health.

development of public health. These subject areas share a fundamental belief that understanding the organization and motivation behind social forces, along with a better understanding of the behavior of individuals, can be used to improve the lives of individuals, as well as those of society as a whole.[1]

The 19th century development of social and behavioral sciences, as well as public health, grew out of the Industrial Revolution in Europe, and later in America. It was grounded in efforts to address the social and economic inequalities that developed during this period and provided an intellectual and institutional structure for what was and is now called social justice. Social justice implies a society that provides fair treatment and a fair share of the rewards of society to individuals and groups of individuals. Early public health reformers advocated for social justice and saw public health as an integral aspect of it.

The intellectual link between social and behavioral sciences and public health is so basic and so deep that it is often taken for granted. As students with opportunities to learn about both social sciences and public health, it is important to understand the key contributions that social sciences make to public health. It is not an exaggeration to view public health as an application of the social sciences, i.e., as an applied social sci-

ence. Table 4–1 summarizes many of the contributions that the social sciences make to public health.

Let us start with a key question that needs to be addressed to understand the relationship between social forces and health.

How Does Socioeconomic Status Affect Health?

Beginning in the 19th century, social scientists developed the concept of **socioeconomic status**. They also developed elaborate systems to operationalize the definition of socioeconomic status and classify individuals. In the United States, the definition has generally included measures that are primarily economic including:[b]

- family income
- educational level or parents' educational level
- professional status or parents' professional status

Let us examine how socioeconomic status has been shown to affect health. Then, we will examine additional social factors that affect health and the response to disease.

[b] A more formal social hierarchy has traditionally existed in Europe. European social scientists utilized the concept of social class when categorizing individuals by socioeconomic status. In Europe, economics alone was not thought to be adequate to explain socioeconomic status or categorize individuals.

Health status, at least as measured by life expectancy, is strongly associated with socioeconomic status.[2, 3] Greater longevity is associated with higher social status with a gradient of increasing longevity from lowest to highest on the socioeconomic scale.

It is also important to recognize that socioeconomic impact are not solely related to a person's income Above an annual threshold income level of about $10,000 per person, the association of longevity with income is best explained by the disparities in income, rather than the absolute level. Thus, developed countries with smaller disparities of income, such as Japan, Sweden, and Canada, have greater average longevity and smaller disparities in longevity between their richest and poorest citizens than compared to a country like the United States. In the United States, greater disparities in income and longevity exist between the richest and poorest citizens. However, the enormous diversity of the population of the United States in terms culture and religion as well as socioeconomic level may also help explain the disparities in longevity.[c]

We understand many, but not all, of the ways that socioeconomic factors affect health. Greater economic wealth usually implies access to healthier living conditions. Improved sanitation, less crowding, greater access to health care, and safer methods for cooking and eating are all strongly associated with higher economic status in developed, as well as developing countries.

Education is also strongly associated with better health. It may change health outcomes and increase longevity by encouraging behaviors that provide protection against disease and likewise reduce exposure to behaviors that put individuals at risk of disease. Higher education levels, coupled with the increased resources that greater wealth can provide, may increase access to better medical care and provide greater ability to protect against health hazards.

---

[c] The association between socioeconomic status and longevity is most strongly associated with an individual's socioeconomic status as an adult. The socioeconomic status of an individual's parents has a much weaker association. This suggests that genetic factors have little to do with the association between socioeconomic status and life expectancy. Education has a stronger association with health status than income or professional status. Lower socioeconomic status leads to poor health rather than poor health leading to lower socioeconomic status. Socioeconomic factors are associated with an increase in relative risk of death of 1.5 to 2.0 when comparing the lowest and highest socioeconomic groups. This means that those in the lowest group have more than a 50 percent increase in the death rate compared to the highest group. This relative risk steadily increases as the socioeconomic level decreases. The relationship has a dose-response relationship, that is, there is an increase in longevity with every increase in socioeconomic status. Thus, the impact is not limited to those with the lowest status. The largest contributors to the differences in the death rate are: cardiovascular disease, violence, and increasingly AIDS; however the death rate is impacted in general by a wide range of diseases—most being malignancies and infectious diseases.[3]

Individuals of lower socioeconomic status are more likely to be exposed to health hazards at work and in the physical environment through toxic exposure in the air they breathe, in the water they drink, and in the food they eat. Table 4–2 outlines a number of mechanisms by which socioeconomic status can directly and indirectly influence health.

These factors, while important, explain only about half of the observed differences in life expectancy among individuals of different socioeconomic status. For instance, the rates of coronary heart disease are considerably higher among those of lower socioeconomic status—even after taking into account cigarette smoking, high blood pressure, cholesterol levels, and blood sugar counts.[3]

Considerable research is now being directed to better understand these and other effects of socioeconomic status. One theory suggests that social control and social participation may help explain these substantial differences in health. It contends that control over individual and group decision making is much greater among individuals of higher socioeconomic status. The theory holds that the ability to control one's life may be associated with biological changes that affect health and disease.[3] Additional research is needed to confirm or reject this theory and/or provide an adequate explanation for these important, yet unexplained, differences in health based upon socioeconomic status.

What Other Social Factors Explain Differences in Health and Response to Disease?

Culture and religion have effects on health above and beyond socioeconomic status as measured by income, education, and professional status. They can be viewed as behaviors, values, and beliefs that are learned from others and shared with others.

Culture

Culture, in a broad sense, helps people make judgments about the world and decisions about behavior. Culture defines what is good or bad, and what is healthy and unhealthy. This may relate to lifestyle patterns, beliefs about risk, and beliefs about body type—for example, a large body type in some cultures symbolizes health and well-being, not overweight or other negative conditions.

Culture directly affects the daily habits of life. Food choice and methods of food preparation and preservation are all affected by culture, as well as socioeconomic status. The Mediterranean diet, which includes olive oil, seafood, vegetables, nuts, and fruits, has been shown to have benefits for the heart even when used in countries far removed from the Mediterranean.

There are often clear-cut negative and/or positive impacts on disability related to cultural traditions as diverse as feet

TABLE 4-2 Examples of Ways that Socioeconomic Status May Affect Health

Type	Examples
Living conditions	Increases in sanitation, reductions in crowding, methods of heating and cooking
Overall educational opportunities	Education is the strongest association with health behaviors and health outcomes.
	May be due to better appreciation of factors associated with disease and greater ability to control these factors
Educational opportunities for women	Education for women has an impact on the health of children and families
Occupational exposures	Lower socioeconomic jobs are traditionally associated with increased exposures to health risks
Access to goods and services	Ability to access goods, such as protective devices and high quality foods and services, including medical and social services to protect and promote health
Family size	Large family size affects health and is traditionally associated with lower socioeconomic status and with lower health status
Exposures to high risk behaviors	Social alienation related to poverty may be associated with violence, drugs, other high risk behaviors
Environmental	Lower socioeconomic status associated with greater exposure to environmental pollution, "natural" disasters, and dangers of the "built environment"

binding in China and female genital mutilation in some parts of Africa. Some societies reject strenuous physical activity for those who have the status and wealth to be served by others.

Culture is also related to an individual's response to symptoms and acceptance of interventions. In many cultures, medical care is exclusively for those with symptoms and is not part of prevention. Many traditional cultures have developed sophisticated systems of self-care and self-medication supported by family and traditional healers. These traditions greatly affect how an individual responds to symptoms, how they communicate the symptoms, and the types of medical and public health interventions that they will accept.

Many cultures allow and even encourage the use of traditional approaches alongside Western medical and public health approaches. In some cultures, traditional healers are considered appropriate for health problems whose causes are not thought to be biological, but related to spiritual and other phenomena. Recent studies of alternative, or complementary, medicine have provided evidence that specific traditional interventions, such as acupuncture and specific osteopathic and chiropractic manipulation, have measurable benefits. Thus, cultural differences should not be viewed as problems to be addressed, but rather as practices to be understood. Table 4-3 summarizes a number of the ways that culture can affect health.

Religion

Social factors affecting health include religion along with culture. Religion can have a major impact on health particularly for specific practices that are encouraged or condemned by a particular religious group. For instance, we now know that male circumcision reduces susceptibility to HIV/AIDS. Religious attitudes that condone or condemn the use of condoms, alcohol, and tobacco have direct and indirect impacts on health as well.

Some religions prohibit specific healing practices, such as blood transfusions or abortion, or totally reject medical interventions altogether, as is practiced by Christian Scientists. Religious individuals may see medical and public health interventions as complementary to religious practice or may substitute prayer for medical interventions in response to symptoms of disease. Table 4-4 outlines some of the ways that religion may affect health.

We have examined a number of ways that socioeconomic, cultural, and religious factors may affect health and the response to disease. Many, but not all, of these factors ultimately influence the health-related behavior of individuals. Thus, we need to look at the relationship between behavior and health and the ways that we can use knowledge from the social sciences to improve health.

TABLE 4-3 Examples of Ways that Culture Can Affect Health

Ways that culture may affect health	Examples
Culture is related to behavior—social practices may put individuals and groups at increased or reduced risk	Food preferences—vegetarian, Mediterranean diet Cooking methods History of binding of feet in China Female genital mutilation Role of exercise
Culture is related to response to symptoms, such as the level of urgency to recognize symptoms, seek care, and communicate symptoms	Cultural differences in seeking care and self-medication Social, family, and work structures provide varying degree of social support—low degree of social support may be associated with reduced health-related quality of life
Culture is related to the types of interventions that are acceptable	Variations in degree of acceptance of traditional Western medicine including reliance on self-help and traditional healers
Culture is related to the response to disease and to interventions	Cultural differences in follow-up, adherence to treatment, and acceptance of adverse outcome

TABLE 4-4 Examples of Ways that Religion May Affect Health

Ways that religion affects health	Examples
Religion may affect social practices that put individuals at increased or reduced risk	Sexual: circumcision, use of contraceptive Food: avoidance of seafood, pork, beef Alcohol use: part of religion versus prohibited Tobacco use: actively discouraged by Mormons and Seventh-Day Adventists as part of their religion
Religion may affect response to symptoms	Christian Scientists reject medical care as a response to symptoms
Religion may affect the types of interventions that are acceptable	Prohibition against blood transfusions Attitudes toward stem cell research Attitudes toward abortion End-of-life treatments
Religion may affect the response to disease and to interventions	Role of prayer as an intervention to alter outcome.

Can Health Behavior Be Changed?

Much of the preventable disease and disability today in the United States and other developed countries is related to the behavior of individuals. From cigarette smoking to obesity, from intentional to unintentional injuries, from sexual behavior to drug abuse, health issues can be traced to the behavior of individuals. At times, we hear discouraging messages that behavior cannot be changed. However, if we take a relatively long-term view, we find that there are many examples of behavioral change that have occurred for the better. For instance:

- Cigarette smoking in the United States among males has been reduced from approximately 50 percent in the 1960s to less than 25 percent today.
- Infants today generally are placed on their backs for sleeping and napping and not on their stomachs, as was the usual practice in the 1980s and earlier. "Back-to-sleep" campaigns are believed to have reduced Sudden Infant Death Syndrome (SIDS) by nearly 50 percent in the United States.
- Seat belt use in the United States has increased from less than 25 percent in the 1970s to over 80 percent currently.
- Drunk driving in the United States has been dramatically reduced with a resulting decline in automobile-related fatalities.
- Mammography use increased by approximately 50 percent during the 1990s and has been credited with beginning to reduce the previously-rising mortality rates from breast cancer.

The potential to change behavior can make health worse as well. The following changes for the worse have also occurred in the United States in recent years:

- Over the last three decades, Americans have increased their caloric intake and reduced their average amount of exercise, resulting in a doubling of the obesity rate to approximately one-third of all adults.
- Between the 1960s and the 1990s, teenage girls and young adult women increased their cigarette smoking, subjecting their unborn children to additional hazards of low birthweight.

Thus, behaviorial change is possible for the better and for the worse. Some behaviors, however, are easier to change than others. Let's take a look at why this is.

Why Are Some Individual Health Behaviors Easier to Change Than Others?

Some behaviors are relatively easy to change, while others are extremely difficult. Being able to recognize the difference is an important place to start when trying to alter behavior. It is relatively easy when one behavior can be substituted for a similar one and results in a potentially large payoff. In these situations, knowledge often goes a long way. For instance, the substitution of acetaminophen (Tylenol) for aspirin to prevent Reye's Syndrome was relatively easy. Similarly, the "back-to-sleep" campaign was quite successful in reducing the rate of death from SIDS. In both of these cases, an acceptable and convenient substitute was available making the needed behavioral change much easier to accomplish.

Along with knowledge, incentives—such as reduced cost, increased availability, or improvements in ease-of-use—can encourage rapid acceptance and motivate behavioral change. For instance, easier-to-install child restraint systems have increased their use. Greater insurance coverage and widespread availability of modern mammography equipment has led to an increase in the number of mammograms performed.

The most difficult behaviors to change are those that have a physiological component, such as obesity, or an addictive element, such as cigarette smoking. Individual interventions aimed at smoking cessation or long-term weight control generally succeed less than 30 percent of the time—even among motivated individuals. Even intensive interventions with highly-motivated individuals cannot be expected to be successful more than 50 percent of the time, as was illustrated by the Multiple Risk Factor Intervention Trial (MRFIT), which attempted intensive interventions to reduce risk factors for cardiovascular disease.

In addition, physical, social and economic barriers can stand in the way of behavior change, even if individuals themselves are motivated. If health care is not accessible, or if survival needs require individuals to engage in risks they might not take otherwise, change in behavior may be impeded.

Successful behavioral change requires that we understand as much as we can about how behavior can be changed and what we can do to help.

How Can Individual Behavior Be Changed?

The behavior of individuals is often the final common pathway through which disease, disability, and death can be prevented. The fact that individual behavior has a clearly observable connection with these factors does not necessarily imply that the best or only way to address the behavior of individuals is to focus exclusively on individuals. The forces at work to mold individual behaviors are sometimes referred to as **downstream factors**, **mainstream factors**, and **upstream factors**. Downstream factors are those that directly involve an individual and can potentially be altered by individual interventions, such as an addiction to nicotine. Mainstream factors are those that result from the relationship of an individual with a larger group or population, such as peer pressure to smoke or the level of taxation on cigarettes. These factors require attention at the group or population level. Finally, upstream factors are often grounded in social structures and policies, such as government-sponsored programs that encourage tobacco production. These require us to look beyond traditional health care and public health interventions to the broader social and economic forces that affect health.

Thus, changes in behavior often require more than individual motivation and determination to change. They require encouragement and support from groups ranging from friends and families to work and peer groups. Behavioral change may also require social policies and expectations that reinforce individual efforts. It also requires us to examine the stages that individuals experience as they struggle to change behaviors, especially those habits with physiological challenges.

What Stages Do Individuals Go Through in Making Behavioral Changes?

The process of individual behavioral changes can be described using what has been called the **Stages of Change model**.[4-6] This model provides a useful longitudinal description of five steps that individuals go through in changing behavior. It also suggests steps that can be taken to help individuals make changes.[d]

The first stage, called **precontemplation**, implies that an individual has not yet considered changing their behavior. At this stage, efforts to encourage change are not likely to be successful. However, efforts to educate and offer help in the future may lay the groundwork for later success.

The second phase, known as **contemplation**, implies that an individual is actively thinking about the benefits and barriers to change. At this stage, information focused on short- and immediate-term gains, as well as long-term benefits, can be especially useful. In addition, the contemplation stage lends itself to developing a baseline—that is, establishing the current severity or extent of the problem in order to measure future progress.

The third phase is called **preparation**. During this phase the individual is developing a plan of action. At this point, the individual may be especially receptive to setting goals, considering a range of strategies, and developing a timetable. Help in recognizing and preparing for unanticipated barriers can be especially useful to the individual during this phase.

The fourth phase is the **action** phase when the change in behavior takes place. This is the time to bring together all possible outside support to reinforce and reward the new behavior and help with problems or setbacks that occur.

The fifth—and hopefully final phase—is the **maintenance** phase in which the new behavior becomes a permanent part of an individual's lifestyle. The maintenance phase requires education on how to anticipate the long-term nature of behavioral change, especially how to resist the inevitable temptations to resume the old behavior. Using the cigarette smoking as illustration again, Table 4–5 summarizes the stages of behavioral change and the specific actions that can be helpful at each of the stages.

Notice that individual behavioral change is made easier when group and social efforts are also brought to bear. Higher taxes on cigarettes, peer attitudes and support, and enforcement of laws restricting the permissible locations for smoking, all can be effective social interventions that increase the chances of entering the precontemplation phase, reinforce individual efforts to change behavior, and assist with the maintenance phase. Thus, when looking at how to change individual behavior, we also need to consider how group behaviors can be changed.

How Can Group Behaviors Be Changed?

In recent years, public health has begun to apply marketing approaches to try to better understand and change the health behaviors of groups of people—especially those like cigarette smokers who are at high risk of health impacts of their behavior. **Social marketing**, a use and extension of traditional product marketing, has become a key component of a public health approach to behavioral change.[7] Social marketing campaigns were first successfully used in the developing world for promoting a range of products and behaviors, including family planning and pediatric rehydration therapy. In recent years, social marketing efforts have been widely and successfully used in developed countries, including such efforts as:

- The truth® campaign—Developed by the American Legacy Foundation, it aims to redirect smoking from being seen as a teenage rebellion to not smoking being a rebellion against the alleged behavior-controlling tobacco industry.
- The National Youth Anti-Drug campaign—It uses social marketing efforts directed at young people, including the "Parents. The anti-drug." campaign.
- The VERB™ campaign—It focused on 9 to 13 year olds, or "tweens," with a goal of making exercise fun and "cool" for everyone, not just competitive athletes.

---

[d]Designing interventions based upon the Stages of Change model has not been uniformly successful. One potential reason for this may be that individuals are often in different stages of change for different types of interventions. With complex interventions, such as those required to address obesity, an individual may be in one stage of change for exercise, another for adding fruits and vegetables to his/her diet, and in a different stage in terms of calorie reduction.

TABLE 4-5 Stages of Behavioral Change

Stages of change	Actions	Example—Cigarette Smoking
Precontemplation	**Prognosticate**	
Individuals not considering change	Assessing readiness for change—timing is key	Determine individual's readiness to quit. If not ready, indicate receptivity to help in the future
		Look for receptive timing such as during acute respiratory symptoms
		Social factors, such as workplace and indoor restriction on smoking and taxation, increase likelihood of entering precontemplation phase
Contemplation	**Motivate change**	
Individual thinks actively about the health risk and action required to reduce that risk	Provide information focused on short and intermediate gains from behavioral change, as well as long-term benefits	Reinforce increase in exercise level, reduction in cough, financial savings, serving as example to children, protection of fetus, etc.
Issue of change is on the individual's agenda but no action planned	Doubtful, dire, and distant impacts are less effective	Also continue to inform of longer term effects on health
	Establish baseline to assess severity of the problem; focus attention on the problem and provide basis for comparison	Develop log of timing, frequency, and quantity of smoking, as well as associated events
Preparation	**Plan change**	
Prepare for action including developing a plan and setting a timetable	Set specific measurable and obtainable goals with deadlines	Quit date or possible tapering if heavy smoker
	Two or more well chosen simultaneous interventions may maximize effectiveness	Family support, peer support, individual planning, medication, etc.—may reinforce and multiply impacts
	Recognize habitual nature of existing behavior and remove associated activities	Remove cigarettes, ashtrays, and other associated smoking equipment
		Remove personal and environmental impacts of past smoking, such as teeth cleaning and cleaning of drapery
		Anticipate temptations, such as associations with food, drink, and social occasions
Action	**Reinforce change**	
Observable changes in behavior with potential for relapse	Provide/suggest tangible rewards	Provide rewards, such as alternative use of money—focus on personal hygiene or personal environment
	Positive feedback encouragement of new behavior	Focus on measurable progress toward new behavior
		Provide receptive environment, but avoid focus on excuses
	Anticipate adverse effects and frustrations	Take short term one-day-at-a-time approach
		Recognize cravings and have plan including use of medications
		Recognize potential for symptoms to worsen at first before improvement occurs
		Anticipate potential for weight gain and encourage exercise and other behaviors to reduce potential for weight gain
	Utilize group/peer support	Family and peer reinforcement critical during action phase

continues

TABLE 4-5 Stages of Behavioral Change (continued)

Maintenance	Maintain change	
New behavior needs to be consolidated as part of permanent lifestyle change	Practice/reinforce methods for maintaining new behavior	Avoid old associations and prepare/practice response when encountering old circumstances
	Recognize long term nature of behavioral change and need for supportive peers and social reinforcement	Negative social attitudes toward smoking among peers and society along with social restrictions, such as limiting public indoor smoking and social actions, such as taxation, help prevent smoking and reinforce maintenance of cessation

Source: Data from Prochaska JO, DiClemente CC. Stages and processes of self-change of smoking: toward an integrative model of change. *J Consult Clin Psychol.* 1983;51:390–395.

Social marketing incorporates the "4 Ps," which are widely used to structure traditional marketing efforts. These are:

- **Product**: Identifying the behavior or innovation that is being marketed
- **Price**: Identifying the benefits, the barriers, as well as the financial costs
- **Place**: Identifying the target audiences and how to reach them
- **Promotion**: Organizing a campaign or program to reach the target audience(s)

Social marketing has incorporated concepts from the **diffusion of innovation theory**. This theory, like the stages of behavioral change, contends that adoption of new behaviors requires a series of phases or steps. These move from knowledge of the innovation, to persuasion of its benefits, to the decision to adapt, to implementation, and confirmation.[1] The diffusion of innovation theory has contributed the concept of different types of adopters including: **early adopters**—those who seek to experiment with innovative ideas; **early majority adopters**—often opinion leaders whose social status frequently influences others to adopt the behavior; and **late adopters** (or laggards)—those who need support and encouragement to make adoption as easy as possible.

A different approach is often needed to engage each of these groups. For instance, marketing efforts may initially target early adopters with an approach encouraging innovation and creativity. This may be followed by an approach to opinion leaders who can help the innovation or behavior change become mainstream. A different approach emphasizing ease-of-use and widespread acceptance may be most helpful for encouraging late adopters.

Social marketing, like product marketing, often relies on what marketers call **branding**. Branding includes words and symbols that help the target audience identify with the service; however, it goes deeper than just words and symbols. It can be seen as a method of implementing the fourth "P," or promotion. It also builds upon the first three "Ps":

- Branding requires a clear understanding of the product or the behavior to be changed (product).
- Successful branding puts forth strategies for reducing the financial and psychological costs (price).
- Branding identifies the audience and segments of the audience and asks how each segment can be reached (place).

Thus, branding is the public face of social marketing, but it also needs to be integrated into the core of the marketing plan.[e]

Social marketing efforts in developing and developed countries have demonstrated that it is possible to change key

---

[e] Social marketing has not only incorporated traditional product marketing approaches, it has extended them to address the special circumstances of not-for-profit and government organizations. The use of social marketing in public health has required modifications and enhancements that have been described using four more "Ps": publics, partnerships, policies, and purse strings. "Publics" refers to the need to reach not only a target audience whose behavior we seek to change, but also those people who influence the target audience—be they parents, employers, or opinion leaders. For example, a campaign to address obesity, cigarettes, or high-risk sexual behavior in schools, requires support from parents. "Partnerships" refers to the need for collaborations to achieve most public health goals. The VERB™ campaign, for instance, partnered with television stations appealing to "tweens" and schools to help get its message out. Successful efforts to reduce adolescent smoking, increase exercise, and reduce drug use, also require changing institutional policies, which means reaching adult decision makers. Finally, the "purse string" aspect is money—few public health social marketing campaigns have adequate resources to do the job. Funding issues may require public health marketing teams to incorporate a long-term approach and look for nontraditional sources of funding.

BOX 4-1 VERB™ Campaign.

The VERB™ social marketing campaign was funded through the Centers for Disease Control and Prevention (CDC), which worked with advertising agencies to reach "tweens" to make exercise "cool." After a series of focus groups and other efforts to define and understand the market, they concluded that the message should not be one of improving health, but rather of having fun with friends, exploring new activities with a sense of adventure, and being free to experiment without being judged on performance.

Marketing efforts also identified barriers including time constraints and the attraction of other activities from social occasions to television to computers. Barriers included lack of access to facilities, as well as negative images of competition, embarrassment, and the inability to become an elite athlete.

The VERB™ campaign implied action and used the tagline "It's what you do." Initial messages used animated figures of children covered with verbs being physically active. Later, messages turned these animated verb-covered kids into real kids actively playing. Widely-used logos were developed and promoted as part of the branding effort. The VERB™ campaign partnered with television channels that successfully reach "tweens," sponsored outreach events, and distributed promotional materials.

During the four years of the VERB™ campaign, "tweens" developed widespread recognition of the program and rated it highly in terms of "saying something important to me" and "makes me want to get more active" with maximum levels of recognition of 64 percent and 68 percent, respectively. Despite the documented success of VERB™, it was discontinued because of cuts in the federal budget.

---

health behaviors of well-defined groups of people, including adolescents, which are often regarded as the hardest to reach. An example of the use of social marketing to reach young people, the VERB™ campaign, is examined in Box 4-1.[8]

To be most successful, behavior-changing efforts need to include individual, group, and social aspects. Let us look at some approaches to combining these efforts.

How Can We Combine Individual, Group, and Social Efforts to Implement Behavioral Change?

As we have seen, behavioral change is most successful when it combines efforts aimed at the individuals, the at-risk group, and the population, or society as a whole. It can be useful to look again at the Stages of Change model to see how interventions can be successfully combined at each stage in the behavior change process. Let us return to cigarette smoking as an example.

In the precontemplation and contemplation stages, individual interventions are focused on education, assessing readiness to change, and offering help. Interventions targeting at-risk groups and populations, such as taxation on cigarettes and restriction on public and workplace smoking, can be very useful in smoking cessation preparation and preventing individuals from starting smoking in the first place.

The preparation stage requires individual action, but it can be encouraged and reinforced by family and friends, as well as via national efforts, such as the American Cancer Society's annual Great American Smokeout®, which encourages smokers to quit for a lifetime by starting with just one day. The action phase may appear to be exclusively based on individual action; however, it can be supported and encouraged by family and peers and reinforced by social efforts, such as health insurance polices that provide payment for support groups and medications.

The maintenance phase also relies on individual, group, and population/social interventions. Individual interventions often focus on education about the long-term nature of behavioral change and the efforts necessary to resist the temptation to resume smoking. Group support and reinforcement continue to be important in encouraging maintenance of the new behavior. The same types of social interventions that encourage individuals to stop cigarette smoking, such as taxation and restrictions on public and workplace smoking, also help encourage them to continue their smoke-free behavior. Table 4-6 summarizes the roles that individual, group, and population intervention can play in changing cigarette smoking behavior.

We have now looked at how health informatics and health communications, as well as social and behavioral interventions, can be used in population health. In Chapter 5, we will turn our attention to another set of key tools of population health: law, policy, and ethics.

TABLE 4-6 Stages of Change—Individual, Group and Population/Social Interventions to Change Cigarette Smoking Behavior

Stage of change	Individual	At-risk group	Population/society
Precontemplation	Assess readiness for change and offer future help	Social marketing aimed at specific groups Restriction on smoking at work	Cost affected by taxes, restrictions on smoking in public places, warning labels on packages
Contemplation	Information on hazards of smoking and gains from quitting	More receptive to social marketing aimed at specific groups Restriction on smoking at work	More receptive to costs of cigarettes, restrictions on smoking in public places, and warning labels
Preparation	Set individual goals and develop strategy Medication may be helpful	Support group/friends and family reinforce individual preparation; telephone "quit lines"	National efforts, e.g., American Cancer Society National Quit Day
Action	Remove connections between cigarettes and pleasurable activities Use of medications if needed	Public commitment to action—announce to family, friends, and work colleagues	Pay for medication and other assistance with cessation as part of insurance
Maintenance	Education regarding long term physical addiction and potential for relapse	Continued reinforcement at work and by peer and social groups	Continued reinforcement by social marketing, taxes, and restriction on public smoking

Key Words

- Stages of Change model
- Social marketing
- Diffusion of innovation theory
- Branding
- Downstream factors
- Mainstream factors
- Upstream factors
- Precontemplation
- Contemplation
- Preparation
- Action
- Maintenance
- Product
- Price
- Place
- Promotion
- Early adopters
- Early majority adopters
- Late adopters

Discussion Questions

Take a look at the questions posed in the following scenarios, which were presented at the beginning of this chapter. See now whether you can answer these questions.

1. You travel to a country in Asia and find that their culture affects most parts of life. From the food they eat and their method of cooking to their attitudes toward medical care to their beliefs about the cause of disease and the ability to alter it through public health and medical interventions, this country is profoundly different from the United States. You ask: how does culture affect health?

2. You are working in a country with strict Islamic practices and find that religion like culture can have major impacts on health. Religious practices differ widely—from beliefs about food and alcohol; to sexual practices, such as male circumcision and female sexual behavior; to acceptance or rejection of interventions aimed at women's health. You ask: how does religion affect health?

3. You're trying to help your spouse quit smoking cigarettes and your kids from starting. You know that gentle encouragement and support on a one-on-one basis are essential, but often are not enough because cigarettes are an addiction that produces withdrawal and long-term cravings. Like most addictions, it requires a combination of individual motivation, support from family and friends, and sometimes the use of medications; but you wonder: do warning labels on cigarettes, taxes on cigarettes, and "no smoking" zones in public places make any difference?

4. Your efforts to convince your friends to avoid smoking (or at least stop smoking) focus on giving them the facts about how cigarettes cause lung cancer, throat cancer, and serious heart disease. You are frus-

trated by how little impact you have on your friends. You wonder, whether you would be more successful by focusing on the immediate negative impacts, such as stained teeth and bad breath, as well as the loss of control that goes along with addiction to nicotine?

5. As a new parent, you hear from your pediatrician, nurses in the hospital, and even from the makers of your brand of diapers, that babies should sleep on their backs. They call it "back-to-sleep." You're surprised to find that it's part of the class on babysitting given by the local community center and a required part of the training for those who work in registered day care centers. You find out that it's all part of a social marketing campaign that has reduced in half the number of deaths from sudden infant death syndrome. You ask: why has the "back-to-sleep" campaign been so successful?

REFERENCES

1. Edberg M. *Essentials of Health Behavior: Social and Behavioral Theory in Public Health.* Sudbury, MA: Jones and Bartlett Publishers; 2007.
2. Commission on Social Determinants of Health. *Closing the Gap in a Generation: Health Equity through Action on the Social Determinants of Health. Final Report of the Commission on Social Determinants of Health.* Geneva, Switzerland: World Health Organization; 2008.
3. Marmot M. *The Status Syndrome: How Social Standing Affects Our Health and Longevity.* New York: Henry Holt and Company; 2004.
4. DiClemente CC, Prochaska JO. Self-change and therapy change of smoking behavior: a comparison of processes of change in cessation and maintenance. *Addict Behav.* 1982;7:133–142.
5. Prochaska JO, DiClemente CC. Stages and processes of self-change of smoking: toward an integrative model of change. *J Consult Clin Psychol.* 1983;51:390–395.
6. Jenkins CD. *Building Better Health: A Handbook of Behavioral Change.* (Technical Publication No. 590). Washington, DC: Pan American Health Organization; 2003.
7. Weinreich NK. What is social marketing? Available at: http://www.social-marketing.com/Whatis.html. Accessed March 12, 2009.
8. Wong F, Huhman M, Asbury L, Mueller RB, McCarthy S, Londe P, et al. VERB™—A social marketing campaign to increase physical activity among youth. *Prev Chronic Disease.* 2004;3(1):1–7.

Health Law, Policy, and Ethics

A new statute and subsequent administrative regulations give only a temporary license to newly-licensed drivers, prohibiting late night driving, the use of cell phones and limiting the number of passengers. You ask: should elderly drivers be subject to these same types of regulations, such as being required to take a driver's test?

You decide not to enroll in the health plan offered by your employer because it seems so expensive and you are young and healthy. Shortly thereafter, your car is struck by a hit-and-run driver and you find yourself on the way to the nearest hospital. After stabilizing you as required by law, they transfer you to the public hospital, which is the only one in town that will take care of you without insurance. You ask: do you have a right to health care?

You hear that a new drug has shown extremely promising results, but will not be available for a least a couple of years. You wonder: why do you have to wait so long to take the newest prescription medicine while your e-mail fills up with promotions for

the untested ways to enhance your energy, beauty, and sexual performance?

You hear that a neighbor has TB and refuses treatment. You wonder: what if he has the type of TB that can't be cured with drugs? You ask: can't they make him take his medicine or at least get him out of your neighborhood?

You hear an advertisement about participating in a new research study. It sounds like you're eligible, so you check into it. You're surprised to find that even if you participate you may not receive the new drug and won't even be told which treatment you are receiving. Despite your willingness to take your chances, you're told that you are not eligible for the study due to conditions that put you at increased risk of developing side effects. You ask: why can't I participate if I'm willing to take the risks?

These are the types of issues that are part of health law, policy, and ethics. Let us begin by examining the scope of these issues.

WHAT IS THE SCOPE OF HEALTH LAW, POLICY, AND ETHICS?

Health law, policy, and ethics reflect a wide range of tools that society uses to encourage and discourage behaviors by individuals and groups. These tools apply to health care, as well as to traditional public health. In addition, in recent years a field called **bioethics** has been defined, which includes elements of both health care and public health and focuses on applying morals or values to areas of potential conflict.[1]

Health law, policy, and ethics affect the full range of issues that confront us in population health. They address such things as the access to and the quality and cost of health care. They also address the organizational and professional structures designed to deliver health care. Health law, policy, and ethics are also key tools for accomplishing the goals of traditional public health ranging from occupational safety to drug and highway safety and from control of communicable diseases to non-communicable and environmental diseases. Bioethics lies at the intersection of health law and policy and attempts to apply individual and group values and morals to controversial issues, such as abortion, stem cell research, and end-of-life care. Table 5-1 outlines a range of issues that are addressed by health law, policy, and ethics.

The scope of health law, policy, and ethics is so vast that we will focus on first defining key principles and philosophies that underlie our society's approach to these issues. Then, we will focus on three examples that illustrate key issues confronted in the healthcare, public health, and bioethics arenas. These are:

1. Is there a right to health care?
2. How does public health balance the rights of individuals and the needs of society?
3. How can bioethical principles be applied to protecting individuals who participate in research?[1]

Let us start by taking a look at key legal principles that underlie the approach to public health and health care in the United States.

What Legal Principles Underlie Public Health and Health Care?

In order to better appreciate the issue of health policy and law, it is important to understand some key legal principles that underlie both public health and healthcare law in the United States.[1] First, the U.S. Constitution is a fundamental document that governs the issues of public health and healthcare law. However, the U.S. Constitution does not mention health. As a result, public health and health care are among those issues that are left primarily to the authority of the states unless delegated by the state-to-local jurisdictions, such as cities or counties. The use of this authority, known as **police power**, allows states to pass legislation and take actions to protect the common good. The authority to protect the common good may justify a wide range of state actions including: the regulation of healthcare professionals and facilities; the establishment of health and safety standards in retail, as well as other occupational settings; and the control of hazards ranging from requiring use of car restraint systems to vaccinations to restricting the sale of tobacco products.[1, 2]

The use of state police power is limited by the protections afforded to individuals. These protections are known as **rights** and are created either through the U.S. Constitution, through a state's constitution, or through laws passed at the federal or state levels. The U.S. Constitution allows, but does not require, governments to act to protect public health or to provide healthcare services. This has been referred to as the **negative constitution**. Thus, while governments often have the authority to act, they are not required to do so. For instance, the Supreme Court has not found an obligation on the part of states to act to prevent child or spousal abuse even when the state is fully aware of specific circumstances or a court has issued a restraining order.[1]

Second, the Interstate Commerce Clause of the U.S. Constitution is the major source of federal authority in public health and health care. It provides the federal government

TABLE 5-1 Components of Health Law, Policy, and Ethics

Component	Scope	Examples of issues
Health care	Access, quality, and cost of health care. Organizational and professional structures for the delivery of care	Rules governing Medicare and Medicaid, as well as laws governing private insurance. Hospital governance and professional licensure
Public health	Population health and safety, including governmental efforts to provide services to entire populations, as well as vulnerable groups	Food and drug laws and procedures, environmental laws and procedures, regulations for control of communicable diseases
Bioethics	Application of individual and group values and morals to controversial areas	End-of-life care, stem cell research, abortion, protection of research subjects

with authority to tax, spend, and regulate interstate commerce.[2] This authority has been used to justify a wide range of federal involvement in health care and public health. Federal authority is often exerted through incentives to the states. For instance, states may be offered federal funding or matching funding if they enact specific types of legislation, such as the rules governing Medicaid or definitions of blood-alcohol levels for driving under the influence.[3] The U.S. Constitution's supremacy clause declares that legitimate federal laws are the supreme laws of the land and they preempt or overrule state laws that conflict with them.[a] This provision has been used by federal public health agencies, such as the Food and Drug Administration and the Environmental Protection Agency, to justify national standards that overrule and limit state rules and regulations ranging from quality controls on drugs to levels of permissible exposures to toxic substances.[1, 2]

Third, the U.S. Constitution grants individual rights. Some of them, such as freedom of speech, religion, assembly, and the right to bear arms, are explicit in the document. Others have been inferred by the U.S. Supreme Court, such as the right to procreation, privacy, bodily integrity, and travel. These inferred rights are often the basis for individual protections in public health and health care, including the right to utilize contraception, have an abortion, and limit the state and federal authority to use quarantine and other travel restrictions.[1, 2] Unless the U.S. Constitution explicitly includes a right or one has been "found" by the Supreme Court of the United States, no right exists. However, federal and state legislatures may create rights through legislation ranging from access to education to access to medical care. The existence of a right implies that state and/or federal courts are expected to uphold and enforce the right.[b]

Health law is based upon these rules governing the authority of federal and state governments and also the rights of individuals. It is derived from four sources that are summarized in Box 5-1.[1]

Thus, health law refers to a vast array of legal issues that influence much of what goes on in public health and health care. However, the influence of health policy often extends beyond that of the formal legal system. Let us take a look at what we mean by health policy.

What Do We Mean by Health Policy?

Within the constraints set by law, there is considerable latitude for governments, as well as private groups, to develop policies that affect the ways that public health and health care are conducted. Health policy is a subset of the larger arena of public policy. According to Teitelbaum and Wilensky, "when deciding on whether something is a public policy decision, the focus is not only on who is making the decision, but also on what kind of decision is being made."[4] They define individuals or groups that make public policy based on the ability of the individual or group to make an **authoritative decision**. An authoritative decision is a decision made by an individual or group that has the power to implement the decision. A range of governmental and private groups make public policy decisions in areas such as cigarette smoking. In government, authoritative decisions might be made by an executive branch official, such as the president or a governor, or administrative officials, such as federal, state, or local health officers. These may range from policies that discourage the growing of tobacco to policies that encourage the sale of tobacco products abroad to policies that restrict smoking in public places or tax tobacco sales. These polices may or may not be incorporated into laws or statutes.

At times, health policy may be made by private groups, including professional societies, such as the American Public Health Association, or commercial trade associations representing hospitals, the drug industry, the insurance industry, etc. Policies that affect large numbers of people, such as those that restrict smoking in hospitals, encourage clinicians to incorporate smoking prevention and cessation programs, compensate clinicians' efforts through insurance, and encourage the development of new drugs to assist with smoking cessation, are all examples of health polices that may be set by groups outside of government. Thus, the "public" in public policies does not necessarily imply that the policies were developed or implemented by government.

According to Teitelbaum and Wilensky, in addition to being authoritative, a public policy decision must be one that "goes beyond the individual sphere and affects the greater community."[4] Decisions to seek vaccination or screenings, to smoke

---

[a] Another implication of constitutional law is the supremacy of the U.S. Constitution even over international law. Human rights and standards incorporated into international documents are not directly enforceable in the United States. These rights and standards are only enforceable in the United States through enactment of federal or state laws.[1]

[b] Enforcement is required by law to occur based on due process. Due process includes **substantive due process**, which refers to the grounds for depriving an individual of a right, as well as **procedural due process**, which refers to the processes that must be undertaken to deprive an individual of a right. The former implies that state and federal governments must justify depriving an individual of life, liberty, and property. When fundamental rights are involved or laws are based on suspect classifications, such as gender or race, the court applies strict criteria that place difficult burdens of proof on the government to justify these types of actions. Procedural due process implies that when a right exists, governments may not deny individuals the right in an arbitrary or unfair way. This process requires that acceptable legal processes be followed before an individual can be deprived of a right. The Supreme Court has considered a fundamental right as one that is explicit in the U.S. Constitution, that has been "found" in the U.S. Constitution by the Supreme Court, or that is rooted in the nation's history and traditions.[1, 2]

BOX 5-1 Types of Law.

To appreciate the complex relationship between the law and public health and health care, it is important to appreciate that there are four sources of law. These may be classified as **constitutional law, legislative statutes, administrative regulations**, and **judicial law** (also called case law or common law).

Constitutional law includes not only the United States Constitution, but the constitutions of the 50 states. The provisions of state constitutions are important because the responsibilities for health lie with the states unless the federal constitution grants authority to the federal government. As we have seen, the commerce clause and the due process clauses of the constitution have been the basis for extensions of federal authority into areas of health. State constitutions are often easier to amend than the federal constitutions, and thus can and do change more frequently. Constitutions often limit the role of government and define its processes. Constitutional law, however, does not usually directly mandate roles for government in the area of health.

Legislative law, or statutes, is/are written by legislative bodies at local, state, and federal levels. Federal statutes preempt, that is they over-rule, conflicting state statutes, as long as they are consistent with the limitation placed on the federal government by the U.S. Constitution. Statutes often directly address health issues. Legislative law may place requirements or prohibition on future activities. Statutes may authorize governmental regulation, such as professional or institutional licensure; require specific activities, such a restaurant inspections; prohibit other activities, such as smoking in public places; or provide funding to pay for governmental services or reimburse those who provide the services, such as health care.

Administrative law is produced by executive agencies of the federal, state, and local governments in order to implement legislative statutes, which are often written in quite general language. Executive agencies must follow legally-defined processes and stay within what is called the legislative intent of the statute. Administrative law can be seen as operationalizing statutes passed by legislative bodies. These types of laws may define who is eligible for services, how these services may be provided, the levels of reimbursement received, and a large number of other important details that affect the day-to-day operations of government services and programs. Administrative law affects public health in many ways from the regulation of septic tanks to requirements for immunization to enroll in public education. Executive agencies often set up quasi-judicial processes to review contested cases. These judicial processes usually provide for limited access to the court system to contest their decisions.

Judicial, case, or common law, is law made by courts when applying constitutional, statutory, or administrative law to specific cases. In addition, common law may fill in the holes when statutory law does not provide guidance. For instance case law may be the basis for addressing environmental health issues which the law defines as "nuisances" ranging from excess noise to disposal of garbage. Judges' primary responsibility is to apply previous rulings or precedence to new cases that come before them; however, they may take into account existing traditions and customs of society when applying the law to specific cases. Higher courts including appellate courts, and ultimately the U.S. Supreme Court, and in some instances, state Supreme Courts may decide that a statute violates the relevant constitutions. That is, they can rule a statute unconstitutional.

cigarettes at home, or to purchase a particular type of health insurance are individual decisions. Public policy issues revolve around incentives or requirements to encourage or discourage these actions by groups of individuals or the society as a whole. Health policy often rests upon the attitude or philosophy that a group takes toward the role that different types of institutions should play in public health and health care. Specifically, the appropriate role of government is often a controversial subject.

How Do Philosophies Toward the Role of Government Affect Health Policies?

One of the most fundamental differences within our society is the attitude or philosophy about the roles that government

and the economic market should play in advancing health. To appreciate this issue, it is useful to look at two contrasting philosophies regarding the government's role in health care and public health. These philosophies are called **social justice** and **market justice**.

Understanding these quite different approaches is helpful because our current system of health care and public health borrows from both of these basic approaches to varying degrees. Table 5-2 outlines the contrasting characteristics of market justice and social justice. Table 5-3 examines many of the implications of the two different philosophies.[5]

Market and social justice approaches are useful for understanding the structure of healthcare systems, as we will see

TABLE 5-2 Characteristics of Market and Social Justice

Market Justice	Social Justice
Views health care as an economic good	Views health care as a social resource
Assumes free market conditions for health services delivery	Requires active government involvement in health services delivery
Assumes that markets are more efficient in allocating resources equitably	Assumes that the government is more efficient in allocating health resources equitably
Production and distribution of health care determined by market-based demand	Medical resource allocation determined by central planning
Medical care distribution based on people's ability to pay	Ability to pay inconsequential for receiving medical care
Access to medical care viewed as an economic reward for personal effort and achievement	Equal access to medical services viewed as a basic right

Source: Shi L, Singh D. *Delivering Health Care in America.* 3rd ed. Sudbury, MA: Jones and Bartlett Publishers; 2004: 59.

TABLE 5-3 Implications of Market and Social Justice

Market Justice	Social Justice
Individual responsibility for health	Collective responsibility for health
Benefits based on individual purchasing power	Everyone is entitled to a basic package of services
Limited obligation to the collective good	Strong obligation to the collective good
Emphasis on individual well-being	Community well-being supersedes that of the individual
Private solutions to social problems	Public solutions to social problems
Rationing based on ability to pay	Planned rationing of health care

Source: Shi L, Singh D. *Delivering Health Care in America.* 3rd ed. Sudbury, MA: Jones and Bartlett Publishers; 2004: 59.

in Chapter 11. They are also useful in understanding the evolution of public health approaches and institutions, such as those of the United States Food and Drug Administration[6] illustrated in Box 5-2.

We have now looked at key principles and approaches of health law and health policy that underlie our approach to health care and public health. To see how these principles operate in practice, let us review the three questions introduced earlier:

1. Is there a right to health care?
2. How does public health balance the rights of individuals and the needs of society?

3. How can bioethical principles be applied to protecting individuals who participate in research?

Is There a Right to Health Care?

In 1948, a right to health care was incorporated into the Universal Declaration of Human Rights and the Constitution of the World Health Organization. The former states that "(e)veryone has the right to a standard of living adequate for the health and well-being of himself and his family, including…medical care…and the right to security in the event of…sickness…."[7] Most developed countries have incorporated a right to health

BOX 5-2 The United States Food and Drug Administration and Market Justice versus Social Justice.

The arguments over the use of the market mechanism and the governmental regulatory mechanism in public health are well illustrated by the history of the U.S. Food and Drug Administration. These opposing philosophies are highlighted as we as a nation have attempted to balance market approaches versus regulatory or social justice approaches.

Until the early years of the 20th century, the market controlled the availability of drugs. Narcotics and other addictive substances were widely sold in the marketplace totally within the law. Drugs were falsely advertised to produce miraculous cures. There were few limitations on what could be advertised or what substances the miracle cures of the day could contain.

The "muckrakers," aggressive journalists of the early 20th century, brought to public attention many abuses, from the sale of drugs laced with narcotics, cocaine, and alcohol, to the abuses in the meatpacking industry so vividly portrayed in Upton Sinclair famous novel, *The Jungle*. In 1906, these efforts finally resulted in the passage of federal legislation establishing the Food and Drug Administration (FDA). The FDA act is often considered a key accomplishment of what has been called the Progressive Era of American politics.

Though this legislation creating the FDA provided the foundation for modern food and drug regulation, the original law only required that products be accurately labeled indicating their ingredients. The burden was on the FDA to demonstrate safety problems before a drug could be removed from the market. It was not until the late 1930s that the authority of the FDA was expanded. This expansion was justified by use of the interstate commerce clause since most drugs are part of commerce between two or more states.

In 1937, a Tennessee drug company producing a pediatric liquid form of sulfa, the first antibiotic precipitated the changes in FDA law. The solvent in this untested product was a highly toxic chemical related to antifreeze. Over 100 people died, mostly children. The public outcry brought Congress to action with the passage of the 1938 FDA amendments. These amendments required safety testing prior to making a new drug available to the market. The process of safety regulation soon resulted in an additional requirement that certain drugs be prescribed only by a physician, while others were available over-the-counter.

Over the years, the FDA's authority has been repeatedly increased in the wake of highly-publicized tragedies. The production and distribution of a batch of polio vaccine that itself caused polio led to the regulation of vaccines in the 1950s. The Dalkon Shield, an intrauterine device (IUD) that produced thousands of cases of infection and subsequent infertility, brought about regulations of medical devices in the mid-1970s. Perhaps the most famous U.S. disaster was the one that did not happen. In the early 1960s, FDA safety regulations resulted in a delay in approving a new, very effective sleeping pill called thalidomide. In Europe, the drug produced thousands of grossly-deformed newborns, an event which did not occur in the United States. Ironically, the thalidomide case resulted in the Kefauver-Harris Drug Amendments, which focused on efficacy, not safety, and mandated efficacy testing before a drug could be approved and marketed. This landmark legislation laid the groundwork for today's process of drug approval and for the evolution of evidence-based medicine and public health.

The authority of the FDA, however, has not continued to expand. The 1980s and 1990s produced a social movement that sought smaller government and less authority over the lives of individuals. In 1994, Congress created a new category of substances—carved from the definition of drugs—dietary supplements. These included not only vitamins and minerals, but also herbal remedies. Dietary supplements, as opposed to drugs, were subject to far less regulation. As long as they did not claim therapeutic value for specific diseases, dietary supplements could be advertised and sold without demonstrating either safety or efficacy. In parallel with the 1906 legislation, only accurate labeling was required and the burden was on the FDA to prove problems with safety.

The move back to market control also resulted from an early 1990s Supreme Court decision that allowed advertising of prescription drugs. The enormous expansion of prescription drug promotion produced a flood of direct advertisement to consumers and a rapid expansion of the quantity of prescription drugs marketed and prescribed. During this period of rapid expansion, the FDA focused on premarket regulation of the safety and efficacy of drugs. However, once approved, the FDA did not have the authority to further evaluate the drug's safety. Rare, but often serious, side effects of drugs were evident only after the drugs were prescribed to large numbers of patients in clinical practice. The short period of premarket observation also hid side effects that only appeared after longer term use. In addition, individuals included in premarket trials often had one disease and were not taking other medications. Patients with multiple diseases on multiple medications often experienced far more side effects.

Most recently, a widely-publicized tragedy has led to new legislation and approaches to regulation. Vioxx®, one of a new class of medications for pain relief and reduction in inflammation, was widely advertised and used by tens of millions of people before it was recognized that it increased the incidence of heart disease. The drug was estimated to have caused tens of thousands of deaths from heart disease. The FDA amendments of 2007 aimed to address safety issues by giving the FDA authority for the first time to require pharma-

(continues)

> **BOX 5-2** continued.
>
> ceutical companies to perform postmarket data collection; by authorizing programs to utilize large national prescription databases to search for adverse drug effects; and by encouraging FDA review of direct-to-consumer drug advertising before it is seen by consumers.
>
> The history of the FDA reflects the tension in American society between governmental efforts to regulate and efforts to allow market regulation through the choices made by individuals. This tension has been a part of the regulation of drugs, vaccines, and medical devices for over 100 years and is likely to continue to be important in coming years.

care in their constitution or have created rights to health care as part of the legislative process, usually as part of a healthcare system that provides universal coverage. This internationally recognized right to health care cannot be enforced in the United States unless it is found to be recognized by the U.S. Constitution or a state constitution or has been incorporated into federal, state, or local statutes. Therefore, we need to examine what has happened within the legal system of the United States.

As we have discussed, the U.S. Constitution does not mention the word health. Rights, however, can be "found" or created by the Supreme Court through their interpretation of the Constitution. Rights to travel and privacy, for example, have been "found" by the Supreme Court, while a right to health care has not been. State courts, such as the Supreme Court of Indiana, have addressed the meaning of a license to practice medicine in *Hurley v. Eddingfield*. In the case, a licensed physician refused services to a pregnant woman despite being offered prepayment and despite the fact that the physician knew that no other qualified physician was available. As a result, the woman did not receive medical care and both she and her unborn child died.[1] The court established what has been called the **no-duty principle**. This principle holds that healthcare providers (whether they are individuals or institutions) do not have an obligation to provide health services. A right to health care can be created within a state via its constitution. It can also be created in the United States or within a state by legislative action.[1]

Limited rights to health care have been established by legislative action. For instance, federal law includes the 1986 Treatment for Emergency Medical Conditions and Women in Labor Act, which provides a right to emergency medical care usually provided through hospital emergency departments.[c] This act establishes a right to health care by those seeking emergency services and establishes a duty on the part of hospital emergency department to provide these services.

This right and the corresponding duty, however, are quite limited. Patients have the right to receive care and the hospital has a duty to provide an "appropriate" examination. The institution also has the duty to stabilize an emergency situation by providing as much treatment as possible within its capacity. When a hospital does not have the capacity to treat the emergency condition, it is required to transfer the patient to another facility in a medically-appropriate fashion. These rights and duties are limited to emergency conditions in hospital emergency departments and do not provide more general rights to health care.[d]

Thus, a right to health care in the United States has not been generally established. As with health law and policies in general, this issue has not been definitively settled. As the state and federal governments struggle with the problems of providing health care for everyone, the right to health care is again emerging as an issue for debate and consideration. Let us now take a look at another fundamental issue that is at the core of public health law and policy—the balance between the rights of the individual and the needs of society.

How Does Public Health Balance the Rights of Individuals and the Needs of Society?

Public health interventions often create a level of tension between the concerns of individuals and the needs of society. This is the situation even when individual rights are not involved. For instance, the courts have been clear that a driver's license is a privilege and not a right. Thus, it can be regulated by states without having to justify that individuals who are denied a driver's license are being denied a right. The regulation of driver's licenses is a state responsibility and as such there is

---

[c] This act is often referred to as EMTALA which is an acronym for the law's original name—the Emergency Medical Treatment and Active Labor Act.

[d] Another example of legislation that has established rights to health care is the Medicaid program. Medicaid establishes defined criteria for eligibility to enroll that are partially governed by federal law and partially by state law, as we will discuss in Chapter 11. During the time that an individual is qualified for Medicaid, they have certain rights to health care that can be enforced by individuals in the courts.

enormous variation in factors such as age requirement, the length and requirement for learning permits, the type of examination required, the rules for suspension of a driver's license, and requirements for renewal of a driver's license.

Motor vehicle injuries remain a major cause of death and disability. It is widely accepted that there are two age groups at highest risk of death and disability from motor vehicles. The first are adolescents during their initial years of driving and the second are elderly individuals. Until recently, most states imposed minimum or no barriers to either group once an initial driver's license had been issued. In many states, these limitations have now been imposed for one or both age groups. Possible public health interventions include raising the driving age, requiring stricter standards for licensure, and placing initial limitations on new drivers including restricting night time driving, the number of passengers, and the use of cell phones. Common restrictions on older drivers include vision and hearing tests and reexamination including road testing.

The tension level between the individual and society is even greater when fundamental rights are denied as is the case with the use of quarantine. Box 5-3 examines the historical and current uses of quarantine.[8]

The dynamic between individual and societal needs is also key to understanding most bioethical issues. The modern field of bioethics grew out of the efforts to protect participants in research, while ensuring that society can benefit from the results of ethical human research. Let us look at how these standards developed and how research subjects are protected today.

How Can Bioethical Principles Be Applied to Protecting Individuals Who Participate in Research?

Ethical issues pervade nearly every aspect of public health and medical practice. However, ethical considerations have had an especially strong impact on the conduct of research. The mod-

---

BOX 5-3   Quarantine as a Public Health Authority.

Quarantine, the compulsory physical separation of those with a disease—or at high risk of developing a disease—from the rest of the population goes back to ancient times when it was used to restrict entry of ships into ports where epidemic diseases threatened. Attempts to control epidemics of yellow fever, smallpox, and other infectious disease by quarantine were very much a part of the early history of the United States.

In the 19th century, tuberculosis (TB) sanatoriums often isolated those afflicted on a voluntary basis. Laws existed and were occasionally used that allowed quarantine of patients who felt well though were thought to be carriers of TB and other contagious diseases, such as typhoid. The infamous "Typhoid Mary" was quarantined on an island in New York after she refused to voluntarily refrain from working as a food handler.

Quarantine was only occasionally used to control disease in the 20th century. However, in the early 21st century it again became a public health issue precipitated by the recognition of SARS and the fear of rapid global spread of SARS and other communicable diseases. The spread of resistant and extremely resistant tuberculosis has again made use of quarantine for TB an ongoing important public health issue.

Quarantine laws are in the process of revision. The issues of quarantine reflect many of the tensions between the right of the individual and the rights of society. For instance, a recent *New England Journal of Medicine* article on use of quarantine for control of extremely resistant TB states:

> In recent decades, courts have clarified the legal rights of patients with tuberculosis who are subject to compulsory isolation. Drawing an analogy between isolation orders and civil commitment for mental illness, courts have affirmed that patients who are isolated by law have many procedural due-process rights, including the right to counsel and a hearing before an independent decision maker. States must also provide "clear and convincing" evidence that isolation is necessary to prevent a significant risk of harm to others. Most important, some courts have held that isolation must be the least restrictive alternative for preventing such a risk. If the government can protect public health without relying on involuntary detention, it must and should do so."[8]

The use of quarantine is thus likely to be restricted and used very infrequently in the future. Increasingly, the emphasis on the rights of the individual outweighs any value that quarantine might have in protecting the public's health.

ern field of bioethics in general and research ethics in particular grew out of the Nuremberg trials of German physicians who performed experiments on prisoners in Nazi concentration camps. These crimes included exposure to extremes of temperature, mutilating surgery, and deliberate infection with a variety of lethal germs. The report of the Nuremberg trials established internationally-accepted principles known as the Nuremberg Code shown in Box 5-4.[9]

Abuse of individuals participating in research has not been limited to victims of Nazi concentration camps. In the United States from the late 1930s through the early 1970s, the Tuskegee Syphilis Study used disadvantaged, rural black men to study the untreated course of syphilis. These men were recruited to a study of "bad blood," and were misled into believing that they were receiving effective treatment; in addition, they were provided deceptive information in order to retain them in the study. These subjects were deprived of penicillin treatment in order not to interrupt the research, long after such treatment became generally available for syphilis. The Tuskegee Study was a major reason for the creation of The National Commission for the Protection of Human Subjects of Biomedical and

Behavioral Research, which produced what has come to be called the **Belmont Report.** The Belmont Report focused on the key issues of defining informed consent and selection of participants and led to the development of **Institutional Review Boards** (**IRBs**), which now must approve most human research. The report remains a vital part of the framework for defining the rights of research subjects.[10] The followed excerpts outline three basic ethical principles:

1. **Respect for Persons**—Respect for persons incorporates at least two ethical convictions: first, individuals should be treated as autonomous agents, and second, that persons with diminished autonomy are entitled to protection. The principle of respect for persons thus divides into two separate moral requirements: the requirement to acknowledge autonomy and the requirement to protect those with diminished autonomy.

2. **Beneficence**—Persons are treated in an ethical manner not only by respecting their decisions and protecting them from harm, but also by making efforts to secure their well-being. Such treatment falls under the

---

BOX 5-4   The Ten Principles Contained in the Nuremberg Code.

1. The voluntary consent of the human subject is absolutely essential....
2. The experiment should be such as to yield fruitful results for the good of society, unprocurable by other methods or means of study, and not random and unnecessary in nature.
3. The experiment should be so designed and based on the results of animal experimentation and knowledge of the natural history of the disease or other problem under study that the anticipated results will justify the performance of the experiment.
4. The experiment should be so conducted as to avoid all unnecessary physical and mental suffering and injury.
5. No experiment should be conducted where there is an a priori reason to believe that death or disabling injury will occur; except, perhaps, in those experiments where the experimental physicians also serve as subjects.
6. The degree of risk to be taken should never exceed that determined by the humanitarian importance of the problem to be solved by the experiment.
7. Proper preparations should be made and adequate facilities provided to protect the experimental subject against even remote possibilities of injury, disability, or death.
8. The experiment should be conducted only by scientifically qualified persons. The highest degree of skill and care should be required through all stages of the experiment of those who conduct or engage in the experiment.
9. During the course of the experiment the human subject should be at liberty to bring the experiment to an end if he has reached the physical or mental state where continuation of the experiment seems to him to be impossible.
10. During the course of the experiment the scientist in charge must be prepared to terminate the experiment at any stage, if he has probable cause to believe, in the exercise of the good faith, superior skill and careful judgment required of him that a continuation of the experiment is likely to result in injury, disability, or death to the experimental subject.

Source: United States Government. Trials of War Criminals before the Nuremberg Military Tribunals under Control Council Law No. 10, Vol. 2. Washington, DC: U.S. Government Printing Office; 1949: 181–182.

principle of beneficence. . . . Two general rules have been formulated as complementary expressions of beneficent actions in this sense: (1) do no harm and (2) maximize possible benefits and minimize possible harms.

3. **Justice**—Who ought to receive the benefits of research and bear its burdens? This is a question of justice, in the sense of fairness in distribution or what is deserved. An injustice occurs when some benefit to which a person is entitled is denied without good reason or when some burden is imposed unduly. Another way of conceiving the principle of justice is that equals ought to be treated equally.

Institutional Review Boards were created to ensure the ethical conduct of research. The code of federal regulations outlines the following key roles that the Institutional Review Board is expected to play. In order to approve research, the IRB shall determine that all of the following requirements are satisfied:[11]

1. Risks to subjects are minimized.
2. Risks to subjects are reasonable in relation to anticipated benefits.
3. Selection of subjects is equitable.
4. Informed consent will be sought from each prospective subject or the subject's legally-authorized representative.
5. The research plan makes adequate provision for monitoring the data collected to ensure the safety of subjects.
6. When appropriate, there are adequate provisions to protect the privacy of subjects and to maintain the confidentiality of data.
7. When some or all of the subjects are likely to be vulnerable to coercion or undue influence, such as children, prisoners, pregnant women, mentally disabled persons, or economically or educationally disadvantaged persons, additional safeguards have been included in the study to protect the rights and welfare of these subjects.

We have come a long way from the days when human research was conducted without informed consent on individuals who could be coerced to participate. The standards of research, however, continue to evolve and will most likely continue to change through identification of ethical limitations of current studies.[e]

We have now examined key principles of health law, policy, and ethics and their applications to issues in health care, public health, and bioethics. These principles are key tools, along with health informatics, health communications, as well as the social and behavioral sciences, and can be considered options for implementation when striving to achieve the goals of public health. They are especially powerful tools because they often carry with them the compulsory authority of government. The police powers of public health are increasingly being used cautiously and with careful consideration of the rights of individuals. In many ways, the use of laws is seen as a last resort when provision of information and incentives for change has not been successful. Now that we have examined key tools of population health, let us turn our attention in Section III to efforts to prevent disease, disability, and death for non-communicable diseases, communicable disease, and environmental health and safety.

---

[e] Recent changes in research ethics include limitations on the use of placebos and requirements to register randomized clinical trials before they begin. Placebos are now considered ethical only when no effective active intervention is accepted as the standard of care. The requirement to register randomized clinical trials before they begin was put into effect after randomized clinical trials came to public attention that were never submitted for publication because the results were in conflict with the interests of the trial's sponsor.

Key Words

- Bioethics
- Police power
- Rights
- Negative constitution
- Substantive due process
- Procedural due process
- Authoritative decision
- Social justice
- Market justice
- No-duty principle
- The Belmont Report
- Institutional Review Boards (IRBs)
- Respect for Persons
- Beneficence
- Justice

Discussion Questions

Take a look at the questions posed in the following scenarios which were presented at the beginning of this chapter. See now whether you can answer them.

1. *A new statute and subsequent administrative regulations give only a temporary license to newly-licensed drivers, prohibiting late night driving and the use of cell phones and limiting the number of passengers. You ask: should elderly drivers be subject to these same types of regulations, such as being required to take a driver's test?*

2. *You decide not to enroll in the health plan offered by your employer because it seems so expensive and you are young and healthy. Shortly thereafter, your car is struck by a hit-and-run driver and you find yourself on the way to the nearest hospital. After stabilizing you as required by law, they transfer you to the public hospital, which is the only one in town that will take care of you without insurance. You ask: do you have a right to health care?*

3. *You hear that a new drug has shown extremely promising results, but will not be available for a least a couple of years. You wonder: why do you have to wait so long to take the newest prescription medicine while your e-mail fills up with promotions for the untested ways to enhance your energy, beauty, and sexual performance?*

4. *You hear that a neighbor has TB and refuses treatment. You wonder: what if he has the type of TB that can't be cured with drugs? You ask: can't they make him take his medicine or at least get him out of your neighborhood?*

5. *You hear an advertisement about participating in a new research study. It sounds like you're eligible, so you check into it. You're surprised to find that even if you participate you may not receive the new drug and won't even be told which treatment you are receiving. Despite your willingness to take your chances, you're told that you are*

not eligible for the study due to conditions that put you at increased risk of developing side effects. You ask: why can't I participate if I'm willing to take the risks?

REFERENCES

1. Teitelbaum JB, Wilensky SE. *Essentials of Health Policy and Law.* Sudbury, MA: Jones and Bartlett Publishers; 2007.

2. Gostin LA. *Public Health Law: Power, Duty, Restraint.* Berkeley and New York: University of California Press and Milbank Memorial Fund; 2000.

3. Turnock BJ. *Public Health: What It Is and How It Works.* 4th ed. Sudbury, MA: Jones and Bartlett Publishers; 2009.

4. Teitelbaum JB, Wilensky SE. *Essentials of Health Policy and Law.* Sudbury, MA: Jones and Bartlett Publishers; 2007: 12.

5. Shi L, Singh D. *Delivering Health Care in America.* 3rd ed. Sudbury, MA: Jones and Bartlett Publishers; 2004.

6. United States Food and Drug Administration. FDA History. Available at: http://www.fda.gov/oc/history/default.htm. Accessed March 18, 2009.

7. United Nations General Assembly. The Universal Declaration of Human Rights. Available at: http://www.un.org/Overview/rights.html. Accessed March 18, 2009.

8. Parmet WE. Legal power and legal rights—isolation and quarantine in the case of drug-resistant tuberculosis. *New England Journal Medicine* 2007; 357: 434.

9. United States Government. Trials of War Criminals before the Nuremberg Military Tribunals under Control Council Law No. 10, Vol. 2. Washington, DC: U.S. Government Printing Office; 1949: 181–182.

10. The National Commission for the Protection of Human Subjects of Biomedical and Behavioral Research. The Belmont Report: Ethical Principles and Guidelines for the Protection of Human Subjects of Research. Available at: http://ohsr.od.nih.gov/guidelines/belmont.html. Accessed March, 2009.

11. United States Department of Health and Human Services. Title 45 Public Welfare Department of Health and Human Services, Part 46 Protection of Human Subjects. Available at: http://www.hhs.gov/ohrp/humansubjects/guidance/45cfr46.htm. Accessed March 18, 2009.

Section II:
Cases and Discussion Questions

Don's Diabetes

Don had been a diabetic for over a decade and took his insulin pretty much as the doctor ordered. Every morning, after checking his blood sugar levels, he would adjust his insulin dose according to the written instructions. From the beginning, Don's doctor worried about the effect of the diabetes—he ordered tests, adjusted dosages and prescriptions, and sent his patient to the ophthalmologist for assessment and laser treatment to prevent blindness.

It was the amputation of his right foot that really got Don's attention. Don wasn't exactly athletic, but he did play a round of golf once in a while. He first noticed a little scratch on his foot after a day on the golf course. It wasn't until a week later that he noticed the swelling and the redness in his foot and an ulceration that was forming. He was surprised that his foot didn't hurt, but the doctor informed him that diabetic foot ulcers often don't cause pain. That's part of the problem with diabetes—you lose your sensation in your feet.

After six months of receiving treatment on a weekly basis, a decision had to be made. "There isn't any choice," his doctor said, "the foot infection is spreading and if we don't amputate the foot, we might have to amputate to the knee or even higher." So after describing the potential benefits and harms of the surgery and asking whether there were any questions, the doctor asked Don to sign a form. The next morning, Don's leg was amputated above the ankle leaving him with a stump in place of a foot.

The surgeon came to Don's room the day after surgery to take a look at his amputation. "Beautiful work," he said with a big smile on his face. Maybe it was a beautiful stump, Don thought to himself, but it doesn't work like my old foot. At first, he felt sorry for himself—thinking of what lay ahead to literally get back on his feet.

The physical therapist who visited Don in the hospital told him, "You got off lucky—now, are you going to take control or let diabetes control you?" But, diabetes was already controlling him, Don thought to himself—daily insulin, blood sugar testing, weekly trips to the doctor, and now despite it all—an amputated foot. "Diabetes is a bad disease," his doctor told him. "We're doing everything we can do and you're still experiencing complications."

Maybe the doctors were doing everything they could, but Don wondered what else was possible. He enrolled in a self-help group for diabetics. They shared stories of medical care, new advances in diabetes management, and their own frustrations with the disease and with their medical care. Don realized he had received good medical care, but he also acknowledged that good care by good doctors is not enough. There needs to be a system that makes the pieces work together, but there also needs to be a patient who takes charge of his care.

So take charge, he did. He worked closely with the practice's physician assistant and nurse practitioner, who were experts in diabetic management. He learned how to interpret his blood tests and how they were useful for day-to-day monitoring of his disease. He also learned about hemoglobin A1c blood tests, which measure how well his diabetes is doing over periods of months. After several months, his clinicians taught him how to adjust his dose of insulin to accommodate for changes in his routine or during minor illnesses. They always let him know that care was available and that he did not need to make decisions all by himself. Don also learned to examine his feet and how to prevent minor injuries from turning into major problems. His sporadic eye doctor appointments turned into regular question-and-answer sessions comparing the most recent photographs of his retina to those from the past.

Don found himself keeping his own records to be sure that he had them all in one place—fearing that one doctor would not talk to another and that the records in one office or one hospital would never make their way to the next. Don's fears were well-founded when his kidney function began to deteriorate and his primary care doctor sent him to a kidney specialist, who sent him to a transplant surgeon, and then to a vascular surgeon to prepare him for dialysis. Sure enough, the only records the dialysis doctors could rely upon were the ones that Don had kept on his own.

Soon the dialysis doctor told Don that he had a tough decision to make. Did he want to come into the dialysis center for half a day twice a week where they take care of everything or did he want to learn home dialysis and take care of this treatment on his own? Don had lots of questions. He needed to understand what each dialysis scenario entailed and the advantages and disadvantages of both options, including the costs and discomforts. He also wanted to know about any other potential treatments. Don asked questions of his doctors, learned as much as he could about dialysis on the Internet, and outlined the pros and cons of home dialysis. After that, is was an easy decision for Don. "Sure, I'll learn how to do it myself. I want to be in charge of my own care. I want to stand on my own two feet," he told the doctor without a moment's hesitation.

Discussion Questions

1. What type of decision-making process was going on during the early stages of Don's diabetes? Explain.
2. What type of decision-making process was used to reach the decision to have an amputation? Explain.
3. What type of decision-making process occurred in the decision about dialysis? Explain.
4. In Don's case, what are the advantages and disadvantages of each of these approaches to decision making from both the patient and the clinician's perspective? Explain.

José and Jorge—Identical Twins without Identical Lives

José and Jorge were identical twins separated at birth. José grew up in a large family in an impoverished slum in the middle of a crime-ridden and polluted district of a major city. Jorge grew up in an upper-middle-class professional family with one other brother in a suburban community in the same city. Despite the fact the José and Jorge were identical twins, their lives and health could not have been more different.

José had few opportunities for medical care or public health services as a child. His nutrition was always marginal and he developed several severe cases of diarrhea before he was one year of age. He received a polio vaccine as part of a community vaccination program, but never received vaccinations for measles, mumps, rubella, or other childhood illnesses. At age four, he developed measles and was so sick his mother was sure he would not make it.

As a child, José developed asthma which seemed to worsen when he played outdoors on hot smoggy days. Dropping out of school at age 14, José went to work in a factory, but quit when he found himself panting for breath at the end of the day.

As a teenager José was repeatedly exposed to crime and drugs. Once, he was caught in the crossfire of gangs fighting for control of drugs in his community. Experimenting with drugs with his teenage friends, José contracted HIV from use of contaminated needles. José did not know he had HIV until he was nearly 30 years old and developed tuberculosis (TB). He did receive treatment for the TB free-of-charge from the health department, but once he felt better he didn't follow-up with treatment.

By the time the TB returned, José had lost 30 pounds and could barely make it into the emergency room of the public hospital because of his shortness of breath. He was hospitalized for the last two months of his life, mostly to prevent others from being exposed to what was now drug-resistant tuberculosis. No one ever knew how many people José exposed to HIV or TB.

Jorge's life as a child was far less eventful. He received "well child" care from an early age. His family hardly noticed that he rarely developed diarrhea and had few sick days from "diseases of childhood." He did well in school, but like José, he developed asthma. With good treatment, Jorge was able to play on sports teams at least until he began to smoke cigarettes at age 14.

Jorge soon began to gain weight and by the time he graduated from college was rapidly becoming obese. In his twenties, he developed high blood pressure, and in his 30s he had early signs of diabetes. Jorge had a heart attack in his mid 40s and underwent bypass surgery a few years later. The treatments for diabetes, hypertension, and high cholesterol worked well and Jorge was able to lead a productive professional life into his 40s.

By the time that Jorge turned 50, his diabetes began to worsen and he developed progressive kidney disease. Jorge soon needed twice-a-week dialysis, which kept him alive as he awaited a kidney transplant.

Discussion Questions

1. How do social and economic factors contribute to the different disease patterns of José and Jorge?
2. How do factors in the physical environmental explain differences in the health of José and Jorge?
3. What role does medical care play in the differences between the health outcomes of José and Jorge?
4. What roles do public health services play in the health outcomes of José and Jorge?

Changing Behavior—Cigarette Smoking

It wasn't going to be easy for Steve to stop smoking. He had been at it for 30 years—ever since he took it up on a dare at age 16 and found that it was a good way to socialize. In his 20s, it seemed to make dealing with the work pressure easier and in those days you could smoke in your office and didn't even need to shut the door—much less deal with those dirty looks he was getting now.

Steve always was confident that he could take them or leave them. He'd quit when he was good and ready and a few cigarettes couldn't hurt. But, then he talked to some friends who had quit for a decade or more and said they'd go back in a minute if they thought cigarettes were safe. Maybe for some people those cravings just never go away, he worried to himself. However, there was that bout of walking pneumonia and then the cough that just didn't seem to go away. The cough was so bad that he had trouble smoking more than a few cigarettes a day. The physician assistant let him know that these symptoms were early warning signs of things to come, however Steve just wasn't ready to stop. So, the physician assistant gave him a fact sheet and let Steve know there was help available when he was ready.

It might have been his fears about his 10-year-old son that finally tipped the scales. "Daddy, those cigarettes are bad for you," or maybe it was when he found cigarette butts in the backyard after his 16-year-old daughter's birthday party. Steve knew enough to believe that a father who smokes has a child who smokes. So this time he would do it right.

Steve's physician assistant recognized that Steve was finally ready to quit. He let him know in no uncertain terms that it was important to quit totally, completely, and forever. He also informed Steve that he could rely on help—that he was not alone. With the encouragement of his physician assistant, Steve joined a support group and set a quit date and announced it to his friends and family. The new medication he was prescribed seemed to relieve the worst cravings and the feeling he called "crawling the walls."

His wife Dorothy was supportive. She cleared the cigarette butts and ashtrays out of the house and dealt with the smell by having all the drapes cleaned. She also helped by getting him up after dinner and taking a walk, which kept him from his old habit of having a cigarette with dessert and coffee. It also helped keep him from gaining too much weight, which she confided was her greatest fear. Dorothy's quiet encouragement and subtle reinforcement without nagging worked wonders when Steve needed them the most.

Saving a couple of dollars a day didn't hurt. Steve collected those dollars and put them in a special hiding place. On his first year anniversary of quitting, he wrapped up the dollar bills in a box and gave them to Dorothy as a present. The note inside said: "A trip for us for as long as the money lasts." Dorothy was delighted, but feared the worst when Steve began to open up his present to himself. As he unwrapped a box of cigars, he smiled a big smile and said, "I'm congratulating myself on quitting smoking."

Discussion Questions

1. How are each of the phases of the stages of behavioral change model illustrated in Steve's case?
2. Which techniques for successful cigarette cessation are illustrated in Steve's case?
3. Which effective public health (or population) approaches does this case illustrate?
4. What is the impact of combining individual clinical approaches and public health (or population) approaches?

The Elderly Driver

It was late in the afternoon on a sunny April day. Maybe it was the sun in her eyes, but 82-year-old Janet found herself in her car in a ditch at the side of the road, unsure of how she got there. Once at the hospital, her son and daughter joined her and heard the good news that Janet had escaped with just a broken arm. The police report strongly suggested that she had swerved off the road, but it was not clear why.

This was not Janet's first driving "episode"; in fact, her driving had been a constant worry to her daughter for over two years. Her daughter often offered to take her Mom shopping and insisted that she do the driving when they were together. "Don't you trust me?" was the only thanks the daughter received. When alone, Janet continued to drive herself, staying off the freeway and increasingly driving only during the day. She knew it wasn't as easy as it used to be, but it was her lifeline to independence.

Then, a few months after the April accident, the form for Janet's license renewal arrived. A vision test and a physical exam were required, along with a doctor's certification that Janet was in good health and capable of driving; however, no road test was required. So Janet made a doctor's appointment and at the end of it she left the forms with a note for the doctor saying, "To the best doctor I've ever had. Thanks for filling this out. You know how much driving means to me."

On Janet's way home from the doctor's office, it happened. She was driving down the road when suddenly she was crossing that yellow line and heading toward an oncoming car. The teenage driver might have been going a little fast, but Janet was in the wrong lane and the head-on collision killed the 16-year-old passenger in the front seat who was not wearing a seatbelt. The 18-year-old driver walked way from the accident unharmed, thanks to an inflated airbag.

Janet was never the same emotionally. And despite escaping the accident with just a few bruises, the loss of her driver's license symbolized the end for her. Those lost weekly shopping trips and the strangers in the Assisted Living Center were not the same as living in her own home. The young man in the accident screaming for help woke her up almost every night. It was only a year after the accident when Janet died, and it was just like she had said: "Take my license away and it will kill me."

Discussion Questions

1. How does this case reflect the important issue of balancing the legal rights of the individual and the rights of society as a whole?
2. What role do you believe healthcare providers should play in implementing driving laws and regulations?
3. Identify any changes you would make to prevent the types of outcomes that occurred in this case study.
4. How would you communicate the lessons learned in this case to new and inexperienced drivers?

SECTION III

Preventing Disease, Disability, and Death

As we saw in Chapter 1, in public health we are increasingly identifying disease, disability, and death as being produced by underlying determinants, which we organized using the BIG GEMS mnemonic. While these determinants are useful in thinking about basic reasons for disease and disability, it is often difficult to link the underlying determinants with the diseases and disabilities that result. As we discussed in chapter 1 with asthma, at times many or most of the determinants of disease play a role in the development of a disease.

The concept of **actual causes** is more closely connected with the development of disease. It provides a way of organizing what we know about the prevention of disease and disability into categories that we can measure. Thus, it allows us to ask a key question: how much disease and disability can be prevented?[1] Actual causes of disease can then be linked to three basic categories: non-communicable diseases, communicable diseases, and environmental diseases and injuries. Figure 3-A illustrates the framework we will use in this section to connect determinants of disease, actual causes, and categories of disease and injury.

The concept of actual causes of disease is a relatively new concept which has been successfully applied to the causes of death, though not to disability. Table 3-A provides the most recent data on the actual causes of death. It indicates that nearly half of all deaths in the United States are related to nine potentially preventable actual causes.[a]

The concept of actual causes of disease provides us with a framework for thinking about the underlying problems that lead to death. As indicated in the table, nearly half of all deaths can be ascribed to one of these actual causes. Actual causes can help guide us in placing priorities on where we should put our attention and spend our money to prevent disease.

FIGURE 3-A Public health framework for diseases and injuries

---

[a] Causes of death on death certificates have traditionally been defined in terms of specific diseases that have been formally incorporated with thousands of listings in the International Code of Diseases (ICD codes). This coding system includes a wide range of specific diseases, as well as injuries and other conditions. These items are then categorized based upon organ system or another biological framework.

TABLE 3-A Actual Causes of Death in the United States

Actual Cause	Number of Deaths
Tobacco	435,000
Diet and Physical Inactivity	400,000
Alcohol consumption	85,000
Microbial agents (infections)	75,000
Toxic agents	55,000
Motor vehicles	43,000
Firearms	29,000
Sexual behavior	20,000
Illicit drug use	17,000
Total	**1,159,000 (total deaths = 2,403,351)**

Source: Data from: Mokdad AM, Marks JS, Stroup DF, Gerberding JL. Actual causes of death in the United States 2000. *JAMA.* 2004; 291: 1238–1245.

A substantial portion of the actual causes of death are related to the development of non-communicable disease including tobacco, diet and physical inactivity, alcohol and illicit drug use. Communicable disease remains an important category related not only to microbial agents, but also to sexual behavior. Finally, a broad range of environmental diseases and injuries are related to toxic agents, motor vehicle- and firearm-related injuries. In Chapters 6, 7, and 8, we will address non-communicable and communicable diseases, and environmental health and injury and examine the public health strategies that have been used to address them. We will aim to better understand the burden of disease and strategies for addressing it. Let us begin with the largest category of disease in the United States today—non-communicable diseases.

Key Words

- Actual causes

REFERENCES

1. Mokdad AM, Marks JS, Stroup DF, Gerberding JL. Actual causes of death in the United States 2000. *JAMA*. 2004; 291: 1238–1245.

Non-Communicable Diseases

Sasha didn't want to think about the possibility of breast cancer, but as she turned 50 she agreed to have a mammography which, as she feared, was positive or "suspicious," as her doctor put it. Waiting for the results of the follow-up biopsy was the worst part, but the relief she felt when the results were negative brought tears of joy to her and her family. Then she wondered: is it common to have a positive mammography when no cancer is present?

The first sign of Michael's coronary heart disease was his heart attack. Looking back, he had been at high risk for many years since he smoked, had high blood pressure, and high cholesterol. His lack of exercise and obesity only made the situation worse. Michael asked: what are the risk factors for coronary heart disease and what can be done to identify and address these factors for himself and his family?

John's knee injury from skiing continued to produce swelling and pain, greatly limiting his activities. His physician informed him

that the standard procedure today is to look inside with a flexible scope and do any surgery that is needed through the scope. It's simpler, cheaper, and does not even require hospitalization. "We call it 'cost-effective,' " his doctor said. John wondered: what does cost effective really mean?

Jennifer and her husband George were tested for the cystic fibrosis gene and both were found to have it. Cystic fibrosis causes chronic lung infections and greatly shortens the length of life. They now ask: what does this mean for our chances of having a child with cystic fibrosis? Can we find out whether our child has cystic fibrosis early in pregnancy?

Fred's condition deteriorated slowly, but persistently. He just couldn't remember anything and repeated himself endlessly. The medications helped for a short time, but before long he didn't recognize his family and couldn't take care of himself. The diagnosis was Alzheimer's and he was not alone. Almost everyone in the nursing home seemed to be affected. No one seems to understand the cause of Alzheimer's disease. The family asked: what else can be done, not only for Fred, but for those who come after Fred?

Alcohol use is widespread on your campus. You don't see it as a problem as long as you walk home or have a designated driver. Your mind changes one day after you hear about a classmate who nearly died from alcohol poisoning as a result of binge drinking. You ask yourself: what should be done on my campus to address binge drinking?

Each of these scenarios represents one of the approaches to non-communicable diseases that we will examine in this chapter.

WHAT IS THE BURDEN OF NON-COMMUNICABLE DISEASE?

Non-communicable disease represents a wide range of diseases from cardiovascular disease, to cancers, to depression, Alzheimer's, and chronic arthritis. Together, they represent the majority of causes of death and disability in most developed countries. Today, cardiovascular diseases and cancer alone each represent nearly 25 percent of the causes of death as reflected on death certificates in the United States.

The impact of non-communicable diseases on death only reflects part of the impact. Chronic disabilities, largely due to non-communicable diseases, are now the most rapidly growing component of morbidity in most developing as well as developed countries. As populations age, non-communicable diseases increase in frequency. The presence of two or more chronic diseases makes progressive disability particularly likely. The consequences of the rapidly growing pattern of disability due to non-communicable diseases has enormous economic implications. The great increase in direct costs for health care is in part due to the increased burden of non-communicable diseases. The impact extends beyond healthcare costs as it affects the quality of life and may limit the ability of those who wish to work to continue to do so.

Non-communicable diseases have not always dominated the types of diseases which impact a society. Box 6-1 discusses the **epidemiological transition**[1] and provides a perspective on where we stand today.

There are a wide range of preventive, curative, and rehabilitative approaches to non-communicable diseases. However, there are a limited number of basic strategies being used that are part of the population health approach including:

- screening for early detection and treatment of disease
- multiple risk factor interventions
- identification of cost effective treatments
- genetics counseling and intervention
- research

We will take a look at each of these approaches. Finally, we will see how many of these approaches can be combined using the population health approach. Let us begin with what we call **screening** for disease.

BOX 6-1   The Epidemiological Transition and Non-Communicable Diseases

Disease patterns have not always been the same and will continue to evolve. To gain a big picture understanding of this process of change, it is useful to understand the concept known as the epidemiological or public health transition.

The epidemiological transition describes the changing pattern of disease that has been seen in many countries as they have experienced social and economic development. Its central message is that prior to social and economic development, communicable diseases—or microbial agents using the term from actual causes—represent the dominant cause of disease and disability. In countries in early stages of development, infections are a key cause of mortality either directly or indirectly. For instance, in undeveloped countries maternal and perinatal conditions, as well as nutritional disorders, are often identified as the causes of death. Microbial agents play a key role in maternal and perinatal deaths, as well as deaths ascribed to nutrition. Most maternal deaths are due to infection not necessarily transmitted from others, but related to exposure to microbial agents at the time of birth and in the early postpartum period.

Similarly, most deaths among young children in undeveloped countries are related directly or indirectly to infection. Inadequate nutrition predisposes children to infection and interferes with their ability to fight off infection when it does occur. Many of the deaths among children with malnutrition are related to acute infections, especially acute infectious diarrhea and acute respiratory infections.

As social and economic development progresses, non-communicable diseases including cardiovascular diseases, diabetes, cancers, chronic respiratory ailments, and neuropsychiatric diseases, such as depression and Alzheimer's, predominate as the causes of disability and death. Depression is rapidly becoming one of the major causes of disability and the World Health Organization (WHO) estimates that it will produce more disability than any other single condition in coming years. In addition, illicit drug use has become a major cause of death among the young and includes not only illegal use of drugs, but also abuse of prescription drugs.

In much of the developing world, the same basic patterns are occurring in the developing regions within these countries. Often, earlier distributions of disease dominated by communicable diseases coexist with patterns of non-communicable disease typical of developed countries. Thus, is it not unusual to find that malnutrition and obesity are often present side-by-side in the same developing country.

The epidemiologic transition does not imply that once countries reach the stage where non-communicable diseases dominate that this pattern will persist indefinitely. Newly-emerging diseases, such as HIV/AIDS, pandemic flu, and drug-resistant bacterial infections, raise the possibility that communicable diseases will once again dominate the pattern of disease and death in developed countries.

HOW CAN SCREENING FOR DISEASE ADDRESS THE BURDEN OF NON-COMMUNICABLE DISEASES?

Screening for disease implies the use of tests on individuals who do not have symptoms of a specific disease. These individuals are **asymptomatic**. This implies that he or she does not have symptoms related to the disease being investigated. He or she may have symptoms of other diseases. Screening for disease can result in detection of disease at an early stage under the assumption that early detection will allow for treatment that will improve outcome. Screening has been successful for a range of non-communicable diseases including breast cancer and colon cancer, as well as childhood conditions, including vision and hearing impairments. In all of these conditions, screening has resulted in reduced disability and/or deaths. Not all non-communicable diseases, however, are good candidates for screening and in some cases screening programs have yet to be devised and studied for some non-communicable diseases for which early detection could be useful.

Four criteria need to be fulfilled for an ideal screening program.[2] While few, if any, health conditions completely fulfill all four requirements, these criteria provide a standard against which to judge the potential of a screening program. These criteria are:

1. The disease produces substantial death and/or disability.
2. Early detection is possible and improves outcome.
3. There is a feasible testing strategy for screening.
4. Screening is acceptable in terms of harms, costs, and patient acceptance.

The first criterion is perhaps the easiest to evaluate. Conditions, such as breast and colon cancer, result in substantial death and disability rates. Breast cancer is the second-most common cancer in terms of causes of death and is the most common cancer-related cause of death among women in their 50s. Colon cancer is among the most common causes of cancer death in both men and women. Childhood conditions, such as hearing loss and visual impairment, are not always obvious, however they cause considerable disability.

Determining whether early detection is possible and will improve outcomes is not as easy as it might appear. Screening may result in early detection, but if effective treatment is not available it may merely alert the clinician and the patient to the disease at an earlier point in time without offering hope of an improved outcome. Screening cigarette smokers for lung cancer using X-rays would seem reasonable because lung cancer is the number one cancer killer of both men and women. However, X-ray screening of smokers has been beneficial only in terms of early detection. By the time lung cancer can be seen via chest X-ray, it is already too late to cure. This early detection without improved outcome is called **lead-time bias**.[a]

As indicated in the third criteria, in order to implement a successful screening program, there must be a feasible testing strategy.[b] This usually requires identification of a high-risk population. It also requires a strategy for using two or more tests to distinguish what are called **false positives** and **false negatives** from those who truly have and do not have the disease. False positives are individuals who have positive results on a screening test but do not turn out to have the disease. Similarly, false negatives are those who have negative results on the screening test but turn out to have the disease.

How can we develop feasible testing strategies?[3] To understand the need for and use of feasible testing strategies, it is important to recognize that screening for diseases is usually conducted on groups that are at an increased risk for the condition. For instance, screening men and women for colon cancer and women for breast cancer is often conducted on people aged 50 years and older. This type of group is considered high-risk usually with a chance or risk of having the disease being 1 percent or more. Use of high-risk groups like these allows tests that are less than perfect to serve as initial screening tests.

For instance, mammography has a substantial number of false positives and false negatives. A 50-year-old woman with a positive mammography has only about a 10 to 15 percent chance of having breast cancer. That is, most of the initial positive results will turn out to be false positives.[c]

Therefore, screening for diseases such as breast cancer almost always requires two or more tests. These tests need to be combined using a testing strategy. The most commonly used testing strategy is called **sequential testing** or **two-stage testing**. This approach implies that an initial screening test is followed by one or more definitive or diagnostic test. Sequen-

---

[a] The concept of lead time implies that screening produces an earlier diagnosis that may be effectively used to intervene prior to diagnosis without screening.

[b] A prerequisite to use of tests in screening and other situations is establishing the cut-off line that differentiates a positive test and a negative test. Often this is done by using what is called a **reference interval**. This range is often established by utilize populations that are believed to be free of a disease. The central 95 percent of the range of values (or the mean plus or minus two standard deviations) for this population is then used as the reference interval or range of normal. This approach has a number of limitations including equating existing levels on a test with desirable levels. When data is available on the desirable levels, it is preferable to utilize these levels to establish a reference interval and to define a positive and negative test result. Establishing the desirable level for a test result requires long term follow-up. For such measurements as blood pressure, cholesterol, and fasting blood sugar, desirable levels are now available.

[c] This assumes a 1 percent pretest probability and a **sensitivity** and **specificity** of 90 percent. A moderately accurate test, such as a mammography, may have a sensitivity of about 90 percent and a similar specificity. Sensitivity implies that the test is about 90 percent accurate in the presence of disease (i.e., present in disease) while specificity tells us the mammography is about 90 percent accurate in the absence of disease (i.e., negative in health).

tial testing is used in breast cancer, hearing and vision testing, and most other forms of screening for non-communicable diseases. It is generally the most cost-effective form of screening because only one negative test is needed to rule out the disease.

Sequential testing by definition misses those who have false negative results because a negative test occurs and the testing process is over at least for the immediate future. Thus, a testing strategy needs to consider how to detect those missed by screening. We need to ask: is there a need for repeat screening and if so, when should it occur?[d]

Finally, an ideal screening test should be acceptable in terms of harms, costs and patient acceptance. Harms must be judged by looking at the entire testing strategy—not just the initial test. Physical examination, blood tests, and urine tests often are used as initial screening tests. These tests are virtually harmless. The real question is: what needs to be done if the initial test is positive? If invasive tests such as catheterization or surgery are required, the overall testing strategy may present substantial potential harms.

Screenings and diagnostic tests themselves can be quite costly. In addition, costs are related to the length of time between testing. Testing every year will be far more costly than testing every five or ten years. The frequency of testing depends on the speed at which the disease develops and progresses, as well as the number of people who can be expected to be missed on the initial test. Mammographic screening is traditionally conducted every year because breast cancer can develop and spread rapidly. In the case of colon cancer, however, longer periods between testing are acceptable because the disease is much slower to develop. Thus, cost considerations may be taken into account when choosing between technologies and when setting the interval between screenings.[e]

Finally, patient acceptance is key to successful screening. Many screening strategies present little problem with patient acceptance. However, colon cancer screening has had its challenges with patience acceptance because many consider it an invasive and uncomfortable procedure. Far less then half the people who qualify for screening based upon current recommendations currently pursue and receive colon cancer screening. This contrasts dramatically with mammography where a substantial majority now receives the recommended screening.

The screening tests that completely fulfill these ideal criteria are few and many more are successfully used despite not fulfilling all these criteria. Screening may still be useful as long as we are aware of its limitations and prepared to accept its inherent problems. Table 6-1 illustrates how commonly-used screening tests for risk factors for cardiovascular disease and common cancers perform based upon the four criteria we have outlined.

These criteria do help identify types of screening that should not be done. In general, we do not screen for disease when early detection does not improve outcome. We do not screen for rare diseases, such as many types of cancer, especially when the available tests are only moderately accurate. Finally, we do not screen for diseases when the testing strategy produces substantial harms. Screening for disease is not the only population health approach that can be used to address the burden of non-communicable disease. Multiple risk factor reduction is a second strategy that we will examine.

HOW CAN IDENTIFICATION AND TREATMENT OF MULTIPLE RISK FACTORS BE USED TO ADDRESS THE BURDEN OF NON-COMMUNICABLE DISEASE?

As we have seen, the concept of risk factors is fundamental to the work of public health. Risk factors ranging from high levels of blood pressure and LDL cholesterol to multiple sexual partners and anal intercourse help us identify groups that are most likely to develop a disease. Evidence-based recommendations often focus on addressing risk factors and implementation efforts often address the best way(s) to target high-risk groups. Thus, identifying and reducing risk factors is an inherent part of the population health approach to non-communicable diseases.

A special form of intervention aimed at risk factors is called **multiple risk factor reduction**. As the name implies, this strategy intervenes simultaneously in a series of risk factors all of which contribute to a particular outcome, such as cardiovascular disease or lung cancer. Multiple risk factor reduction is most effective when there are constellations or groups of risk factors that cluster together in definable groups of people. It may also be useful when the presence of two or more risk factor increases the risk more than would be expected by adding together the impact of each risk factor.

The success of the last half century in addressing coronary artery disease exemplifies multiple risk factor reduction. Box 6-2 discusses the impact of the strategy on coronary

---

[d] A sequential testing strategy also requires a decision on the order of administering the tests. Issues of cost and safety are often the overriding consideration in determining which test to use first and which to use to confirm an initial positive test. At times, a testing strategy known as **simultaneous testing** or **parallel testing** is used. In this scenario, two tests are used initially if one test can be expected to detect one type of disease and the other test can be expected to detect a different type of disease. Traditionally, flexible sigmoidoscopy, which examines the lower approximately 35 cm of the colon, has been used along with tests for occult blood in the stool. Tests for occult blood attempt to screen for cancer in the large section of colon proximal to the sigmoid region. Using both of these tests has been shown to be more accurate for screening than use of either test alone because each attempts to find cancer in different anatomical sites.

[e] Today, there is a wide range of methods for screening for colon cancer including colonoscopy, which examines the entire colon, and virtual colonoscopy, which does not require an internal examination. These newer tests are much more costly than sigmoidoscopy and occult stool testing. Which is the most accurate and cost-effective test remains controversial. However, the need for and benefits of screening for colon cancer are widely accepted.

TABLE 6-1 Examples of Screening Tests for Heart Disease and Cancer and Ideal Criteria

	Substantial mortality and/or morbidity	Early detection possible and alters outcome	Screening is feasible (can identify a high-risk population and a testing strategy)	Screening acceptable in terms of harms, costs, and patient acceptance
Hypertension	Contributory cause of strokes, myocardial infarctions, kidney disease	High blood pressure precedes bad outcomes often by decades and effective treatment is available	Test everyone—desirable range has been established	Screening itself is free of harms, low cost, and acceptable to patients Treatments, however, may be complicated and have harms, costs, and side effects
LDL cholesterol	Contributory cause of strokes, myocardial infarctions, and other vascular diseases	Precedes the development of disease by decades and treatment is effective in altering outcome	Test everyone—desirable range has been established	Screening itself is free of harm, low cost, and acceptable to patients Treatment has rare side effects, which can be detected by symptoms and low-cost blood tests
Breast cancer	2nd most common fatal cancer among women and most common for women under 70	Early detection improves outcome	For those 50 and over, combination of mammography and follow-up biopsy shown to be feasible	Harm may occur due to false positives, low risk of harm from radiation, patient acceptance good, but test can be somewhat painful Screening younger women increases costs and false positives
Cervical cancer	If undetected and untreated—may be fatal	Early treatment dramatically reduces the risk of death	Pap smear and follow-up testing have been extremely successful	Pap results in substantial number of false positives New DNA testing may be used to separate true and false positives
Colon cancer	2nd most common fatal cancer in men and third in women	Early detection of polyps reduces development of cancer and early detection of cancer improves chances of survival	Men and women 50 and older, plus those with high risk types of colon disease Options for screening include: fecal occult blood testing, plus flexible sigmoidoscopy, colonoscopy, and virtual colonoscopy	Patient acceptance has been major barrier, small probability of harm from procedure, substantial cost for colonoscopy and virtual colonoscopy

BOX 6-2 Coronary Artery Disease and Multiple Risk Factor Reduction.

An epidemic of coronary artery disease and subsequent heart attacks spread widely through mid-20th century America. Sudden death, especially among men in their 50s and even younger, became commonplace in nearly every neighborhood in suburban America. To better understand this epidemic, which caused nearly half of all deaths in Americans in the 1940s and 1950s, the National Institutes of Health began the Framingham Heart Study in the late 1940s.[4]

In those days, there were only suggestions that cholesterol and hypertension contributed to heart disease and little, if any, recognition that cigarettes played a role. The Framingham Heart Study enrolled a cohort of over 7000 individuals in Framingham, Massachusetts: questioning, examining, and taking blood samples from them every other year to explore a large number of conceivable connections with coronary artery disease—the cause of heart attacks. Now well into its second half-century after thousands of publications and hundreds of thousands of examinations, the Framingham Heart Study continues to follow the children and grandchildren of the original Framingham cohort.

The study has provided us with extensive long-term data on a cohort of individuals. These form the basis for many of the numbers we use to estimate the strength of risk factors for coronary artery disease. It has helped demonstrate not only the risk factors for the disease, but also the protective or resilience factors. The use of aspirin, regular exercise, and modest alcohol consumption have been suggested as protective factors despite the fact that no one ever thought of them in the 1940s.[f]

The Framingham Heart Study demonstrated that high blood pressure preceded strokes and heart attacks by years and often decades. It took the Veterans Administration's randomized clinical trials of the early 1970s to convince the medical and public health communities that high blood pressure needed and benefited from aggressive detection and treatment. Through a truly joint effort by public health and medicine, high blood pressure detection and treatment came to public and professional recognition as a major priority in the 1970s.

The impact of elevated levels of low-density lipoprotein (LDL), the bad cholesterol, were likewise suggested by the Framingham Heart Study, but it was not until the development of a new class of medications called statins in the mid-1980s that treatment of high levels of LDL cholesterol took off. These drugs have been able to achieve remarkable reductions in LDL and equally remarkable reductions in coronary artery disease with only rare side effects. These drugs have been so successful that some countries have made them available over-the-counter. Clinicians are using them more and more aggressively to achieve levels of LDL cholesterol that are less than half those sought a generation ago.[g]

Although diabetes has been treated with insulin since the 1920s and oral treatments beginning after World War II, the treatment of diabetes to prevent its consequences—including coronary artery disease—was not definitely established as effective until the 1990s. Our current understanding of diabetes has come from a series of randomized clinical trials and long-term follow-ups that demonstrate the key role that diabetes can play in diseases of the heart and blood vessels and the impressive role that aggressive treatment can play in reducing the risks of these diseases.

Efforts aimed at early detection and treatment of heart attacks and prevention of second heart attacks through the use of medications have become routine parts of medical practice. Medical procedures, including angioplasty and surgical bypass of diseased coronary arteries, have also been widely used. Widespread availability of defibrillators in public areas is one of the most recent effort to prevent the fatal consequences of coronary artery disease.

Between the 1950s and the early years of the 21st century, the death rate from coronary artery disease has declined by over 50 percent. The impact is even greater among those in their 50s and 60s. Sudden death from coronary artery disease among men in their 50s is now a relatively rare event.

For years medicine and public health professionals debated whether public health and clinical preventive interventions or medical and surgical interventions deserved the lion's share of the credit for these achievements. The evidence suggests that both prevention and treatment have had important impacts.[6] When medicine and public health work together, the public's health is the winner.

---

[f] The data developed for the Surgeon General's Reports on Smoking and Health in the 1960s and beyond, strongly pointed to substantial effects of cigarettes not only on lung disease, but on coronary artery disease as well. In fact, given the large number of deaths from coronary artery disease compared to lung disease, it became evident that in terms of number of deaths the biggest impact of cigarette smoking is on heart disease, not lung disease.

[g] Recent data even suggests that for individuals with levels of LDL cholesterol within the currently accepted range of normal, statins may be beneficial in the presence of evidence of inflammation as measured by a test called C-reactive protein.[5]

artery disease. Multiple risk factor reduction strategies are being attempted for a range of diseases from asthma to diabetes.

Multiple risk factor reduction is most successful when a number of risk factors are at work in the same individual. As we have seen with asthma, factors like indoor and outdoor air pollution, cockroaches and other allergens, and a lack of adherence to medications, tend to occur together and may be most effectively addressed together. Similarly, obesity and lack of exercise tend to reinforce each other often requiring a comprehensive multiple risk factor reduction approach.[h]

Screening for disease and multiple risk factor reduction are key approaches to using testing as part of secondary intervention.[i] The enormous burden of non-communicable disease cannot be totally prevented even by maximizing the use of these strategies. It is important to couple them with cost-effective treatment. Thus, a third population health strategy for addressing the burden of non-communicable disease is to develop cost-effective interventions to treat common diseases.

HOW CAN COST-EFFECTIVE INTERVENTIONS HELP US ADDRESS THE BURDEN OF NON-COMMUNICABLE DISEASES?

Clinicians today have a wide range of interventions to treat disease. Many of these interventions have some impact on the course of a disease. The proliferation of interventions means that it is especially important to identify which provide the greatest benefits at the lowest cost. In order to understand how cost-effective interventions can help address the burden of non-communicable disease, we need to understand what we mean by cost-effective.

Cost-effectiveness is a concept that combines issues of benefits and harms with issues of financial costs. It starts by considering the benefits and harms of an intervention to determine its **net-effectiveness**. Net-effectiveness implies that the benefits are substantially greater than the harms even after the value (or utility), as well as the timing of the harms and benefits, are taken into account. Only after establishing net-effectiveness do we take into account the financial costs.

Cost-effectiveness compares a new intervention to the current or standard intervention. It usually asks: is the additional net-effectiveness of an intervention worth the additional cost? At times it may also require us to ask: is a small loss of net-effectiveness worth the considerable savings in cost? Figure 6-1 is a tool for categorizing interventions in order to analyze their costs and net-effectiveness.

Box 6-3 provides more details on the use of cost-effectiveness analysis.[7]

Preventive interventions often undergo cost-effectiveness analysis. Many interventions, ranging from mammography to most childhood vaccinations to cigarette cessation programs, get high or at least passing grades on cost-effectiveness. However, many widely-used treatment interventions do not or would not meet the current standards of cost-effectiveness. The application of cost-effectiveness criteria to common clinical interventions is considered a population health intervention aimed at getting maximum value for the dollars spent.

The results of cost-effectiveness analysis have already had an impact on a number of common clinical procedures. For instance, cost-effective treatments include: the use of minimally-invasive orthopedic surgery, such as knee surgery; the reduced length of intensive care and hospitalization for coronary artery disease; and the use of home health care for intravenous administration of antibiotics and other medications. These efforts to

---

[h] In some situations the existence of multiple risk factors does more than add together to produce disease. At times, the existence of two or more factors multiply the risk. In these situations addressing even one of the factors can have a major impact on disease. For instance, it is now well established that asbestos exposure and cigarette smoking multiply the risks of lung cancer. Thus, if the relative risk for cigarettes is 10 and the relative risk for asbestos exposure is 5, then the relative risk if both factors are present is approximately 50. If an individual who has previously been exposed to both risk factors stops smoking cigarettes and the effects of cigarette smoking are immediately and completely reversible, we can expect the relative risk of lung cancer to decline from approximately a fifty-fold increase to a five-fold increase. We will take up this issue again in Chapter 8 because this type of interaction is increasingly central to addressing complex public health issues.

[i] The principles of testing discussed here are not limited to screening for disease and identification of risk factors. They are also useful as part of a cost-effective approach to diagnosis of symptomatic diseases. In addition, testing is often used for a range of applications in medicine and public health, including monitoring response to treatment, identifying side effects, identifying genetic predictors of disease, and establishing baseline levels for future testing. Public health applications include the use of environmental testing and testing for disease prevalence.

FIGURE 6-1 The four quadrants of cost and net-effectiveness

BOX 6-3   Cost-Effectiveness and Its Calculations.

Cost-effectiveness is often judged by comparing the costs of a new intervention to the cost of the current, standard, or state-of-the-art intervention. A measure known as the **incremental cost-effectiveness ratio** is then obtained. This ratio represents the additional cost relative to the additional net-effectiveness.

Net-effectiveness may measure a diagnosis made, a death prevented, or a disability prevented, etc. To operationize the concept of net-effectiveness requires us to define, measure, and combine the probabilities and utilities of benefits with the probabilities and utilities of harm and take into account the timing of the benefits and the harms. Thus, the process of calculating net-effectiveness can be quite complex.

Similarly, calculating costs can be challenging. Most economists argue that the costs are not limited to the costs of providing the intervention and the current and future medical care, but should also include the cost of transportation, loss of income, and other expenses associate with obtaining health care and being disabled. Thus, calculating a cost-effectiveness ratio has become a complex undertaking.

The criteria for establishing cost effectiveness have changed over time. Most experts in cost-effectiveness prefer the use of a measurement called **quality-adjusted life years** or **QALYs.** QALYs ask about the number of life-years saved by an intervention, rather than the number of lives. Thus, one QALY may be thought of as one year of life at full health compared to immediate death.

In cost-effectiveness analysis, a financial value is usually placed on a QALY reflecting what a society can afford to pay for the average QALY as measured by its per capita gross domestic product (GDP). In the United States, where the GPD is approaching $50,000 there is a general consensus that a QALY currently should be valued at $50,000. Thus, when you hear that a formal cost-effectiveness analysis has shown that an intervention is cost-effective, it generally implies that the addition cost is less than $50,000 per QALY.[j]

The ideal intervention is one in which the cost goes down and the effectiveness goes up. Cost-saving, quality-increasing interventions have a negative incremental cost-effectiveness ratio. That is, QALYs go up while the costs go down. These cost-reducing, QALY-increasing interventions, while highly desirable, are very rare. Usually we need to spend more to get additional QALYs. One example of an intervention that reduces costs and at the same time produces additional QALYs is treatment of hypertension in high risk individuals, such as those with diabetes.[k]

[j] An increase of one QALY may be the result of obtaining small improvements in utility from a large number of people. For instance, if ten people increase their utility from 0.1 to 0.2, the result is an increase of one QALY. The value of a QALY is often set slightly above the average gross domestic product (GDP) or sum of all goods and services produced per person. In the United States, the GDP now exceeds $40,000 per person per year. Thus, setting the value of a QALY at $50,000 reflects how much we can afford to pay rather than strictly reflecting how much we think a QALY is worth.

[k] Another example is the use of influenza vaccine among the elderly and those with chronic disease predisposing them to the complications of influenza. It is important to distinguish these types of interventions from those that reduce the costs, but also reduce the QALYs, because at times both are referred to as cost-saving measures.

increase the cost-effectiveness of routine healthcare procedures are becoming key to maximizing the benefits obtained from the vast amount of money spent on health care as we will discuss in Chapter 11.

Applying cost-effectiveness analysis to routine clinical interventions is often coupled with efforts to better predict the outcome of disease and treatment. Improving the ability to predict the outcome of diseases and interventions can help us know when, how, and if to intervene. Improved prediction holds out the hope of increased effectiveness, as well as reduced costs by tailoring the treatment to the individual patient.[l]

In addition to screening, multiple risk factor reduction, and cost-effective intervention using prediction rules, the revolution in genetics has opened up another possible strategy for addressing the burden of non-communicable diseases.

HOW CAN GENETIC COUNSELING AND INTERVENTION BE USED TO ADDRESS THE BURDEN OF CHRONIC DISEASES?

Interventions based upon genetics have been part of medical and public health practice since at least the 1960s, when it was recognized that abnormalities of single genes for such condi-

[l] Research designed to develop **prediction rules** has become a major focus of clinical, as well as public health research. This challenging type of research may be able to improve evidence-based recommendations by providing different recommendations for groups with different prognoses and/or different responses

to treatment. Efforts to improve the effectiveness of breast cancer treatments, for instance, are now focused on testing patients to determine the best type of chemotherapy to use to treat their particular cancer. This approach shows promise of producing greater benefit and less harm at reduced cost.

tions as Tay-Sachs disease (found among Ashkenazi Jews) and sickle cell anemia (found among African-Americans) could be detected by testing potential parents who could then be counseled on the risks associated with childbearing.

It was also recognized that chromosomal abnormalities that produce Down Syndrome, the most commonly-recognized cause of mental retardation, could be detected at an early stage in pregnancy. In addition, certain genetic defects such as phenylketonuria (PKU) can be recognized at birth and relatively simple dietary interventions can prevent the severe retardation of mental development that would otherwise occur.

In light of all this valuable knowledge, today genetic testing and counseling are often offered to prospective parents. Testing for Down Syndrome is a standard part of prenatal care; and testing for a wide range of rare, but serious disorders is a population health intervention. In fact, in most states these tests are legally required soon after birth. The triumph of the human genome project in the early years of the 21st century has sparked interest in expanding the applicability of genetic interventions in medicine and public health. For instance, the gene for cystic fibrosis, the most common genetic disorder among whites in the United States, has been identified and screening of large numbers of couples is now possible. Even among whites without a history of cystic fibrosis, the chance of carrying the gene is about three percent. If both the mother and the father carry the gene, the chances of having a child with cystic fibrosis is 25 percent with each pregnancy. The fetus can be tested for the disease early in pregnancy.

There are a wide range of current and developing applications of genetics including:[8]

- **Genetic prevention**—This approach incorporates efforts to prevent the occurrence of single genes or multiple gene combinations that are likely to produce disease. This includes: expanded use of genetic counseling, prenatal testing, and early abortion or fetal therapies. Knowledge of the human genome holds promise for expanding this approach beyond diseases caused by single-gene defects to diseases that depend on multiple genes. It is important to recognize that diseases that are dependent on multiple genes will be more difficult to predict than resulting from a single-gene.
- **Genetic detection prior to disease**—This approach includes efforts aimed at detection of genetic defects and implementation of early intervention to prevent what is called the **phenotypic expression of genes**. Building on the success of treatment of PKU and other inborn errors of metabolism, risk factors for common diseases, such as high cholesterol, high blood sugar, or obesity might be detected early and aggressively managed during childhood.
- **Gene-environmental protection**—Genetic testing holds out the possibility of defining combinations of genes that identify individuals who are especially likely to develop disease when they experience specific environmental exposures, such as those interactions that occur in occupational settings where workers are exposed to specific chemicals often at low doses. Identification of gene-environment interactions may lead to identification of those who are at high risk if they work in certain occupational settings.
- **Genotypic-based screening for early disease**—Combinations of genes may identify groups that are at high risk of common diseases and that can be targeted for screening. For instance, studies suggest that for certain common cancers, such as those of the breast, prostate, and colon, genetic factors are associated with 30–40 percent of these diseases. Finding predisposing genetic patterns early in life may be useful for identifying those who need earlier or more intensive screening for early detection.

Each of these potential uses of genetics in public health present ethical as well as technological issues. Questions to consider include: Should we identify diseases when little can be done to prevent or treat them? How can we identify genetic risk factors without stigmatizing or putting those with the genes at a disadvantage? Will screening programs be improved by identifying groups at genetic risk of disease or will high risk groups without genetic risk factors unfairly be passed over for screenings?

These and other approaches based on the rapidly accumulating knowledge of genetics are likely to become routine medical and public health strategies for primary, secondary, and tertiary interventions for non-communicable disease in the coming years. Their successful adoption, however, will require careful attention by those in the fields of public health and medicine to ensure that benefits are gained and harms minimized. Despite the enormous advances that have occurred in public health and medicine in recent decades, there is still much to be learned. A final strategy for non-communicable diseases addresses the question: what can we do when highly-effective interventions don't exist?

WHAT CAN WE DO WHEN HIGHLY-EFFECTIVE INTERVENTIONS DON'T EXIST?

Alzheimer's disease reflects the challenge of what to do when the cause of a disease is not known and the treatment is not highly effective.[9] Alzheimer's is among the most rapidly increasing condition among those that we classify as non-communicable diseases. The aging of the population has been and is expected to be associated with many more cases of Alzheimer's, which primarily affects the quality of life with its progressive damage to memory—especially short-term memory.[m]

Today we have limited treatment options for those afflicted with Alzheimer's. Several drugs are available that have modest positive impacts on memory. Efforts to stimulate mental activity through keeping active mentally and physically have also been shown to have positive, yet modest impacts. Public health efforts have encouraged the use of these existing interventions especially when there is evidence that they allow individuals to function on their own or with limited assistance for longer periods of time.

The population health approach to Alzheimer's disease, however, also stresses the need for additional research. Epidemiological research has helped produce the modest advances in preventing progression and treating the symptoms of the disease. A population health approach, however, needs to acknowledge the need for a basic biological understanding of what causes Alzheimer's. As we learned in Chapter 2, the P.E.R.I. process asks us to address the etiology as the basis for evidence-based recommendations and intervention. Thus, the population health approach to Alzheimer's, as with other diseases of unknown etiology, requires us to ask basic questions about the biology of the disease and to learn more about its cause(s). Fortunately, an increasingly sophisticated and well-financed effort is being directed at understanding the etiology of Alzheimer's. We can now have hope and increasing confidence that the epidemic being faced by many of your grandparents will be brought under control in the not-too-distant future.

We have now explored the major population health strategies for addressing non-communicable diseases. These include screening, multiple risk factor reduction, cost-effective treatments, genetic counseling, and more research. A complex problem often requires us to combine many of these approaches.

HOW CAN WE COMBINE STRATEGIES TO ADDRESS COMPLEX PROBLEMS OF NON-COMMUNICABLE DISEASES?

Multiple interventions combining health care, traditional public health approaches, and social interventions are often needed to address the complex problems presented by non-communicable diseases. The combined and integrated use of

---

[m] Not all cases of memory loss or dementia are due to Alzheimer's. Additional causes include: strokes and cerebral vascular disease, chronic alcoholism, thyroid disease, specific infectious diseases (such as syphilis and AIDS), as well as the effects of drugs and a long list of rare diseases. Today, however, Alzheimer's is the most common and the most important cause of memory loss and dementia. We tend to classify a disease as non-communicable unless there is convincing evidence that it can be transmitted or that it is due in large part to environmental exposures or injuries. Despite the fact that we do not yet know the etiology of Alzheimer's disease, it is generally classified as non-communicable.

BOX 6-4   Alcohol Abuse and the Population Health Approach.

Alcohol has been a central feature of American society and American medicine and public health since the early days of the country. It was among the earliest painkillers and was used routinely to allow surgeons to perform amputations during the Civil War and earlier conflicts. The social experiment of alcohol prohibition during the 1920s and early 1930s ended in failure as perceived by a great majority of Americans.

Efforts to control the consequences of alcohol took a new direction after World War II. Americans began to focus on the consequences of the disease, including liver disease, fetal alcohol syndrome, automobile accidents, and intentional and unintentional violence.

Population health interventions became the focus of alcohol control efforts. For instance, taxation of alcohol based upon 1950s legislation raised the price of alcohol enough to substantially reduce consumption. Restrictions on advertising and higher taxes on hard liquor with its greater alcohol content eventually contributed to greater use of beer and wine. Despite the continued growth in alcohol consumption, the number of cases of liver disease and other alcohol-related health problems have declined. In recent years, efforts to alert pregnant women to the health effects of drinking through product labeling and other health communications efforts have had an impact.

The highway safety impacts of alcohol use have led to population health efforts in cooperation with transportation and police departments. Greatly increased police efforts to catch drunk drivers and stripping of the licenses of repeat offenders have become routine and have been attributed to impressive reductions in automotive accidents related to alcohol. Efforts such as the designated driver movement originated by Mothers Against Drunk Drivers (MADD) have demonstrated the often-critical role that private citizens can play in implementing population health interventions.

(continues)

BOX 6-4 continued.

Focusing on high-risk groups, as well as using what we have called "improving-the-average" strategies, has had an important impact. Alcoholics Anonymous (AA) and other peer support groups have focused on encouraging individuals to acknowledge their alcohol problems. These groups often provide important encouragement and support for long-term abstinence.

Medical efforts to control alcohol consumption have been aimed primarily at those with clear evidence of alcohol abuse—often those in need of alcohol withdrawal or "drying out." Drugs are available that provide modest help in controlling an individual's alcohol consumption. Screening for alcohol abuse has become a widespread part of health care. These interventions have been aimed at those with the highest levels of risk. The combination of individual, group, and population interventions has reduced the overall impact of alcohol use without requiring its prohibition. In fact, modest levels of consumption, up to one drink per day for women and two for men, may help protect against coronary artery disease.

The issue of alcohol and public health has not gone away. The focus today has returned to identifying high-risk groups and intervening to prevent bad outcomes. A key risk factor today is binge drinking with its risk of acute alcohol poisoning, as well as unintentional and intentional violence. College students are among the highest risk group. One episode of binge drinking dramatically increases the probability of additional episodes suggesting that intervention strategies are needed to reduce the risk. We've made a great deal of progress controlling the impacts of alcohol, but we clearly have more to do.

multiple interventions is central to the population health approach. Box 6-4 looks at what we can learn about the population health approach to non-communicable diseases from the long history of alcohol use and abuse, as well as the substantial recent success in addressing disease due to alcohol.[10]

We have now taken a look at strategies to control non-communicable diseases that are currently the most common reason for disability and death in most developed countries. Now, let us look at a second category—communicable disease—which has been central to the history of public health and threatens to become central to its future.

Key Words

- Epidemiological transition
- Screening
- Asymptomatic
- Lead-time bias
- Watchful waiting
- False positives
- False negatives
- Reference interval
- Sensitivity
- Specificity
- Sequential testing (or two-stage testing)
- Simultaneous testing (or parallel testing)
- Multiple risk factor reduction
- Cost-effectiveness
- Net-effectiveness
- Prediction rules
- Phenotypic expression of genes

Discussion Questions

Take a look at the questions poised in the following scenarios which were presented at the beginning of this chapter. See now whether you can answer them.

1. *Sasha didn't want to think about the possibility of breast cancer, but as she turned 50 she agreed to have a mammography which, as she feared, was positive or "suspicious," as her doctor put it. Waiting for the results of the follow-up biopsy was the worst part, but the relief she felt when the results were negative brought tears of joy to her and her family. Then she wondered: is it common to have a positive mammography when no cancer is present?*

2. *The first sign of Michael's coronary heart disease was his heart attack. Looking back, he had been at high risk for many years since he smoked, had high blood pressure, and high cholesterol. His lack of exercise and obesity only made the situation worse. Michael asked: what are the risk factors for coronary heart disease and what can be done to identify and address these factors for himself and his family?*

3. *John's knee injury from skiing continued to produce swelling and pain, greatly limiting his activities. His physician informed him that the standard procedure today is to look inside with a flexible scope and do any surgery that is needed through the scope. It's simpler, cheaper, and does not even require hospitalization. "We call it 'cost-effective,' " his doctor said. John wondered: what does cost effective really mean?*

4. *Jennifer and her husband George were tested for the cystic fibrosis gene and both were found to have it. Cystic fibrosis causes chronic lung infections and greatly shortens the length of life. They now ask: what does this mean for our chances of having a child with cystic fibrosis? Can we find out whether our child has cystic fibrosis early in pregnancy?*

5. *Fred's condition deteriorated slowly, but persistently. He just couldn't remember anything and repeated himself endlessly. The medications helped for a short time, but before long he didn't recognize his family and couldn't take care of himself. The diagnosis was Alzheimer's and he was not alone. Almost everyone in the nursing home seemed to be affected. No one seems to understand the cause of Alzheimer's disease. The family asked: what else can be done, not only for Fred, but for those who come after Fred?*

6. *Alcohol use is widespread on your campus. You don't see it as a problem as long as you walk home or have a designated driver. Your mind changes one day after you hear about a classmate who nearly died from alcohol poisoning as a result of binge drinking. You ask yourself: what should be done on my campus to address binge drinking?*

REFERENCES

1. Omran AR. The epidemiologic transition: a theory of the epidemiology of population change. *The Milbank Memorial Fund Quarterly.* 1971; 49(4): 509–538.

2. Riegelman RK. *Studying a Study and Testing a Test: How to Read the Medical Evidence.* Philadelphia: Lippincott, Williams & Wilkins; 2005.

3. Gordis L. *Epidemiology.* 4th ed. Philadelphia: Elsevier Saunders; 2009.

4. Framingham Heart Study. History of the Framingham Heart Study. Available at: http://www.framinghamheartstudy.org/about/history.html. Accessed March 18, 2009.

5. Ridker PM, Danielson E, Fonesca FAH, Genest J, et al. Rosuvastatin to prevent vascular events in men and women with elevated C-reactive protein. *N Engl J Med.* 2008; 259(21): 2195–2207.

6. Critchley J, Capwell S, Unal B. Life-years gained from coronary heart disease mortality reduction in Scotland—prevention or treatment? *J Clin Epi.* 2003; 56(6): 583–590.

7. Gold MR, Siegel JE, Russell LB, Weinstein MC. *Cost-Effectiveness in Health and Medicine.* New York: Oxford University Press; 1996.

8. Khoury MJ, Burke W, Thomson EJ. *Genetics and Public Health in the 21st Century: Using Genetic Information to Improve Health and Prevent Disease.* New York: Oxford University Press; 2000.

9. National Institute on Aging. Alzheimer's Disease Fact Sheet. Available at: http://www.nia.nih.gov/Alzheimers/Publications/adfact.htm. Accessed March 18, 2009.

10. Room R, Babor T, Rehm J. Alcohol and public health. *Lancet.* 2005; 365(9458): 519–530.

CHAPTER 7

Communicable Diseases

LEARNING OBJECTIVES

By the end of this chapter, the student will be able to:

- describe the burden of disease caused by communicable diseases.
- identify the roles that barrier protections play in preventing communicable diseases.
- identify the roles that vaccinations can play in preventing communicable diseases.
- identify the roles that screening, case finding, and contact treatment can play in preventing communicable diseases.
- identify the conditions that make eradication of a disease feasible.
- describe a range of options for controlling the HIV/AIDS epidemic.

Your college roommate went to bed not feeling well one night and early the next morning you had trouble arousing her. She was rushed to the hospital just in time to be effectively diagnosed and treated for meningococcal meningitis. The health department recommends immediate antibiotic treatment for everyone that was in close contact with your roommate. They set up a process to watch for additional cases to be sure an outbreak is not in progress. Fortunately, no more cases occur. You ask yourself: should your college require that all freshmen have the meningococcal vaccine before they can register for classes?

As a health advisor to a worldwide HIV/AIDS foundation, you are asked to advise on ways to address the HIV and developing tuberculosis (TB) epidemics. You are asked to do some long-range thinking and to come up with a list of potential approaches to control the epidemics, or at least ways reduce the development of TB. The first recommendation you make is to forget about eradicating HIV/AIDS. How did you come to that conclusion?

Your hometown of 100,000 is faced with a crisis as an airplane lands containing a passenger thought to have a new form of severe influenza that has recently gained the ability to spread from person to person through airborne spread. As the mayor of the city, what do you decide to do?

You are a principal at a local high school. One of your top athletes is in the hospital with a spreading bacterial infection due to a staphylococcus bacteria resistant to all known antibiotics. The infection occurred after what appeared to be a minor injury during practice. As the principal, what do you decide to do?

Diseases due to infection form a large part of the history of public health and are again a central part of its present and its future. Infections of public health importance may be caused by a wide variety of organisms ranging from bacteria, to viruses, to a spectrum of parasites including malaria and hookworm. Let us examine the burden of disease due to infections.[a]

---

[a] The term **infectious disease** is intended to include both communicable disease and disease caused by organisms that are not communicable. The central feature that distinguishes **communicable disease** from other diseases caused by organisms is its ability to be transmitted from person to person or from animals or the physical environment to humans by a variety of routes: from air and water, from contaminated articles (fomites), or from insect and animal bites. Other **infections** of public health interest are caused by organisms, such as pneumococcus (streptococcus pneumoniae), which usually coexist with healthy individuals, but are capable of causing disease when relocated to areas of the body with increased susceptibility or when they are provided opportunities to multiply or invade new areas because of an individual's decreased resistance. It is important to note that the distinction between infectious diseases and communicable diseases is not always made and at times they are considered synonyms.

WHAT IS THE BURDEN OF DISEASE CAUSED BY COMMUNICABLE DISEASES?

For many centuries, communicable diseases were the leading cause of death and disability among all ages, but especially among the young and the old. Communicable diseases were not only the causes of great epidemics, but they were the causes of routine deaths. These included a key role in maternal deaths associated with childbirth, infant and early childhood deaths, as well as deaths of malnourished infants and children.

The last half of the 20th century saw a brief respite from deaths and disabilities caused by communicable diseases and other infections. This was due in large part to medical efforts to treat infections with drugs and public health efforts to prevent infections (often with vaccines) and to eradicate or control other infections. Even as these great accomplishments were underway, warning signs of bacteria resistant to antibiotics began to appear. Staphylococcus organisms resistant to current antibi-otics began to plague hospitals in the 1950s until new antibiotics were developed. Resistance of gonorrhea and pneumococcus to a range of antibiotics became widespread. World Health Organization (WHO)—and U.S. government-sponsored programs, such as those to promote the eradication of malaria and TB, were not able to have sustained impacts and the goals were trimmed back to control rather than eradication.

The early 21st century has seen the return of infections that were previously under control, as well as an emergence of new diseases. Tuberculosis, the great epidemic of the 18th and 19th centuries, has returned in force partially as a result of HIV/AIDS. Box 7-1 looks at the history of TB and the historical and current burden of disease caused by it.[1, 2]

Over a dozen previously-unknown infections have emerged in recent decades—the majority of which are believed to have originated in animal species. In the United States, the presence of Lyme Disease and West Nile virus were unknown until the late 20th century, but have now spread to extensive

---

BOX 7-1   The Burden of TB.

"If the importance of a disease for mankind is measured by the number of fatalities it causes, then tuberculosis must be considered much more important than those most feared infectious diseases, plague, cholera and the like. One in seven of all human beings die from tuberculosis. If one only considers the productive middle-age groups, tuberculosis carries away one-third, and often more."[1]

Robert Koch, March 24, 1882

The history of tuberculosis (TB) goes back to ancient times, but beginning in the 18th century it took center stage in much of Europe and America. It has been estimated that in the two centuries from 1700 to 1900, tuberculosis was responsible for the deaths of approximately one billion human beings. The annual death rate from TB when Koch made his discovery was approximately seven million people.[1] Today that would be the equivalent of over 30 million people considering today's population.

Robert Koch's discovery of the association between the tuberculosis bacilli, its culture and isolation, and its transmission to a variety of animal species provided a clear demonstration that the bacilli are a contributory cause of the disease. While the tuberculosis bacilli are clearly a contributory cause of the disease tuberculosis, they are not sufficient alone to produce disease. A large percentage of the world's population harbors tuberculosis. Other factors are needed to produce active disease. These factors include reduced immunity and nutrition, as well as genetic factors.[b]

The discovery of the tuberculosis bacilli actually followed the development of what was called the sanitarium movement, which began in Europe and America. Sanitariums isolated tuberculosis victims, while providing good nutrition and clean air. The sanitarium movement was coupled in the early 20th century with the use of the Bacillus Calmette-Guérin (BCG) vaccine, purified protein derivative (PPD) skin tests, and the recently-invented chest X-ray. These three early and rather crude technologies are still in use today and were designed to prevent and diagnose TB. In addition, the understanding of the epidemiology of the tuberculosis bacteria led to a clear victory for public health with the near elimination of TB from the milk supply early in the 20th century.

Thus, even before the ability to actively treat tuberculosis, public health interventions were able to dramatically reduce the frequency of the disease at least in Europe and America. A second round of efforts to control TB began in the 1940s with the discovery of streptomycin, the first anti-TB drug, followed over the next decade by para-aminosalicylic acid (PAS) and isoniazid (INH). Combination drug treatments proved highly effective. In addition, INH was found to be effective on its own to prevent skin-test-positive TB from progressing to active disease. Public health and medical efforts to conduct screening for positive skin tests and selectively treating with INH became widespread.

continues

BOX 7-1 continued.

Thus, by the late 1950s and 1960s, TB was brought under control by the combination of medical and public health advances. The success of this effort resulted in the closing of TB sanitariums, gradual cutbacks in screening and treatment programs, and a general loss of interest in TB. From the mid-1960s on, there was little interest or research on TB. Tuberculosis became a treatable disease usually handled as part of routine medical care. Most medical and public health practitioners regarded it as a disease ready for eradication.

Unfortunately, TB was prematurely pronounced dead. It had never come under control in many parts of the world and approximately one-third of those living in developing countries today are estimated to harbor the TB bacillus. That is, they carry TB organisms which may multiply and spread in the future.

Soon after the beginning of the AIDS epidemic that began in the 1980s, active TB came back with a vengeance. AIDS patients with latent TB often developed active TB quite early in their battle with AIDS. They then became contagious to others. Tuberculosis may be more difficult to diagnose and may progress faster in AIDS patients.

Coupled with the return of TB as a public health problem, resistance to TB drugs began to emerge. The problem was successfully combated in the 1990s by the simple public health intervention known as directly-observed therapy or DOT. DOT helped ensure that patients received all the prescribed treatment, thus greatly increasing adherence to effective treatment.

Nonetheless, in recent years resistance to TB drugs and extreme resistance to drug treatments have increased all over the world. Today, we are faced with a triple threat of limited recent research leaving us without modern diagnostic aids or new drugs; a rapidly emerging threat from multiple-drug-resistant tuberculosis, and a spreading epidemic of HIV/AIDS predisposing patients to active tuberculosis. In the past, TB has been exceptionally responsive to a wide range of public health and medical efforts to control its spread. There is hope that with increased awareness and increased further research this will happen again.[2]

---

[b] Establishing that an organism is a contributory cause of the disease traditionally relied on **Koch's postulates.** Koch's postulates hold that in order to definitely establish a cause-and-effect relationship, the following four conditions must be met: 1) the organism must be shown to be present in every case of the disease by isolation of the organism; 2) the organism must not be found in cases of other disease; 3) once isolated, the organism must be capable of replicating the disease in an experimental animal; and 4) the organism must be recoverable from the animal. Ironically, TB cannot be shown to fulfill Koch's postulates. However, a very useful set of **Modern Koch's posulates** has been developed by the National Institute of Allergy and Infectious Disease. It requires evidence of an epidemiological association, isolation, and transmissions to establish that an organism is a contributory cause of the disease.[3]

---

areas of the country. Long-established diseases, such as malaria, are extending their geographic range and further extension is expected with global warming. Influenza is anticipated to return again in pandemic form, as has occurred repeatedly in prior centuries. A pandemic is most likely to occur when ongoing mutations produce new strains capable of person-to-person transmission. Whether you live in a dorm, are a public health professional, a politician, a high school principal, or in almost any profession, the types of questions illustrated in these cases are part of your present and your future.

History suggests that public health and medical interventions have and will continue to have major impacts on the burden of communicable diseases. Let us look at the tools available to address this burden.

WHAT PUBLIC HEALTH TOOLS ARE AVAILABLE TO ADDRESS THE BURDEN OF COMMUNICABLE DISEASES?

A range of public health tools are available to address the burden of communicable diseases. Some of these are useful in addressing non-communicable diseases as well, but they have special applications when directed toward infections. These include:

- Barrier protections, including isolation and quarantine
- Immunizations designed to protect individuals, as well as populations
- Screening and case finding
- Treatment and contact treatment
- Efforts to maximize effectiveness of treatments and prevent resistance

Let us look at each of these tools.

How Can Barriers Against Disease Be Used to Address the Burden of Communicable Diseases?

Examples of barriers to the spread of infections are as old as hand washing and as new as insecticide-impregnated bed nets that have had a major impact on the rate of malaria. Barrier protection, such as condoms, is believed by many to be the most successful intervention to prevent sexually-transmitted diseases. The use of masks may be effective in reducing the spread of disease in healthcare institutions, such as hospitals. The same measures may be preventative in the community at large and are a routine part of winter weather habits in much of Asia.

A special form of barrier protection consists of separating individuals with disease from the healthy population to prevent exposure. As we discussed previously, sanitariums had a major impact in reducing outbreaks of TB in the 19th and first half of the 20th century. Today, once again, we are faced with issues of isolation and occasionally have to legally enforce quarantine as we saw in our discussion of health law and policy in Chapter 5.

A second traditional public health approach to infections is the use of immunizations. Let us take a look at a range of ways that immunizations can be used to address the burden of infections.

How Can Immunizations Be Used to Address the Burden of Communicable Disease?

Immunization refers to the strengthening of the immune system to prevent or control disease. Injections of antibodies may be administered to achieve **passive immunity**, which may provide effective short-term protection. **Inactivated (dead)** and **live vaccines (attenuated live)** can often stimulate the body's own antibody production. Live vaccines utilize living organisms that also stimulate cell-mediated immunity and produce long-term protection that more closely resemble the body's own response to infection.

Vaccines are now available for a wide range of bacterial and viral diseases and are being developed and increasingly used to prevent infections as varied as malaria and hookworm.[4] Unfortunately, if has been difficult to produce effective vaccines for some diseases, such as HIV/AIDS. Vaccines, like medications, are rarely 100 percent effective and may produce side effects including allergic reactions that can be life threatening. Live vaccines have the potential to cause injury to a fetus and can themselves produce disease particularly in those with reduced immunity. Some vaccines are not effective for the very young and the elderly. Therefore, the use of vaccines requires extensive investigations to define its effectiveness and safety as well as to identify high risk groups for whom it should be recommended.

For instance college students and military recruits who tend to live in close quarters represent two high-risk groups for meningococcal disease. This bacterial infection can be rapidly life-threatening and when present it requires testing and antibiotic treatment of close contacts. Effective vaccination is now a key tool for controlling this disease. Ideally, vaccination oc-

curs before exposure, however when an outbreak occurs, vaccination of large numbers of potentially exposed individuals living in the surrounding area may be key to effective control. Thus public health uses of vaccines need to consider who should receive the vaccine, when it should be administered, and how it should be administered.

Vaccines administration has traditionally been limited to injections as shots or ingestion as pills. New methods of administration including nasal sprays are now being developed. In addition, it is often possible to combine vaccines increasing the ease of administration. Inactivated vaccines may not produce long term immunity and may require follow-up vaccines or boosters. Thus the use of vaccinations requires the development of a population health strategy which gives careful attention to who, when, and how.

Some infections, especially those viruses that are highly contagious, can be controlled by vaccinating a substantial proportion of the population often in the range of 70 to 90 percent. In this situation, those who are susceptible rarely, if ever, encounter an individual with the disease. This is known as **herd immunity**. When a population has been vaccinated at these types of levels for infections—such as chicken pox, measles, and polio—those who have not been vaccinated are often protected. For some vaccines, such as live polio vaccine, herd immunity is facilitated by the fact that the virus in the vaccine can itself be spread from person to person providing protection for the unvaccinated. Thus, public health authorities are interested in the levels of protection in the community, that is the level of protection of the unvaccinated as well as the vaccinated.

In addition to tools for preventing disease in individuals and populations, public health efforts are often directed at screening for disease and conducting what is called case finding.

How Can Screening and Case Finding Be Used to Address the Burden of Communicable Disease?

Ideally, screening for infections fulfills the same criteria for non-communicable diseases, which we discussed in Chapter 6, and has played a role in controlling the spread of a number of infections. For example, screening for tuberculosis and syphilis was an effective part of the control of these infections well before they could be cured with antibiotics. Today, screening for sexually-transmitted diseases, including gonorrhea and chlamydia, are a routine part of clinical care. HIV screening has long been recommended for high-risk individuals and for populations with an estimated prevalence above one percent. Today, universal screening is increasingly being adopted as a basic strategy for control of HIV/AIDS.

Screening for communicable diseases has often been linked with the public health practice known as **case finding**. Case

investigating the case

finding implies confidential interviewing of those diagnosed with a disease and asking for their recent close physical or sexual contacts. Case finding techniques have been key to the control of syphilis and to a large extent TB both before and after the availability of effective treatment. The advent of effective treatment meant that case finding was of benefit both to those diagnosed with the disease and those located through case finding.

Successful case finding aims to maintain confidentiality. However, when following-up sexual contacts confidentiality is difficult to maintain. The potential for public recognition and the attendant social sigma has inhibited the use of case finding in HIV/AIDS in many parts of the world. The reluctance to utilize case finding may change in coming years as early diagnosis and perhaps early treatment become more effective in controlling the epidemic.

In addition to the use of barrier protections, vaccination of individuals and populations, as well as the use of screening and case finding, public health tools also encompass treatment of those with disease and their contacts.

How Can Treatment of Those Diagnosed and Their Contacts Help to Address the Burden of Communicable Disease?

Treatment of symptomatic disease may in and of itself reduce the risk of transmission. Successful treatment of HIV has been shown to reduce the viral load and thereby reduce the ease of transmission. Similarly, treatment of active TB reduces its infectivity. In addition to direct treatment, a public health tool known as **epidemiological treatment** or treatment of contacts has been effective in controlling a number of communicable diseases. Sexual partners of those with gonorrhea and chlamydia are routinely treated even when their infections cannot be detected. This approach presumably works because early and low-level infections caused by these organisms may be difficult to detect. As we saw in the meningococcal scenario, epidemiological treatment may be the most effective way to halt the rapid spread of a disease.

Contact treatment of HIV/AIDS may become a routine part of controlling the disease. It is already recommended and widely used for treatment of needlestick injuries in healthcare settings. Let us look at one additional public health tool being increasingly used to maximize effectiveness of treatment and prevent resistance.

How Can Public Health Efforts Maximize Effectiveness of Treatment and Prevent Resistance?

In recent years, the impact of antibiotic resistance has become painfully obvious—resistant pneumococcus, gonococcus, and tuberculosis have become widespread. In fact, extremely drug-resistant strains of TB exist in many areas of the world today. Efforts to control resistance have been modest compared to the forces encouraging resistance. Forces encouraging drug resistance include: overuse of prescribed antibiotics, over-the-counter sales of antibiotics in many countries, and widespread use of antibiotics to stimulate modest growth in agricultural animals.

As we have seen, one successful effort known as directly observer therapy (DOT) has led to a more effective treatment of TB. As the name implies, DOT aims to ensure complete adherence to TB treatment by observing individuals taking their daily or at less frequent intervals of treatment. This effort has been credited with success even in areas of drug resistance perhaps on the basis that the body can handle resistant TB if most of the organisms are effectively treated. Efforts are now underway to reduce or eliminate the use of antibiotics for animal growth and to place increased restrictions on the prescribing of highly useful new antibiotics.

The recent emergence of methicillin-resistant staphylococcus aureus (MRSA) outside hospitals has drawn long-overdue attention. It is spreading to communities and beginning to affect otherwise healthy individuals, including athletes and others simply in close physical contact. An effective program to control MRSA will require the use of a range of interventions. This is the situation for many of today's increasingly complex communicable diseases.

Let us now turn our attention to strategies that combine many of the specific public health tools designed to address the problems of infection. We will look at two basic strategies for combating complex infections: elimination and control.

HOW CAN PUBLIC HEALTH STRATEGIES BE USED TO ELIMINATE SPECIFIC COMMUNICABLE DISEASES?

Smallpox was the first human disease to be eradicated. An international effort is hopefully nearing completion to eradicate polio. These two viral diseases are the only ones that have been successfully targeted for eradication. As we have discussed, programs to eradicate TB and malaria have never come close to meeting their goals. Talk of the end of HIV/AIDS is even more unrealistic. Let us see what it takes to successfully eradicate a disease and why so few diseases are on the short list for potential eradication.

The history of smallpox has a unique place in public health. The disease goes back thousands of years and it played a prominent role in colonial America where epidemics often killed a quarter or more of its victims, especially children, and left most others, including George Washington, with severe facial scars for life. As we discussed in Chapter 1, the concept of vaccination and the first successful vaccination was developed for smallpox. During the 19th and early 20th centuries, smallpox was largely eliminated from most developed and developing countries through modest improvement on Jenner's basic approach to vaccination, despite the many side effects of this quite crude treatment.[c]

Despite the control of smallpox in most developed countries, there were still over 10 million cases annually of the disease in over 30 countries during the early 1960s. In 1967, the WHO began a campaign to eliminate smallpox. The success of the campaign over the next decade depended on extraordinary organizational management and cooperation, but the prerequisite for success were the unique epidemiological characteristics of smallpox that made it possible. Let us outline the characteristics of smallpox that made eradication possible:[5]

- **No animal reservoir**—Smallpox is an exclusively human disease. That is, there is no reservoir of the disease in animals. It does not affect other species that can then infect additional humans. This also means that if the disease is eliminated from humans, it has nowhere to hide and later reappear in human populations.
- **Short persistence in environment**—The smallpox virus requires human contact and cannot persist for more than a brief time in the environment without a human host. Thus, droplets from sneezing or coughing need to find an immediate victim and are not easily transmitted except by human-to-human contact.
- **Absence of a long-term carrier state**—Once an individual recovers from smallpox, they no longer carry the virus and cannot transmit it to others. Some diseases, like HIV/AIDS and hepatitis B, can maintain long-term carrier states and be infectious to others for years or decades.
- **The disease produces long-term immunity**—Once having recovered from smallpox, very effective immunity is established preventing a second infection.
- **Vaccination also establishes long-term immunity**—As with the disease itself, the live smallpox vaccine produces very successful long-term immunity. Smallpox has not mutated to become more infectious despite the extensive use of vaccination.
- **Herd immunity protects those who are susceptible**—Long-term immunity from the disease or the vaccine makes it possible to protect large populations. At least 80 percent of the population needs to be vaccinated to interrupt the spread of the infection to the remaining susceptible people.
- **Easily-identified disease**—The classic presentation of smallpox is relatively easy to identify by clinicians with experience observing the disease, as well as by the average person. This makes it possible to quickly diagnose the disease and protect others from being exposed.
- **Effective postexposure vaccination**—The smallpox vaccine is effective even after exposure to smallpox. This enables effective use of what is called **ring vaccination**. Ring vaccination involves identification of a case of smallpox, vaccination of household and close contacts, followed by vaccination of all those within a mile radius of the smallpox case. In the past, households within ten miles were typically searched for additional cases of smallpox. These surveillance and containment efforts were successful even in areas without high levels of vaccination.

The presence of these characteristics makes a disease ideal for eradication. While fulfilling all of them may not be necessary for eradication, the absence of a large number of them makes efforts at eradication less likely to succeed. Table 7-1 outlines these characteristics of smallpox and compares them to polio—the current viral candidate for eradication—as well as to measles. Based upon the content of the table, you should not be surprised to learn that the polio campaign has been much more difficult and has taken much longer than that of smallpox. The potential for a successful measles eradication campaign is still being debated.[d]

Finally, take a look at Table 7-2, which applies these characteristics to HIV infection. It demonstrates why the eradication of HIV/AIDS is not on the horizon.

Unfortunately, eradication of most diseases is not a viable strategy. Thus, public health measures are usually focused on control of infections. In order to understand the range of strategies that are available and useful for controlling communicable diseases, we will take a look at three important and quite different diseases—HIV, influenza A, and rabies.

---

[c] While the vaccine against smallpox is very effective, it has many side effects. The live virus contained in the vaccine can itself cause disease in those vaccinated especially if they have widespread skin disease or have compromised immune system. Today, these side effects might have prevented the widespread use of the smallpox vaccine because it could threaten the lives of the large number of HIV positive individuals many of whom are unaware of their HIV infection. Allergic reactions to the vaccine are also quite common. Allergic reactions to the smallpox vaccine, including inflammation of the lining of the heart, prompted discontinuation of a campaign to vaccinate first responders and healthcare professionals soon after the 9/11 attack.

---

[d] Efforts are underway for the eradication of Guinea Worm, which exhibits a number of favorable characteristics for eradication.

TABLE 7-1 Eradication of Human Diseases—What Makes It Possible?

	Smallpox	Polio	Measles
Disease is limited to humans, i.e., no animal reservoir?	Yes	Yes	Yes
Limited persistence in the environment?	Yes	Yes	Yes
Absence of long-term carrier state?	Yes	Yes—Absent, but may occur in immune-compromised individuals	Yes—Absent, but may occur in immune-compromised individuals
Long-term immunity results from infection?	Yes	Yes—But may not be sustained in immune-compromised individuals	Yes—But may not be sustained in immune-compromised individuals
Vaccination confers long-term immunity?	Yes	Yes—But may not be sustained in immune-compromised individuals. Virus used for production of the live vaccine can produce polio-like illness and has potential to revert back to "wild type infection"	Yes—But may not be sustained in immune-compromised individuals
Herd immunity prevents perpetuation of an epidemic?	Yes	Yes	Yes
Easily-diagnosed disease?	Yes—Disease easily identified	Yes/No Disease relatively easy to identify, but large number of asymptomatic infections	No Disease may be confused with other diseases by those unfamiliar with measles
Vaccination effective postexposure?	Yes Postexposure vaccination effective	No Postexposure vaccination not effective	No Postexposure vaccination not effective

WHAT OPTIONS ARE AVAILABLE FOR THE CONTROL OF HIV/AIDS?

HIV/AIDS has been a uniquely difficult epidemic to control. An understanding of the biology of the HIV virus helps us understand many of the reasons for this. The HIV virus attacks the very cells designed to control it. The virus can avoid exposure to treatments by residing inside cells without replicating. Many treatments work by interrupting the process of replication and thus are not effective when replication stops. The virus establishes a chronic carrier state enabling long-term in-

fectivity. High mutation rates reduce the effectiveness of drugs, as well as the effectiveness of the body's own immune system to fight the disease.

Despite these monumental challenges, considerable progress has been made by reducing the load of virus through drug treatment and preventing the transmission of the disease through a variety of public health interventions. To appreciate the efforts to control transmission of HIV/AIDS, it is important to understand the large number of ways that it can be transmitted.

TABLE 7-2 Potential for Eradication of HIV/AIDS

	HIV/AIDS
Disease is limited to humans, i.e., no animal reservoir?	No—Animal reservoirs exist
Limited persistence in the environment?	No—May persist on contaminated needles long enough for transmission
Absence of long-term carrier state?	No—Carrier state is routine
Long-term immunity results from infection?	No—Effective long-term immunity does not usually occur
Vaccination confers long-term immunity?	No—None currently available and will be difficult to achieve
Herd immunity prevents perpetuation of an epidemic?	No—Large number of previously-infected individuals increases the risk to the uninfected
Easily-diagnosed disease?	No—Requires testing
Vaccination effective postexposure?	No—None currently available

HIV is most infectious when transmitted directly by blood. Blood transfusions were an early source of the spread of the virus. The introduction of HIV virus testing in the mid 1980s led to dramatic improvement in the safety of the blood supply. Nonetheless, the safest blood transfusions are those that come from an individual's own blood. Thus, donation of one's own blood for later transfusion when needed has become a routine part of surgery preparation in many parts of the world. The most dangerous forms of transfusions are those that come from blood or blood products pooled from large numbers of individuals. Hemophiliacs in many developed countries used pooled blood products to control their bleeding in the 1980s. They suffered perhaps the world's highest rate of HIV infection before this hazard was recognized and addressed. A more recent pooling of blood products occurred in China and contributed to a surge of the disease.

Unprotected anal intercourse is a highly infectious way to transmit HIV. This may help to explain the early spread of the disease among male homosexuals. Today, however, heterosex-

ual transmission is the most common route of infection; additionally, there is a higher risk of transmission from male to female than from female to male. A series of public health interventions have now been shown to be effective: properly used latex condoms, male circumcision, and abstinence are being promoted in efforts to control the disease throughout the world. Aggressive treatment of AIDS at an early stage reduces the viral load and the ease of transmission to others.[e]

Maternal-to-child transmission of HIV was a common, but not universal event before the advent of effective drug treatment. The use of treatment during pregnancy and at the time of delivery has dramatically reduced the maternal-to-child transmission of the infection. Today, this route of transmission is close to being eliminated, which is an important public health achievement. Breastfeeding represents an ongoing and more controversial route of transmission. Up to 25 percent of HIV-positive breastfeeding women may transmit HIV to their children. In countries where breastfeeding provides an essential defense against a wide range of infections, the issue of whether or not to breastfeed has been very controversial. Drug treatment of HIV infections during breastfeeding has been shown to reduce, but not eliminate transmission.

Finally, HIV can be transmitted through contaminated needles. Thus, the risk of HIV transmission needs to be addressed in two very different populations—healthcare workers and those who abuse intravenous drugs. New needle technologies and better disposal methods have reduced the likelihood of needlestick injuries in healthcare settings. Postexposure treatment with drugs has been quite successful in reducing health care-related HIV infections. Reductions in HIV transmission through intravenous drug use have also occurred in areas where public health efforts have focused attention on this method of transmission. Needle exchange programs have met resistance and remain controversial, but most likely contribute to transmission reductions when the programs are carefully designed and administered.

Thus, a range of existing interventions linked to the method of transmission of HIV have been moderately successful in controlling the disease. New methods of control are needed and are being investigated and increasingly applied. Unfortunately, vaccination is not one of them. In fact, randomized clinical trials so far have demonstrated no substantial degree of protection from vaccinations and have raised the concern that vaccination may actually increase the probability of acquiring HIV.

---

[e] It has been suggested that serial monogamy reduces the risk of HIV transmission in populations compared to having two or more concurrent partners. Serial monogamy contributes to only one chain of transmission at a time and thus may slow, if not halt, the speed or spread of the epidemic in a population.

The recognition that effective vaccinations are not likely in the foreseeable future has brought forth a wide array of ideas on how to control the spread of infection. Antiviral creams, postcoital treatments, and early testing and case finding may become effective interventions. Antiviral creams may become both an adjunct to condom use, as well as a substitute in those situations where condom use is not acceptable. The success of postneedlestick interventions in the healthcare setting has raised the possibility that postexposure treatment may also be effective after high risk sexual contact. Finally, new diagnostic tests for HIV that allow for detection of the disease in the most contagious early weeks of the infection are being investigated for widespread use. To be effective, testing for early disease would need to be coupled with rapid case finding to identify and ideally treat contacts.

It is encouraging to know that existing and emerging interventions for HIV hold out possibility of effective control. Public health and medical intervention complement each other and are both needed if we are to effectively address the most widespread epidemic of the 21st century. Table 7-3 summarizes the routes of transmission and the estimated transmission rates per exposure.[6] Finally, it outlines the potential interventions that we have discussed.

WHAT OPTIONS ARE AVAILABLE FOR THE CONTROL OF INFLUENZA?

Pandemic influenza is not a new problem. The influenza epidemic of 1918 is estimated to have killed an estimated 50 million people in a world populated with 2 billion people. Today, that would translate to over 150 million deaths. The history of the 1918 influenza pandemic is briefly summarized in Box 7.2.[7] The 1958 pandemic of Asian flu caused a similar, if less deadly pandemic. Thus, we should not be surprised if pandemic flu returns in the coming years.

Influenza A is a viral infection that has long been capable of pandemic or worldwide spread.[f] Its ability to be rapidly

[f] Influenza B can also cause epidemics of influenza, however it is not thought to pose the same hazard of pandemic disease that is possible with Influenza A.

TABLE 7-3 Mode and Chances of Transmission of HIV and Existing Interventions

Route of transmission	Estimated transmission rate per exposure	Potential interventions
Blood transfusion Blood and blood products, such as pooled blood products previously used in U.S. by hemophiliacs	Contaminated blood over 90% chance of transmission; pooling of blood dramatically increases infection	Screening of blood to detect HIV early Use of individual's own blood for surgery
Sexual contact—Anal higher than vaginal, which is much higher than oral	Range from 0.1% to 10% with unprotected receptive anal intercourse posing highest risk Vaginal male to female greater than female to male Circumcision reduces risk by half Other sexually-transmitted diseases may increase risk	Latex condom Circumcision Abstinence Serial monogamy reduces spread compared to two or more concurrent partners
Mother-to-child transmission	15% to 40% higher in developing countries Highest rate of transmission at time of vaginal delivery	Cesarean delivery Drug treatment during pregnancy and at time of delivery for mother and child
Breast-feeding	Very low per exposure, but up to 25% over year or more of breast-feeding	Continuation of drug treatment reduces, but does not eliminate transmission
Needlestick exposures Healthcare occupational risk	Less than 0.5% of HIV positive needlesticks result in transmission	Postexposure treatment with drugs established as effective prevention
Injection drug use	Less than 1% per episode of needle sharing	Needle exchange programs

Source: Data from Population Reference Bureau. Facing the HIV/AIDS Pandemic. *Population Bulletin* 2002: 57(3).

BOX 7-2   The Influenza Pandemic of 1918.

The history of the influenza pandemic of 1918 is summarized by the United States National Archives and Records Administration as follows:[7]

World War I claimed an estimated 16 million lives. The influenza epidemic that swept the world in 1918 killed an estimated 50 million people. One fifth of the world's population was attacked by this deadly virus. Within months, it had killed more people than any other illness in recorded history.

The plague emerged in two phases. In late spring of 1918, the first phase, known as the "three-day fever," appeared without warning. Few deaths were reported. Victims recovered after a few days. When the disease surfaced again that fall, it was far more severe. Scientists, doctors, and health officials could not identify this disease which was striking so fast and so viciously, eluding treatment and defying control. Some victims died within hours of their first symptoms. Others succumbed after a few days; their lungs filled with fluid and they suffocated to death.

The plague did not discriminate. It was rampant in urban and rural areas, from the densely populated East coast to the remotest parts of Alaska. Young adults, usually unaffected by these types of infectious diseases, were among the hardest hit groups along with the elderly and young children. The flu afflicted over 25 percent of the U.S. population. In one year, the average life expectancy in the United States dropped by 12 years.

transmitted through the air from person to person and its short incubation period have made it an ongoing public health problem. It often kills the very young, the very old, and those with chronic illnesses, particularly those with respiratory diseases and suppressed immune systems. In addition, the disease continues to mutate creating new types against which previous infections and previous vaccinations have little or no impact. Thus, new vaccines are required every flu season. Seasonal influenza kills over 30,000 people in the United States alone in the average year despite the increasingly widespread use of vaccinations.

A variety of public health and medical interventions have been and continue to be used to address the current and potential threat posed by influenza. They may well all be needed to address future threats. Let us take a look at these interventions.

Inactivated or dead vaccines have been the mainstay of immunization against influenza. Unfortunately, current technology requires approximately six months lead time to produce large quantities of the vaccine. Thus, influenza experts need to make educated guesses about next year's dominant strains of influenza. In some years, they have been wrong and the deaths and disability from seasonal influenza have increased. New technologies for vaccine production are greatly needed and are being extensively researched.

In recent years, live vaccines administered through nasal spray have been developed and increasingly used. These vaccines are more acceptable than shots to most patients and are now considered safe for a wide range of age groups. They raise the hope of greater acceptance and wider use of influenza vaccinations in coming years.

Medications to treat influenza and modestly shorten the course of the disease have also been developed. Influenza experts view these drugs as most useful to temporarily slow the spread of new strains providing additional time for the development of vaccines to specifically target the new strain. Widespread use of influenza drugs has already resulted in resistance raising concerns that these drugs will not be effective when we need them the most. Efforts are underway to develop new drugs and reserve their use solely for potential pandemic conditions.

Despite our best efforts, influenza is expected to continue its annual seasonal epidemic and to pose a risk of pandemic spread. The use of barrier protection such as masks, isolation methods, and even quarantine has been considered part of a comprehensive effort to control influenza. It is clear that we have a variety of public health methods to help control the impact of the disease. It is likely that we will need all of these efforts and new ones if we are going to control the potential deaths and disabilities due to influenza in coming years.[8] Now, let us look at our last example of the development of public health strategies to control communicable diseases—that of rabies.

WHAT OPTIONS ARE AVAILABLE FOR THE CONTROL OF RABIES?

Rabies is an ancient disease that has plagued human beings for over 4000 years. It is caused by a ribonucleic acid (RNA) virus that is transmitted through saliva of infected animals and slowly replicates. It spreads to nerve cells and gradually invades the central nervous system over a 20- to 60-day incubation period. Once the central nervous system is involved, the disease progresses almost inevitably to death within one to two weeks. Any warm-blooded animal can be infected with rabies, but some species are particularly susceptible—most commonly raccoons, skunks, and bats. Cats and dogs can also be infected and transmit the virus.

A multicomponent vaccination strategy has been very successful in preventing the development of rabies in humans. In most recent years, there have been between one and five fatal cases of rabies per year in the United States despite the persistence and periodic increase in rabies among wildlife populations. Let us take a look at how this quite remarkable control effort has occurred.

The ability to successfully vaccinate humans against rabies after the occurrence of a rabies-prone bite has long been a component of the success of rabies reduction among humans. The use of postexposure vaccination was first demonstrated by Louis Pasteur in 1887 and was used to dramatically save the life of a young victim. Early live vaccines had frequent and severe side effects. They were sequentially replaced by inactivated vaccines grown in animal nerve tissue. These replacement vaccines still led to occasional acute neurological complications and gave the treatment a reputation of being dangerous. The development of a vaccine grown in human cell cultures in the 1970s led to safety records comparable to those of other commonly-used vaccines. Today, over 30,000 rabies vaccination series are administered annually in the United States.

The success of rabies control is a result of a series of coordinated efforts to utilize vaccinations in different settings: Vaccines are administered to individuals who are bitten by suspicious species of wild animals including raccoons, bats, skunks, foxes, and coyotes. Victims of suspected rabies bites by dogs and cats may await the results of quarantine of the animal and observation over a 10-day period. When substantial doubt still exists after this time frame, vaccination is recommended. Laws requiring rabies vaccination of dogs and cats have been enforced in the United States for decades and have greatly reduced the number of reported infections in these animals. Today only ten percent or fewer of suspect rabies-prone bites come from dogs and cats.

Wildlife remains the greatest source of rabies—wildlife epidemics occur with regularity. Rabies-prone bites still occur especially from raccoons, which regularly feed from garbage cans in rural, suburban, and occasionally urban America. Recent development of effective oral vaccinations that can be administered to wildlife through baits have been credited with reducing the number of infected animals, especially those residing in close proximity to humans.

Rabies illustrates the variety of ways that a key intervention—vaccination—can be used to address a disease. As with many complex diseases of public health importance, a carefully designed and coordinated strategy is required to maximize the benefit of available technology. In addition, ongoing research is needed to continue to develop new and improved approaches to the control of communicable diseases.[9]

HIV/AIDS, influenza A, and rabies represent three very different communicable diseases. However, they all require the use of multiple interventions, close collaboration between the public health and healthcare systems, and continuing efforts to find new and more effective methods for their control.

Efforts to control infectious diseases have increased in recent years along with the increase in emerging and reemerging infectious diseases. Technological advances have provided encouragement for the future but at times have raised concerns about the safety of our interventions.[g] New technology, new strategies for applying technology, and new ways to effectively organize our efforts are needed to ensure the effectiveness and safety of our efforts to prevent, eradicate and control communicable diseases.

Now let us turn our attention to our third category of disease in chapter 8 that of environmental diseases and injuries.

---

[g] In recent decades the number of vaccinations used in children has increased dramatically. The potential for new side effect from multiple vaccinations has been of recent concern especially the previous use of a mercury containing compound designed to help preserve vaccines. Concerns have been raised that multiple vaccines have increased the risk of autism. Despite investigations which do not support an association, these concerns have persisted.

Key Words

- Infectious disease
- Communicable disease
- Infections
- Immunization
- Passive immunity
- Inactived (dead) vaccine
- Live vaccines
- Herd immunity
- Case finding
- Epidemiological treatment
- Ring vaccination

Discussion Questions

Take a look at the questions posed in the following scenarios which were presented at the beginning of this chapter. See now whether you can answer them.

1. *Your college roommate went to bed not feeling well one night and early the next morning you had trouble arousing her. She was rushed to the hospital just in time to be effectively diagnosed and treated for meningococcal meningitis. The health department recommends immediate antibiotic treatment for everyone that was in close contact with your roommate. They set up a process to watch for additional cases to be sure an outbreak is not in progress. Fortunately, no more cases occur. You ask yourself: should your college require that all freshmen have the meningococcal vaccine before they can register for classes?*

2. *As a health advisor to a worldwide HIV/AIDS foundation, you are asked to advise on ways to address the HIV and developing tuberculosis (TB) epidemics. You are asked to do some long-range thinking and to come up with a list of potential approaches to control the epidemics, or at least ways reduce the development of TB. The first recommendation you make is to forget about eradicating HIV/AIDS. How did you come to that conclusion?*

3. *Your hometown of 100,000 is faced with a crisis as an airplane lands containing a passenger thought to have a new form of severe influenza that has recently gained the ability to spread from person to person through airborne spread. As the mayor of the city, what do you decide to do?*

4. *You are a principal at a local high school. One of your top athletes is in the hospital with a spreading bacterial infection due to a staphylococcus bacteria resistant to all known antibiotics. The infection occurred after what appeared to be a minor injury during practice. As the principal, what do you decide to do?*

REFERENCES

1. Nobelprize.org. Robert Koch and Tuberculosis. Available at: http://nobelprize.org/educational_games/medicine/tuberculosis/readmore.html. Accessed March 18, 2009.

2. New Jersey Medical School Global Tuberculosis Institute. History of TB. Available at: http://www.umdnj.edu/ntbcweb/tbhistory.htm. Accessed March 18, 2009.

3. National Institute of Allergy and Infectious Diseases. The Evidence that HIV causes AIDS. Available at: http://www3.niaid.nih.gov/topics/HIVAIDS/Understanding/HIVcausesAIDS.htm. Accessed March 18, 2009.

4. Centers for Disease Control and Prevention. Vaccines. Available at: http://www.cdc.gov/vaccines/. Accessed March 18, 2009.

5. Sompayrac L. *How Pathogenic Viruses Work*. Sudbury, MA: Jones and Bartlett Publishers; 2002.

6. Lamptey P, Wigley M, Carr D, Collymore Y. Facing the HIV/AIDS pandemic. *Population Bulletin.* 2002; 57(3): 1–3.

7. National Archives and Records Administration. The Deadly Vines: The Influenza Epidemic of 1918. Available at: http://www.archives.gov/exhibits/influenza-epidemic/. Accessed May 12, 2009.

8. World Health Organization. Global Agenda for Influenza Surveillance and Control. Available at: http://www.who.int/csr/disease/influenza/globalagenda/en/index.html. Accessed March 18, 2009.

9. Centers for Disease Control and Prevention. Rabies Home. Available at: http://www.cdc.gov/rabies/. Accessed March 18, 2009.

CHAPTER 8

Environmental Health and Safety

LEARNING OBJECTIVES

By the end of this chapter the student will be able to:

- define the scope of morbidity and mortality caused by the physical environment.
- identify the range of interactions that occur between human beings and the physical environment.
- identify the components of environmental risk assessment and apply them to an environmental hazard, such as lead.
- distinguish between a risk assessment, a public health assessment, and an ecological assessment.
- discuss the meaning of interactions and how they may impact the size of risks.
- illustrate how safety issues, such as motor vehicle injuries, have been addressed using a systems thinking approach.

Joe grew up in an industrial district of town. His family lived in an old apartment building and he played in a playground near a major intersection. By the age of 6, Joe was found to have high lead levels in his blood and was not doing well in school. Where could all that lead come from, his mother wondered?

Jill is pregnant and loves fish, which she has eaten almost daily for years as part of her effort to stay healthy. She hears that fish should not be eaten regularly during pregnancy. Why, she wonders, should I cut down on eating something as healthy as fish?

Ralph and Sonya, a prosperous professional couple, and their two children live in an older suburban home. They feel secure that their environment is safe. They were surprised to find when they wanted to put their house up for sale that it did not pass the safety tests for radon. Where did the radon come from, they wondered, and what can be done about it?

Sandra worked for an international agency that had successfully addressed the danger of radiation due to the hole in the ozone

layer. She was shocked when she was told that she had a life-threatening skin cancer called melanoma. She asked, what could cause melanoma? Could years of sun exposure have played a role?

With your seat belt on, children buckled in, and airbags activated, you head out of the driveway to face the world. You didn't see that truck coming when it hit you from the side. The ambulance responded within minutes and took your family to the nearest emergency room. You all made it through with only minor injuries. You ask yourself, was it just luck or did the system work?

All of these situations are part of what we mean by the burden of environmental disease and injury. In order to understand the impact of the environment on disease, we need to define what we mean by it and appreciate the many ways that we interact with it.

WHAT IS MEANT BY "ENVIRONMENT"?

Environment is an ambiguous term. It is sometimes used to imply all influences other than genetic influences including social, economic, and cultural influences. We will define the environment as the physical environment. The physical environment can be thought of in three categories: unaltered ("natural"), altered, and the built environment.[a] Figure 8-1 diagrams the scope of environmental diseases and injuries.

---

[a] The term "natural" is used in quotations because it can be a misleading term. We often think that the term "natural disasters" implies that human actions had nothing to do with the events. Increasingly, human actions precipitate, worsen, and even cause "natural disasters." Construction on vulnerable lands increases the damage from storms, fires, earthquakes, and even volcanoes. Global warming caused by human activities is also beginning to have its impacts. Our planet has been altered in so many ways that the unaltered environment is becoming difficult to find.

FIGURE 8-1 Scope of environmental diseases and injuries

The health of human beings was affected by the physical environment long before we had the capacity to substantially alter it. Floods, earthquakes, and volcanoes have always been a part of the physical environment. In addition to these intermittent and often isolated impacts, daily exposure to infectious diseases in water and food have always been a part of the unaltered environment.

In recent years, we have recognized more subtle impacts of the **unaltered environment**. Radon, a common naturally-occurring breakdown product of uranium, increases the risk of lung cancer. Exposure to naturally-occurring sunlight increases the chances of skin cancer including melanoma—a potentially lethal skin cancer—especially among light-skinned individuals.

Human activity has altered nearly every aspect of our physical environment. Some alterations to our environment may improve human health—from water treatment, to waste management, to mosquito and flood control. Nonetheless, we need to consider the overall impacts that these changes have on the physical environment. The sheer growth in the number of human beings—we are rapidly approaching a planet population of 7 billion—is likely to magnify our impact on all aspects of our physical environment in the future.

We often think of the **altered environment** as reflecting the impact of chemicals, radiation, and biological products that we introduce into the environment. The list of intentional or unintentional introductions is in fact very long. It ranges from industrial chemicals, such as pesticides, benzene, and chlorofluorocarbons (CFCs), to elements mined from the earth, such as mercury and lead. It also includes radiation from nuclear energy and medical wastes. Biological impacts encompass the introduction of invasive species and the management of biological wastes.

The concept of the **built environment** is a relatively new term that includes all the impacts of the physical environment

as a result of human construction. The impacts of it include injuries and exposures in the home, the transportation system, and where we work and play. It also includes factors ranging from the way we build and heat our buildings and cook our food, to the way we travel from place to place. The built environment influences our safety through its impact on injuries and hazardous exposures. It also influences our activity levels and our social interactions that impact our health.[1]

The impact of the built environment is wide-ranging throughout the world, but differs greatly by geography and stage of social and economic development. Indoor air pollution from cooking is the most prominent source of air pollution in much of the developing world. Motor vehicle injuries are the most deadly consequences of the built environment in most developed countries. The built environment has subtle impacts as well. The way we build our cities affects the amount of exercise we get and the quantity of noise pollution we experience. Construction methods affect air systems in buildings and can increase our exposure to "sick buildings." Let us take a look at the burden of disease that results from the physical environment.

WHAT IS THE BURDEN OF DISEASE DUE TO THE PHYSICAL ENVIRONMENT?

Measuring the impact of the physical environment on health is difficult because of the many types of impacts and the often subtle effects that occur. The impacts we experience today may pale in comparison to what we can expect in the future. Nonetheless, it is useful to appreciate the current estimates of the magnitude of the direct and indirect burden.

As we saw in the introduction to this section, motor vehicle injuries and exposure to toxic substances are two important actual causes of death that represent the largest known impact of the physical environment. Together, these incidents are estimated to cause nearly 100,000 deaths, representing about 20 percent of preventable deaths in the United States and approximately 10 percent of all deaths in the United States according to the Centers for Disease Control and Prevention's (CDC's) calculations.[2] Motor vehicle injuries and other unintentional injuries have especially heavy impacts on the young; in fact, they are the number one cause of death in the United States among those 1 to 24 years of age.[3] As a cause of disability, injuries also rank high especially considering their disproportionate impact on the young.[b]

[b] The role of environmental factors in asthma is difficult to separate from the impact of cigarettes, genetics, and other determinants of health and disease, etc. Subtle, but important impacts are increasingly being recognized. Air pollution, especially very small particle air pollution, is being linked increasingly to coronary artery disease. Attributing a portion of the many deaths from coronary artery disease to air pollution substantially increases the estimates of the environmental burden of disease.

Approximately 5000 deaths due to injuries occur in the occupational setting per year. Certain occupations are particularly vulnerable to injuries including mining, construction, and agriculture. Occupational injuries have been declining in recent years, but remain an important cause of death and disability.[4]

The impact of toxic substances on death and disability is difficult to measure due to the length of time the substances may take to affect the body. It may be years after an exposure before an individual experiences negative health effects on their kidneys, liver, nerves, and other organs. Many toxic exposures occur in occupational settings. Occupational exposures that result in morbidity and mortality include lung diseases caused by exposures to hazardous dusts, hearing loss from loud noises, and back pain from excessive lifting, as well as a wide range of other mechanical problems, including carpal tunnel syndrome often caused by repetitive motion of the hand and wrist.[4]

Cancer caused by occupational exposures has been of particular concern. As much as five percent of cancer deaths in males have been estimated to be due to occupational exposures.[5] Cancers of the lung, bladder, and white blood cells (leukemia), are particularly likely to result from chronic exposures to chemicals, such as formaldehyde, benzene, and organic dyes. Reductions in occupational exposures in the last 25 years have resulted in a declining burden of disease from these exposures in the United States. The opposite is being seen in many newly industrializing countries where current exposures are increasing and may result in more cases of cancer and other diseases in the not-too-distant future.

Finally, we cannot evaluate the impact of toxic exposures solely by tracing them to human deaths and disabilities. The altered environment has impacts on entire ecosystems of plants and animals. The ecological impact of environmental factors can have long-term and largely irreversible consequences. Once chemicals, radiation, and biological products are released into the environment, the process cannot generally be easily reversed. Thus, we need to take a broad and long-term perspective when we address environmental health. To understand how the physical environment—be it the unaltered, altered, or built environment—affects health, we need to explore the myriad ways that we interact with it. Box 8-1 illustrates this concept.

Because of the complexity of the interactions between human beings and the physical environment, a range of approaches has been developed for addressing these issues. We will categorize and examine these approaches as follows:

- **Risk assessment**
- **Public health assessment**
- **Ecological assessment**
- **Interaction analysis**
- **Systems analysis**

We can think of these strategies as a progression of approaches of increasing complexity. We will organize our approach to environmental diseases and injuries starting with risk assessment and proceeding in order to examine each of these strategies.

HOW DOES RISK ASSESSMENT ADDRESS THE IMPACTS OF THE PHYSICAL ENVIRONMENT?

Risk assessment is a formal process that aims to measure the potential impact of known **hazards**. A hazard indicates the inherent danger of an exposure, while a risk assessment aims to take into account not only the inherent danger, but the quantity, route, and timing of the exposure.[6] The risk assessment approach to environmental hazards represents the mainstay of our current approach. The underlying principles have a long history in public health often resulting from the investigation of specific occupational exposures.

One of the earliest occupational investigations occurred among chimney sweeps in 18th-century England. Their high-dose exposure to carbon residues in smokestacks led to early and frequent testicular cancer. Nineteenth century industrializing countries also provided ample opportunities to study the impacts of work-related exposures. For instance, the dangers of radiation came to light after high levels of cancer were detected in workers who painted watches with radiation-containing paint for the purposes of nighttime illumination. The dangers of asbestos became evident after high-dose exposures among ship workers during World War II resulted in cases of lung cancer many years later. The dangers of exposure to polyvinyl chloride (PVC), a common industrial compound, was recognized after five workers from the same manufacturing plant came down with a rare liver tumor in the 1970s.

Risk assessment today has become a complex technical effort requiring quantitative measures of the magnitude of the risk. The history of risk assessment in the United States is closely tied to the investigations and regulations surrounding benzene. Box 8-2 provides an overview of the history of the study and regulation of this chemical hazard.[7, 8]

The formal process of risk assessment represents the current approach to environmental hazards in the United States.[9, 10] Figure 8-2 illustrates the four step risk assessment process as used by the U.S. EPA.

Risk assessment attempts to evaluate the impact of environmental exposures one at a time and to measure the types and magnitudes of the impacts. If a substantial risk is found

BOX 8-1 How We Interact with Our Environment.

We are exposed to the physical environment every minute of our lives through multiple routes. For each of these routes of exposure, the body has mechanisms for protection. We are primarily exposed to the environment via the skin; the respiratory tract (from the nose to the lungs); the alimentary tract or digestive tract (from the mouth to the anus); and the genital-urinary tract.

Each bodily surface that is directly exposed to the physical environment has developed a form of barrier protection. The skin provides direct protection against radiation, organisms, and physical contact, as well as providing some protections against heat and cold. The respiratory tract is guarded by mucous production and by small hair-like structures called cilia, whose motion in conjunction with coughing removes materials that we breathe into our lungs. Cells called phagocytes literally consume organisms and large particles. Antibodies, along with cell-mediated immunity, also protect against access of harmful particles and organisms through the lungs. The alimentary or digestive tract is protected by saliva, mucous membranes, and antibodies, as well as strong acidity in the stomach. The genital-urinary tract is protected by mucous membrane barriers, antibody and cell-mediated immunity, and at times by an acid environment.[c]

Therefore, we need to recognize that the impacts of the environment on health are very complex.[5] We should expect to find that the following issues affect the risk:

* *Route of exposure*—The consequences of exposures to heavy metals including mercury, lead, and cadmium, for instance, depend on whether the exposure is via the skin or the respiratory or gastrointestinal tracts.
* *Timing of exposure*—Short-term high-dose impacts often will not be the same as long-term low-dose impacts even if the total exposure and the routes of exposure are the same. For instance, a small number of severe episodes of sunburn during childhood have been found to greatly increase the risk of skin cancers far more than multiple milder adult sunburns. Chronic low-dose exposures may produce different and more subtle impacts.
* *Stage of life*—The impact on the very young and the very old are likely to be different than the impact for people at other stages of life. We need to be especially concerned about exposures during pregnancy, early childhood, and the later years of life.
* *Other diseases*—The presence of other diseases will affect how the body is impacted by an environmental exposure. We need to be especially concerned about environmental exposures for those with chronic lung diseases and those with suppressed immune systems, such as those living with AIDS.
* *Special sensitivities*—A few individuals will be hypersensitive to specific environmental exposures that have no measurable impact on the vast majority of individuals. We need to be concerned about how to identify and protect these individuals without depriving them of rights or opportunities.

[c]The effectiveness of our bodily defenses depends on a number of factors, for instance, genetic factors. Skin pigmentation reduces the penetration of radiation and reduces the risk of skin cancers, including melanoma, the most serious of skin cancers. Other diseases affect how well our defenses operate—for instance chronic obstructive lung disease and cystic fibrosis can alter the ability of the cilia in the lung to operate effectively. Age can affect the ability of our skin to serve as an effective barrier as well as the ability of the immune system to respond. The elderly are especially prone to the effects of heat and cold. They are also more susceptible to a range of infections and cancers. Our defense mechanisms can overreact to environmental stimuli and themselves produce ailments, including allergies and autoimmune disease. The impacts of environmental exposures may be limited to a small number of susceptible individuals whose immune systems react especially strongly to specific environmental exposures. For instance, allergies to peanuts or household or industrial chemicals can produce unusual, but severe reactions in a small number of susceptible individuals.

to exist, the process then reviews options to protect, detect, and react to the risk to minimize the burden of disease on humans.

The risk assessment process builds in a margin of error designed to provide extra protection for especially vulnerable individuals or populations. Thus those exposed to levels above the recommended maximum levels of exposure will not necessarily experience adverse effects. Table 8-1 outlines the four steps in the risk assessment process and uses a simplified example of how airborne exposure to benzene in occupational settings might be presented in this framework.

Now let us take a look at what is meant by public health assessment.

WHAT IS A PUBLIC HEALTH ASSESSMENT?

Risk assessment is distinguished from what is called a public health assessment. A public health assessment goes beyond a risk assessment by including data on actual exposure in a community.

Public health assessments have the potential for major impacts on large numbers of people because they address the risks not just in a specific location, such as in an occupational

BOX 8-2 Benzene and Risk Assessment.

Benzene is an organic chemical that is used as a solvent in the chemical and pharmaceutical industries. Because it readily becomes a gas at room temperature, airborne exposure is an important concern. Benzene is one of the most widely-used organic chemicals. It is estimated that over 250,000 American workers are exposed to benzene, particularly in the chemical, printing, paint, and petroleum industries.[d]

A range of toxic effects have been documented from benzene over the last 150 years. These include neurological effects of acute and chronic exposure, as well as life-threatening suppression of the production of red blood cells called aplastic anemia.

In the 1960s and 1970s, it was increasingly recognized that benzene caused cancer, particularly leukemia. Early studies of benzene and leukemia were conducted by Muzaffer Aksoy, a Turkish physician, who observed leukemia among many shoemakers in Turkey where benzene was being used as a solvent in the manufacturing of leather products. His large cohort study helped establish the chemical as a presumed cause of leukemia.

Based on a series of studies that documented the risk of leukemia, in 1978 the federal government established a standard for exposure to benzene in the air of 1 part per million (1 ppm), as opposed to the former approach of limiting the exposure to 10 parts per million (10 ppm). One part per million is approximately the equivalent of one drop in 40 gallons of liquid. In 1980, the United States Supreme Court overturned the new standard based upon the argument that the Environmental Protection Agency (EPA) had not documented the impact of the new 1 ppm standard in terms of number of lives saved or compared it to the 10 ppm level. The Supreme Court concluded that "safe" did not mean risk-free, giving the analogies of driving a car and breathing city air. The Supreme Court insisted that standards be set based upon the preponderance of evidence from a formal risk assessment. As a result of this Supreme Court decision, the EPA developed a risk-assessment approach that grew into the current risk-assessment process. The 1 part per million standard was supported by quantitative measures of the impact: the federal government estimated that there would be 14 to 17 excess deaths per 1000 workers exposed to 10 ppm of benzene for a working lifetime, compared to being exposed to the new 1 ppm standard.

Thus, risk assessment today is a highly technical and quantitative activity designed to establish a maximum level of allowed exposure to one particular hazard. The levels set are designed to conform to the Supreme Court's definition of "significant risk," which is characterized by one that is "not acceptable to society" in "ordinary life".[7]

---

[d] Benzene is also a component of gasoline therefore, the entire population has some exposure to benzene. This discussion focuses on the hazard assessment of benzene in the occupational setting.

setting, but risks to large numbers of individuals and often to the population as a whole. These types of risk assessments have been very controversial and have taken years—often decades—to complete. An expert panel for the National Academy of Sciences has recommended a major overhaul of public health assessments.[11] A classic example of the importance and potential impacts of the public health assessment process and its ongoing challenges is discussed in Box 8-3, which looks at the health risks due to lead.[12, 13]

Risk assessments and public health assessments both focus exclusively on the health impacts on human beings. Let us take a look at an additional type of assessment conducted by the EPA that looks at the impact of an exposure on plants and animals.

WHAT IS AN ECOLOGICAL RISK ASSESSMENT?

Environmental health cannot be viewed solely on the basis of current impacts on human health. The impacts of environmental contamination or pollution on plants and animals and

FIGURE 8-2 The 4-step risk assessment process

Hazard Identification — What health problems are caused by the pollutant?

Dose-Response Assessment — What are the health problems at different exposures?

Exposure Assessment — How much of the pollutant are people exposed to during a specific time period? How many people are exposed?

Risk Characterization — What is the extra risk of health problems in the exposed population?

Source: Reprinted from U.S. Environmental Protection Agency. Risk Assessment Portal Available at http://www.epa.gov/risk/hazardousidentification.htm Accessed December 14, 2008.

TABLE 8-1 Four-Step Risk Assessment and Simplified Example—Benzene

Components	Simplified example—benzene
Hazard Identification What health effects are caused by the pollutant?	Benzene causes leukemia Strong evidence from cohort studies and supportive animal data exist
Dose-response Relationship What are the health problems at different exposures?	Strong dose-response relationship among occupational workers with level of 1 ppm over a working lifetime. The impact of exposure at 1 ppm is indistinguishable from unexposed with rapid increase in rates of leukemia above that level
Exposure Assessment How much of the pollutant are people exposed to during a specific time period? How many people are exposed?	Industrial exposures above 1 ppm common in a range of industries at the time the standard was set Over 250,000 workers exposed to benzene
Risk Characterization What is the extra risk of health problems in the exposed population?	14–17 excess cases of leukemia per 1000 workers exposed to 10 ppm throughout a working lifetime

Source: Awofeso N. What's new about the "New Public Health"? *American Journal of Public Health.* 2004; 94(5): 705–709.

the ecosystems in which they exist often has important long-term consequences.

The modern environmental movement in the United States was ignited in large part by Rachel Carson's book, *Silent Spring*, which described how the widespread use of DDT had threatened the American Eagle and other birds as it became deposited in and weakened their eggs.[14] Broader concern about the impacts of contaminants on ecological systems ranging from chemicals, to radiation, to genetically-altered crops has made clear the importance of ecological risk assessments. Human health consequences remain an important, but not necessarily a direct consequence of the impacts of environmental contamination or pollution as described in Box 8-4, which explores the impacts of mercury.[15]

Up to this point, we have addressed the impact of environmental exposures one at a time. Increasingly, we find that the

BOX 8-3 Health Risks Due to Lead.

Knowledge of the potential for lead poisoning goes back to ancient civilizations, where the metal was widely used—for example, it was a component of water pipes and part of the process of making wine. In Rome, lead was used as a method of abortion and high-dose exposures led to a range of mental effects. It is said the Roman emperors were affected by the high levels of lead in Roman wine.

Benjamin Franklin listed every known profession for which lead posed a health hazard and predicted that many years would pass before the public health consequences of lead were addressed. Of course, Benjamin Franklin was right. Things were to get worse before they got better.

In the 1920s, lead was added to gasoline to make for smoother driving. It was highly effective in getting the "knocks" out of early versions of the piston engine, as well as elevating the level of lead in the air. Even today, the lead from gasoline lies in the soil of many playgrounds. High levels of lead also improved the performance of paints. Houses built before the 1970s, and especially before the 1950s, still pose a threat to children who often ingest peeling paint.

It was not until the 1970s that the effect of low-dose lead exposure on the development of intellectual function became clear. The studies of Dr. Herbert Needleman and subsequent investigators documented clear-cut negative effects on the intellectual development of young children even at low levels of exposure. This prompted efforts to remove lead from gasoline, paints, and many other products. In recent years, new sources of lead including toys, pottery, and water have been given increased attention. In short, lead is a well-recognized hazard that is still with us.

continues

BOX 8-3 continued.

Efforts to protect the environment have been coupled with efforts to detect and react to elevated lead levels. It is now standard practice in pediatrics and public health to monitor blood levels in high-risk children, investigate their home environments, and treat persistently-elevated levels. Lead standards for playgrounds, lead abatement programs for homes, and lead monitoring of consumer products, all aim to reduce or eliminate the hazards of lead. The system is by no means foolproof and in recent years elevated levels of the metal have been found from such divergent sources as toys manufactured in China and water in Washington, D.C. Table 8-2 summarizes the potential exposures to lead, including their sources, and offers potential means of reducing or eliminating the hazard.[13]

TABLE 8-2 Where Does Lead in our Bodies Come From and What Can Be Done About It?

How lead enters our bodies	Where it comes from	Ways to reduce exposure
Inhalation	Workers in many lead-exposure industries: including mining, smelting, metal repair, or foundry work. Demolition and renovation activities that generate fumes and dust, including home renovations and hobby activities. Addition of lead to gasoline. Once inhaled deep into the lungs may remain for long periods and be absorbed into blood over time	Occupational controls. Phase-out of lead in gasoline in U.S. from 1976 to 1996
Ingestion	Children—normal ingestion of dirt and dust by infants and young children with up to 5% of children who ingest large quantities—a condition called "pica." Children absorb greater percentage of ingested lead than adults. Children's toys and objects that are placed in the mouth are especially important sources. Soil near old high traffic areas often contaminated from previous lead in gas. Glazed pottery often includes lead that can leach into food	Removal of lead paint from older homes—lead levels in paint in the 1950s and earlier were as much as 50% lead. Enforce elimination of lead paint from children's toys. Monitoring and control of lead levels in soil in young children's play areas. Very high blood levels may require "chelation"—treatment to reduce lead levels in blood
Water	Pipes especially in older water supplies and homes built before the mid-1980s often contain lead. Lead used in pipes outside and within the home can leach into water—especially warm water—over time	Regulation of levels of lead in public water supply. Run home water before use—especially after away for extended period. Use cold water for cooking
In-utero	Pregnant women absorb higher percentage of ingested lead compared to children and can cross placenta. Mother's previous lead exposure stored in her bones can be resorbed into her blood during pregnancy	Special effort to reduce exposure by pregnant women including special care with home renovations during pregnancy especially homes built before 1970

Source: Data from Agency for Toxic Substance and Disease Registry. Case Studies in Environmental Medicine—Lead. Available at: http://www.epa.gov/radon/healthrisks.html. Accessed November 8, 2008.

BOX 8-4 Health Risks of Mercury in the Environment

The impact of high-dose mercury on mental function has been recognized since the 19th century. More recently, it was established that much lower levels of mercury pose risks to the fetus. Neurological damage, including learning disabilities and hearing loss, have been documented at low levels of exposure. The human risks of mercury exposure need to be understood as part of the impact of mercury on an entire ecological system.

For much of the late 19th and 20th centuries, mercury was a common product of industry that heavily contaminated the Great Lakes of the United States. The impacts were not appreciated despite the high levels of contamination and the impacts on animal species. Mercury in bodies of water is filtered by fish species and can concentrate in their fat. Thus, certain fish species can and do accumulate high concentrations of mercury. These species may be eaten by fish-eating birds and pose a risk to a number of endangered avian species. There is no technologically-feasible method for removing mercury from the Great Lakes or other bodies of water. Your children's children will most likely be living with mercury contamination.

Recommendations for limiting the consumption of fish, especially by pregnant women, have been the mainstay of efforts to address this problem. These efforts are complicated by the fact that the consumption of fish also carries health benefits. Today, the challenge is how to minimize the amount of mercury consumed by women without losing the benefits of fish consumption. Because some fish have much higher mercury levels than others, the March of Dimes recommends that pregnant women avoid shark, swordfish, king mackerel, and tilefish. They indicate that "it's ok" to eat a limited amount of fish that contain small amounts of mercury, including salmon, pollock, catfish, and canned light tuna.[16] The details of how much fish is safe for pregnant women to eat remains controversial. For today and many years to come, we will be living with the impacts of past environmental contamination on entire ecosystems.

interactions between exposures produce unexpectedly large impacts. We will take a look at two types of strategies that are being developed to address more than one problem at a time. We will begin by looking at a strategy called an interaction analysis. Finally, we will build upon this approach to see how systems analysis is becoming an important approach for addressing issues of environmental health and safety.

WHAT IS AN INTERACTION ANALYSIS APPROACH TO ENVIRONMENTAL DISEASES?

The term interaction analysis implies that to understand and control the impacts of environmental exposures, it is necessary to take into account the effect of two or more exposures. Risk assessment approaches make the assumption that each exposure stands on its own. Thus, if there is more than one type of exposure, we need to make the assumption that the total impact is the sum of the two impacts. For example, if one exposure has a relative risk of 4 and a second has a relative risk of 6, we assume that exposure to both results in a relative risk of 10. Many times adding together the relative risks does provide an approximation of the risk of two or more exposures. However, in an increasing number of situations we are recognizing that there are interactions between exposures themselves so that the presence of both exposures results in

an overall impact much greater than expected. For instance, we might find that having both exposures results in a relative risk of a bad outcome of 4 times 6 or 24 instead of 10. This type of interaction is called **multiplicative interaction**. Box 8-5 examines the multiplicative interaction between radon and cigarette smoking.[17]

WHAT IS A SYSTEMS ANALYSIS APPROACH TO ENVIRONMENTAL HEALTH AND SAFETY?

As we have seen, the traditional risk assessment approach to environmental hazards assumes that each factor acts on its own without explicitly recognizing the interactions that occur. In addition, traditional risk assessment assumes that more is worse and that a very low exposure has little if any impact. That is, it assumes the existence of a dose-response relationship to estimate the magnitude of the potential harm. Not all environmental hazards conform to these major assumptions. As we have seen, both radon and asbestos exposure interact with cigarette smoking and multiply the risk of disease.

Not all risks for environmental disease require high-level or long-term exposure. In addition to causing lung cancer, asbestos has also been shown to cause a form of cancer called mesothelioma, which originates in the lining of the lung or pleura. Even small and short-term exposures to asbestos may

BOX 8-5 Interaction Between Radon and Cigarettes.

Radon is a naturally-occurring radioactive gas. It is colorless and odorless. Radon is produced by the decay of uranium in soil, rock, and groundwater. It emits ionizing radiation during its radioactive decay. Radon is found all over the country though there are areas of the country with substantially higher levels than other areas. Radon gets into the indoor air primarily by entering via the soil under homes and other buildings at the basement or lowest level.

Today, it is recognized that radon is the second most important cause of lung cancer after cigarettes and the most common cause of cancer among nonsmokers. The EPA estimates that radon accounts for over 20,000 cases of lung cancer, as compared with the over 100,000 cases attributed to cigarettes. The average indoor level in the United States is about 1.3pCi/L. The EPA has set a level of 2pCi/L as an attainable level and a level of 4pCi/L as the maximum recommended level. Approximately 15 percent of homes in the United States have basement radon levels above 4pCi/L.

Cigarette smoking and radon exposure are multiplicative; that is, when both are present, the hazard is multiplied. For instance, using the EPA's figures, the relative risk of lung cancer for the average smoker is approximately nine times the risk compared to a nonsmoker. The relative risk from radon when the level is 10pCi/L compared to 2pCi/L is over 4.5. When both cigarette smoking and a level of radon exposure of 10pCi/L are present, the relative risk of lung cancer increases almost 40 times.

The recognition that radon and also asbestos multiply the impacts of cigarette smoking has had a key impact on the approaches used to address these potential hazards. For smokers with exposure to these hazards the risk can be greatly reduced by reductions in radon and asbestos, as well as by stopping smoking. Because both radon and asbestos are potentially controllable environmental exposures, there has been a great deal of attention and money given to control of these hazards. Thus, the recognition of interactions which multiply or greatly increase the risk have become an important tool for setting priorities and developing approaches to risk reduction.

cause mesothelioma as evidenced by well-documented cases among household members who washed the clothing of those exposed. Low-dose environmental exposures to estrogen-like substances may pose threats to the reproductive health of animal species and could even affect the human rate of breast cancer. New technologies, such as nanotechnology, are raising concerns that the risks of low-level exposure need to be investigated as much as those of high level exposure.

Addressing these types of issues requires us to focus on the interactions between multiple factors which together form a system. Environmental problems often come from multiple sources. A now-classic success story of environmental understanding and collaboration in addressing multiple factors at once is the history of the hole in the ozone layer,[18] which is discussed in Box 8-6.

Systems analysis approaches are an increasingly important strategy for addressing environmental health and safety. A systems analysis approach has been used successfully to address the problem of death and disabilities due to transportation injuries. Vast improvements in motor vehicle safety have occurred in recent decades—from bikes to boats to airplanes. Today, for instance, the commercial airline safety system has become a model. It includes a range of connected interventions from aircraft construction to routine maintenance, from efforts to reduce human error to investigation of near misses and actual crashes. The success of these efforts is evidenced by the fact that the goal of zero deaths per year from commercial airlines is nearing reality in the United States. We have also made great progress in land transportation.[19] Much of this progress has resulted from using a systems analysis approach as discussed in Box 8-7.

We have now taken a look at a series of progressively complex approaches being used to address the issues of environmental disease and injuries. The problems of environmental health and safety require increasingly sophisticated solutions. As we will see in future sections, the lessons learned from these efforts have potential applications to other aspects of public health and health care.

We have now looked at the non-communicable diseases, communicable diseases, and environmental health and safety as the way of organizing the major causes of disability and death. Now, let us turn our attention to the organized systems that have been developed for addressing these problems. First, we will look at the healthcare system in general in Section IV. Section V will explore the traditional public health system.

BOX 8-6   Addressing the Problem of the Hole in the Ozone Layer.

It was first recognized in 1985 that the layer of ozone above Antarctica was being depleted at an alarming rate. Ozone in the upper atmosphere is known to protect against damaging radiation from the sun. Fears were raised that the hole in the ozone would expand progressively and encompass populated areas in the southern hemisphere and involve the northern hemisphere as well.

It was quickly recognized that the problem was linked to multiple interacting human and naturally-occurring systems. The use of chloro-fluorocarbons (CFCs) in such products as refrigerators and air conditioning equipment was quickly identified as a major contributor. In addition, commonly-used aerosol sprays from deodorants to hair sprays contained CFCs. More concerning was the use of CFC in devices to deliver medications.

The timely accumulation of data, the rapid understanding of the multiple contributors to the problem, and a worldwide media campaign soon brought together a remarkably effective response to the problem. By 1987, an international agreement, known as the Montreal Protocol, was developed and quickly implemented by most nations. The agreement and subsequent revisions resulted in the rapid phase-out of most uses of CFC with more graduate elimination of CFCs in medical devices.

The hole in the ozone layer continues to expand due to the extremely long half-life of CFCs. The projections, however, are for a turn-around in the near future and a resolution of the problem by 2050. The coordinated scientific, public health, health communications, and political responses have encouraged future efforts to recognize and jointly address multifactor environmental health problems.

BOX 8-7   A Systems Analysis Approach to Motor Vehicle Injuries.

The approach used to address the complex problem of motor vehicle collisions has been a systems analysis approach. It has incorporated elements of health care, traditional public health, as well as social interventions. Motor vehicle injuries in the United States have been the leading cause of death for children and young adults for at least the last half century. Today, they remain a critical problem, how-ever, the death rates from motor vehicle injuries in the United States over the last half-century have fallen so dramatically that the CDC classified highway safety as one of the ten great public health achievements of the 20th century. This progress has not been due to any one intervention—it is the combination of coordinated interventions that have made the difference. Highway safety can be thought of as a systems analysis success story not only because of the progress that has been made, but because of the potential for continued progress in the future. Interventions have often relied upon engineering solutions or technical innovations. Improvements in automobile design, airbags, and in highway construction have been essential elements in preventing and surviving motor vehicle crashes.

Education has played a role as well. Educational efforts have included instructing parents in the use of child restraints, teaching all driv-ers and passengers to wear seat belts, and encouraging the widespread use of the designated driver concept. Motivational efforts have in-cluded lower insurance rates for safe drivers and progressive stages of licensing for young drivers. Mandatory or obligatory efforts have included enforcement of drunk driver laws and seat belt laws.

Connecting the pieces with an emergency medical system has been key to a successful systems analysis approach. The first hour after a serious injury is often called the golden hour—a period of time when emergency interventions can save many lives. A coordinated emer-gency response, emergency department preparedness, and increased use of modern communications equipment have all helped to create a system out of what was formally a series of disconnected interventions.

The challenge of making transportation safe is by no means over. New innovations and new strategies are needed. The success of the systems analysis approach so far gives us encouragement that more progress is on the way.

Key Words

- Unaltered environment
- Altered environment
- Built environment

- Hazards
- Multiplicative interaction

Discussion Questions

Take a look at the questions posed in the following scenarios which were presented at the beginning of this chapter. See now whether you can answer them.

1. *Joe grew up in an industrial district of town. His family lived in an old apartment building and he played in a playground near a major intersection. By the age of 6, Joe was found to have high lead levels in his blood and was not doing well in school. Where could all that lead come from, his mother wondered?*

2. *Jill is pregnant and loves fish, which she has eaten almost daily for years as part of her effort to stay healthy. She hears that fish should not be eaten regularly during pregnancy. Why, she wonders, should I cut down on eating something as healthy as fish?*

3. *Ralph and Sonya, a prosperous professional couple, and their two children live in an older suburban home. They feel secure that their environment is safe. They were surprised to find when they wanted to put their house up for sale that it did not pass the safety tests for radon. Where did the radon come from, they wondered, and what can be done about it?*

4. *Sandra worked for an international agency that had successfully addressed the danger of radiation due to the hole in the ozone layer. She was shocked when she was told that she had a life-threatening skin cancer called melanoma. She asked, what could cause melanoma? Could years of sun exposure have played a role?*

5. *With your seat belt on, children buckled in, and airbags activated, you head out of the driveway to face the world. You didn't see that truck coming when it hit you from the side. The ambulance responded within minutes and took your family to the nearest emergency room. You all made it through with only minor injuries. You ask yourself, was it just luck or did the system work?*

REFERENCES

1. Prevention Institute. The Built Environment and Health. Available at: http://www.preventioninstitute.org/builtenv.html. Accessed March 19, 2009.

2. Mokdad AM, Marks JS, Stroup DF, Gerberding JL. Actual causes of death in the United States 2000. *JAMA*. 2004; 291: 1238–1245.

3. Centers for Disease Control and Prevention National Center for Health Statistics. Deaths—Leading Causes. Available at: http://www.cdc.gov/nchs/FASTATS/lcod.htm. Accessed March 19, 2009.

4. Friis RH. *Essentials of Environmental Health*. Sudbury, MA: Jones and Bartlett Publishers; 2007.

5. Oncology Encyclopedia. Occupational Exposures and Cancer. Available at: http://www.answers.com/topic/occupational-exposures-and-cancer. Accessed March 19, 2009.

6. Centers for Disease Control and Prevention. Environmental Hazards and Health Effects. Available at: http://www.cdc.gov/vaccines/. Accessed March 19, 2009.

7. Greenberg MR. *Environmental Policy Analysis and Practice*. Piscataway, NJ: Rutgers University Press; 2008.

8. Rom WN, Markowitz SB. *Environmental and Occupational Medicine*. Philadelphia: Lippincott, Williams & Wilkins; 2006.

9. U.S. Environmental Protection Agency. Risk Assessment Portal. Available at: http://www.epa.gov/risk/hazardous-identification.htm. Accessed December 14, 2008.

10. Agency for Toxic Substances and Disease Registry. A Citizen's Guide to Risk Assessments and Public Health Assessments. Available at: http://www.atsdr.cdc.gov/publications/citizensGuidetoRiskAssessments.html. Accessed November 21, 2008.

11. Environmental Health News. EPA must overhaul risk assessments to protect public health, panel says. Available at: http://www.environmental healthnews.org/ehs/news/panel-advises-epa-to-overhaul-risk-assessments. Accessed December 13, 2008.

12. Agency for Toxic Substance and Disease Registry. ToxFAQs™ for Lead. Available at: http://www.atsdr.cdc.gov/tfacts13.html. Accessed November 9, 2008.

13. Agency for Toxic Substance and Disease Registry. Case Studies in Environmental Medicine—Lead. Available at: http://www.epa.gov/radon/healthrisks.html. Accessed March 19, 2009.

14. National Defense Resource Council. The Story of Silent Spring. Available at: http://www.nrdc.org/health/pesticides/hcarson.asp. Accessed March 19, 2009.

15. U.S. Environmental Protection Agency. Mercury Study Report to Congress, Volume I, Executive Summary. Available at: http://www.epa.gov/ttn/oarpg/t3/reports/volume1.pdf. Accessed March 19, 2009.

16. March of Dimes. Pregnancy and Newborn Health Education Center. Available at: http://www.marchofdimes.com/pnhec/159_823.asp. Accessed March 19, 2009.

17. United States Environmental Protection Agency. Radon. Available at: http://www.epa.gov/radon/. Accessed March 19, 2009.

18. National Aeronautics and Space Administration. Ozone Hole Watch. Available at: http://ozonewatch.gsfc.nasa.gov/facts/hole.html#nav_bypass. Accessed March 19, 2009.

19. Pfizer Global Pharmaceuticals. *Milestones in Public Health: Accomplishments in Public Health over the Last 100 Years*. New York: Pfizer Global Pharmaceuticals; 2006.

Section III: Cases and Discussion Questions

High Blood Pressure: A Public Health and Healthcare Success

Elevated levels of blood pressure, or hypertension, have been observed since the development of blood pressure measurements in the 19th century. It was soon recognized that populations with a high frequency of elevated blood pressure were also populations with a high frequency of strokes, yet the dangers of high blood pressure often went unappreciated until recent years.

High blood pressure is a condition that historically has affected both the privileged and the underprivileged in our society. Presidents Woodrow Wilson and Franklin Delano Roosevelt both had high blood pressure and suffered strokes and heart disease. Today, the condition is disproportionately present among African Americans—15 to 20 percent have some degree of elevated blood pressure.

For many years, high blood pressure was considered a consequence of disease rather than its cause. Clinicians seeing a patient with a stroke, for instance, often attributed their elevation in blood pressure to the stroke rather than the other way around. Long-term studies, such as the Framingham Heart Study that followed a large number of individuals for many years, established that the high blood pressure actually preceded strokes and not the other way around. High blood pressure as a contributory cause of strokes, as well as heart and kidney disease, was fully confirmed only after randomized clinical trials in the late 1960s and early 1970s established that lower blood pressure leads to reduced frequency of these afflictions. Screening for high blood pressure became widespread in the same period in large part as a result of these investigations. Elevated levels were initially defined as 140/100 or greater, based upon a range of normal obtained by measuring the blood pressure on large numbers of adult Americans. What were once considered acceptable levels of blood pressure have been redefined as elevated levels in recent years. Today, the desirable level is considered 120/80 or lower. These changing levels are justified by follow-up data from a large number of individuals that demonstrate that even levels of blood pressure only slightly above 120/80 are associated with increased risk of stroke and heart disease.

The fluctuating levels of blood pressure often make it difficult to establish an individual's average level. Electronic monitoring of blood pressure over a 24-hour period has become a feasible and acceptable gold standard for establishing an individual's average level. Early detection and successful treatments have been shown to effectively reduce the consequences of high blood pressure. Weight loss and salt restriction are often prescribed initially with subsequent introduction of one or more drugs. Most, if not all individuals with elevated blood pressure, respond to drug treatment with tolerable or no side effects, but need to continue treatment for many years—usually for the rest of their lives.

A national public health campaign began in the 1970s to encourage individuals to know their blood pressure and to urge clinicians to treat detected elevated levels. In recent decades, national surveys have indicated that a gradually increasing percentage of patients with elevated blood pressures are being successfully treated and that there has been a substantial reduction in strokes and deaths from strokes. Recent evidence showing that reducing the high salt levels in the American diet can reduce the average level of blood pressure has prompted renewed public health efforts to change eating habits and the contents of commercial foods.

Today, treatment of high blood pressure is recognized as one of the most cost-effective interventions. Its cost per quality-adjusted life year saved is only a few thousand dollars a year for the average person. For high-risk groups, such as those with diabetes, it actually saves money to monitor and treat high blood pressure rather than allow it to cause or exacerbate other health problems requiring more expensive treatments.

1. How does this history of high blood pressure demonstrate the problem description and etiology components of the P.E.R.I. process? What different types of studies were used to establish etiology or contributory cause?

2. How does this history of high blood pressure illustrate the evidence-based recommendations and implementation/evaluation components of the P.E.R.I. process?

3. Explain the justification for updating the definition of what is considered a "healthy" blood pressure level.

4. How does this history of high blood pressure demonstrate the application of the four criteria for a successful screening program?

5. Using the four quadrants of cost and effectiveness, how would you classify treatment of hypertension for the average person? For those with diabetes?

Testing and Screening

Ken had just turned 40 and with a little encouragement from his wife, he decided that it was time to have a physical—it would be his first real visit to a doctor since he broke his arm as a kid. Seeing a doctor hadn't made sense to him before. He was in great shape, felt fine, and didn't smoke. Maybe it was his 65-year-old father's sudden death from a heart attack just a few weeks after his retirement that finally convinced Ken to find himself a doctor. He knew that his father had had high cholesterol, but he was told his own cholesterol level and electrocardiogram results were okay when he entered the military at age 18. Besides, Ken wasn't big on desserts and only ate a Big Mac when he took the kids out after their soccer games.

The examination was quite uneventful and Ken was reassured when the doctor couldn't find anything of concern. A few recommendations on nutrition and better ways to exercise were about all that came out of the visit. Then he got the call from the doctor's office—could he make a follow-up appointment to discuss his cholesterol?

His low-density lipoprotein (LDL, or "bad" cholesterol) was 165 and his high-density lipoprotein (HDL, or "good" cholesterol) was 40. "We used to think these levels were okay since they are so common," his doctor began." However, now we consider your LDL cholesterol too high because it increases your chances of developing heart and other blood vessel diseases. There's no evidence of heart disease at this point, but your cholesterol needs attention."

"What do you mean by attention?" Ken replied. "I exercise, don't smoke, and generally keep my fats down." Ken soon learned a lot more about cholesterol. He first tried his best at changing his diet—it helped a little, but just didn't do the trick. Ken's doctor told him: "For some people there is a strong genetic component to high cholesterol levels and while diet is still important, it just can't always reduce LDL cholesterol enough by itself. Exercise helps, especially by increasing the good cholesterol, but it doesn't do much for the

bad cholesterol. Medication may be needed and there is now evidence that if taken regularly, it reduces the chances of having a heart attack or at least delays its occurrence."

Taking medication every day was not so easy for Ken, but he stuck with the plan. His doctor asked him to have his cholesterol levels checked every few months for the first year. Ken was amazed at how well the medicine worked. His LDL fell from 165 to less than 100 on only a modest dose. In addition to routine cholesterol checks, Ken had his blood tested for potential side effects from the medication, such as impacts to his liver, and he was required to report any long-lasting muscle aches and pains. The good news was that he couldn't tell he was taking the medication—he felt just fine.

Now that the cholesterol levels had dropped, he thought maybe he could go off the medication if he just watched his diet closely. His doctor let him try that for a month, but after the 30 days were up his LDL level was back up to 160. "Looks like you're hooked on medication for life," his doctor said with a wry smile, adding, "at least the extra cost is worth the extra benefit." Ken and his wife were told the high cholesterol levels were a genetic condition. Not only did Ken need to take the medication on a permanent basis, but the pediatricians began testing his kids. The doctors said, "we are beginning to understand the genetics behind this condition and would like to do some genetic testing on the children, including that new baby of yours." Ken wondered if the information on his children's cholesterol levels would be part of their medical records for the rest of their lives. "You're not planning to put that on the Internet, are you?" Ken joked nervously as they drew blood from his newborn son.

1. How are the range of normal- and desirable-range approaches to establishing a reference interval and defining a positive and negative test illustrated in this case? Explain.

2. What arguments are presented in this case that fulfill the criteria for screening for high cholesterol? Explain.

3. What definition of cost-effectiveness is being used to justify screening and treatment of elevated LDL cholesterol?

4. What ethical issues need to be considered in screening for conditions such as elevated LDL cholesterol? Explain.

What to Do about Lyme Disease?

You have just moved into a new subdivision—your first home with your young family. The first week you are there, a neighbor tells you that her son has developed Lyme disease and now has chronic arthritis that requires extensive treatment.

Lyme disease is an increasingly common disease that can cause acute and chronic arthritis if not treated early and correctly. In rare instances, it can cause life-threatening heart disease and temporary paralysis often to one side of the face due to nerve damage. The disease is caused by an organism known as a spirochete, which is spread from deer ticks to humans via tick bites. Lyme disease is especially common in communities with large deer populations.

Ticks must remain in place on the human skin at least 12 to 24 hours in order to extract human blood and inject the spirochete organism at the site of the bite. Complete removal of the small, but visible tick within 24 hours usually prevents the disease. Deer ticks are most abundant in the late spring and tend to live on tall grasses from which they can easily move to the bare legs of children and adults. The disease frequently first appears as a circular red rash around the site of the bite. At this stage, early diagnosis and treatment with antibiotics is usually successful. Several weeks or months later, the onset of arthritis may occur and can be difficult to diagnose. A missed diagnosis may result in severe arthritis that is difficult to treat. A vaccine has been developed and briefly marketed to prevent the disease, but it was quite expensive and only partially successful.

In your new hometown, the local health department is charged with developing a plan for control or elimination of Lyme disease. As an informed and concerned citizen, you are invited to give input on the plan identifying possible interventions.

1. What primary interventions would you consider?
2. What secondary interventions would you consider?
3. What tertiary interventions would you consider?
4. What educational interventions do you recommend?
5. Can Lyme disease be eradicated? Can it be controlled?

Sharma's Village

Sharma lives in a small farming village in south Asia, but she could just as well be living in Haiti, Ethiopia, Ghana, or several dozen other countries classified by the World Bank as low-income economies. Her home is a small hut and she works daily with her mother to gather firewood for their small indoor fireplace that acts as the kitchen stove. The smoke often makes her eyes water because there is no chimney or other ventilation. At night, she sleeps with her extended family in a room where mosquitoes bite her regularly. Despite the fact that Sharma lives in a rural community, the villagers live in crowded quarters. The water the family drinks is carried by the women from a well several hundred yards from their home. The water sometimes tastes bad, but it is all they have to drink.

The family farms a small plot of land on the hillside, which had become eroded from years of cutting trees. The last big

monsoon to hit the area created a landslide, which left the village underwater for several weeks creating mold in nearly every home. Most of the adults have goiters from the lack of iodine in the soil. The addition of iodine to salt has prevented goiters in the children. Pesticides are used widely to control mosquitoes and agricultural pests, but the farmers receive little education on their safe use. Recently, a new road was built connecting her village with the neighboring towns. Despite the advantages of having the new road, cars and trucks now speed through her village, rarely stopping to let people cross the road.

In Sharma's village, the life expectancy is 49 years. Babies often die of diarrheal diseases in the first year of life and mothers occasionally die in childbirth. Malaria is widespread and hookworm disease is present among those who farm the fields and in children, whose ability to learn is often affected. Malnutrition is also widespread despite the fact that farming is the major occupation in the village. Chronic lung disease among adults and asthma among the young is surprisingly common even though cigarette smoking is rare. Tuberculosis is widespread and a major cause of death, however there are few cases of HIV/AIDS in the area. Unexplained neurological diseases among farm workers occur regularly. The most common cause of death among teenagers is motor vehicle injuries along the new road even though there is only one truck in the village.

1. What environmental risk factors contributing to disease and other health conditions are illustrated in this case? Classify each as an unaltered, altered, or built environment factor.
2. Discuss at least two examples of how disease or other conditions found in the village can be explained by the environmental risk factors?
3. Identify at least two interventions that would make a large difference in the health of this village.
4. What changes do you expect to occur in this village as social and economic development take place?

Asthma—It's in the Air

Joe had asthma for as long as he could remember. Struggling to keep up with his friends on the playground was among one of his earliest memories. In those days no one worried about it—"you'll outgrow it"—they'd tell him. He grew up not too far from an oil refinery and lots of kids had asthma. He can still remember the debate in town about whether it was worth the costs to reduce the pollution. Asthma kept him out of sports, but turned his attention to schoolwork. He always said the asthma was the key to his academic success. It even kept him from smoking—the wheezing just got too bad whenever he inhaled deeply.

When he left home for college, his asthma seemed to improve. He could now take long walks without discomfort. However, it was more than a little embarrassing for him when he had to stop near the top of a small hill to catch his breath while taking a short hike with his girlfriend. With her encouragement, he finally agreed to go to the clinic to see what could be done. The doctor prescribed an inhaler and told him to work with the physician assistant to see if they "could get down to the bottom of this." The inhaler worked so well and so quickly that Joe decided just to use it whenever he exercised. He even found that he could use it before a cigarette and could now smoke just to be sociable.

Joe didn't return to the clinic again until the prescription ran out. This time, the physician assistant insisted that he learn more about asthma. Joe learned the danger of cigarettes, the need to stay on treatment even when he was doing well, and the importance of rapidly treating worsening symptoms. He also began to understand the importance of getting an annual influenza vaccine and taking that pneumococcal vaccine that he'd originally rejected.

Things went well for a couple of years until despite his best efforts at prevention, he suffered a full-blown asthma attack. The antibiotics he was prescribed didn't do the trick and he ended up in the hospital requiring a ventilator for a couple of days. He couldn't understand what had happened to him—he had tried to do everything right. "It's not your fault," his doctor and physician assistant told him. "Those antibiotics have been used so much that they don't touch some of the bugs anymore. We had to give you some new and expensive drugs that aren't even available as pills."

Joe seemed to understand—there were things he could and should do, but it wasn't all in his control. He now realized that with asthma there were bigger issues—it's in the air, as well as in the lungs, and it can also be in the genes. These words really hit home when his son experienced his first asthma attack before his first birthday. Joe now knew that you don't always outgrow asthma.

1. What does this case illustrate about the relationship of genetics and environmental causes of disease?
2. What preventive efforts are illustrated in this case?
3. What do you think are the advantages and disadvantages of emphasizing better treatment of asthma versus control of air pollution?
4. What do you think is the proper role of cost considerations in addressing environmental issues such as asthma?

Health Professionals, Healthcare Institutions, and Healthcare Systems

In this section, we will take a look at healthcare systems, the people, institutions, and organizational structures that deliver health care to individuals. In the United States, the healthcare system consumes well over $2,000,000,000,000 in resources—that's two TRILLION dollars.

To understand how the U.S. healthcare system functions and is organized, we will start in Chapter 9 by taking a look at the people who provide health services. There are over 15 million people involved in the delivery of health services. We will focus on three of the largest groups: physicians, nurses, and the public health professionals.

In Chapter 10, we will discuss the institutions involved in the delivery of healthcare services and how they interact or do not interact with each other. We will also examine methods for maximizing the quality of health care. Finally, we will examine the healthcare system as a whole in Chapter 11. We will aim to understand how the system is financed and look at the issue of access to care and the costs of that care. These particular issues have become the center of the debate about what needs to be addressed to improve the U.S. healthcare system. To provide perspective, we will also examine the characteristics of some other healthcare systems in developed countries.

Figure 4-A displays the components of a healthcare system that will guide our discussion of this complex subject.

Let us begin in Chapter 9 by turning our attention to the types of clinical and public health professionals that are part of the health workforce.

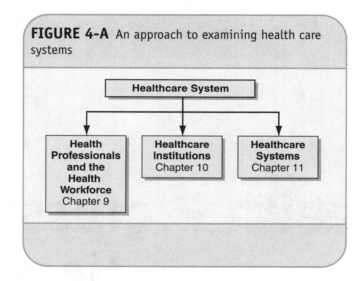

FIGURE 4-A An approach to examining health care systems

Health Professionals and the Health Workforce

LEARNING OBJECTIVES

By the end of this chapter the student will be able to:

- describe roles that education and credentialing play in the development of health professions, such as medicine and nursing.
- describe relationships between clinical health professions and public health.
- identify educational pathways for becoming a public health professional.
- identify components of prevention and public health that are recommended for inclusion in clinical education.
- explain the concept of primary care and differentiate it from secondary and tertiary care.
- identify a range of mechanisms used to compensate clinical health professionals and explain their advantages and disadvantages.

Upon arrival at the hospital, the nurse specialist examines you and consults with the radiologists, the gastroenterologist, and the general surgeon. Your medication is reviewed by the PharmD, and your meals by the clinical nutritionist. Throughout the hospitalization you are followed by a hospitalist. Once you get back home, the home care team comes to see you regularly for the first two weeks and the physician assistant and registered nurse see you in the office. You realize that health care is no longer just about doctors and nurses. You ask yourself: what roles do all of these health professionals play in the healthcare system?

Jenna decides that after college she wants to become a doctor and practice medicine. "I thought there was only one kind of doctor who could diagnose disease and prescribe medicine," she mentions at a career counseling meeting. "Not so, anymore," says her advisor. "There are allopathic and osteopathic physicians. In

addition, there are nurse practitioners who are authorized to diagnose and prescribe medications, and there are physician assistants who do the same under a physician's supervision. The universe of "doctors" now includes doctors of nursing practice, as well as other doctoral degree professionals, such as pharmacists and physical therapists." Understanding careers in health care can be as difficult for students as it is for patients, Jenna thinks to herself. Now she understands why her advisor asked: "what do you mean by 'practice'? What do you mean by 'doctor'?"

Sarah was about to begin medical school and was expecting two years of "preclinical" classroom lectures focusing on the basic sciences, followed by the study of clinical diseases. Then, as she'd heard from her physician father, she expected two years of clinical hospital "rotations" and electives investigating specialties. She is surprised to find that medical school has changed. There are small group problem-based learning sessions where she needs to be able to locate and read the research literature. There is contact with patients and their problems right from the beginning. There is increasingly a four-year approach instead of a preclinical and clinical approach to medical education. She wonders: are these changes for the better? What else needs to be done to improve medical education?

You are interested in clinical care, as well as public health. "I need to make a choice," you think to yourself. "Not necessarily," your advisor says. "There are many ways to combine clinical care with public health." After a little investigation, you find out that undergraduate public health education is increasingly seen as preparation for clinical education and clinical prevention and population health are increasingly becoming part of clinical care. In addition, many careers from health administration, to health policy, to clinical research, combine the individual orientation of clinical care with the population perspective of public health. So what's the best pathway to a public health career for you?

WHAT DO WE MEAN BY A HEALTH PROFESSIONAL?

Until the early years of the 20th century, education and practice for the health professions was an informal process often without standardized admissions requirements, curricula, or even formal recognition of a profession. Throughout the 20th century and into the 21st, there has been an ongoing movement to formalize the education process for health professionals. These formal requirements have come to define what we mean by a health professional and include admission prerequisites, coursework requirements, examinations of competency, official recognition of educational achievements, and granting of permission to practice. Today, the list of formal health professions is very long. Clinical health professions may be classified as physicians, nurses, dentists, pharmacists, optometrists, psychologists, podiatrists, and chiropractors. They also include nurse practitioners, physician assistants, health services administrators, and allied health practitioners.[1] "Allied health practitioner" is a broad category in its own right, ranging from graduate degree trained professionals, such as physical therapists, occupational therapists, and medical social workers, to technical specialists often with an associate's degree, such as dental assistants, sonographers, and laboratory technicians.

Within public health, there is a growing array of health specialties. Some specialties require associate or bachelor's degrees, such as environmental health technicians, environmental health specialists, and health educators. However, many public health roles require graduate degrees that focus on disciplines including: epidemiology, biostatistics, environmental sciences, health administration and policy, and social and behavioral sciences.

Education and training are central to the development and definition of most health professions. Education implies that a student is pursuing a degree or certificate from an accredited educational institution. Training is often organized and directed outside of educational institution. Hospitals, health departments, and large group practices often have the responsibility of training new health professionals.

Before we take a look at specific health professions, let's step back and ask the more general question: how do education and training serve to define health professions?

HOW DO EDUCATION AND TRAINING SERVE TO DEFINE HEALTH PROFESSIONS?

Defining and enforcing educational requirements is central to creating and maintaining a profession. This can be accomplished using two basic approaches: **accreditation** and **credentialing**.

Accreditation implies a process of setting standards for educational and training institutions and enforcing these standards using a regularly-scheduled institutional self-study and an outside review. Accreditation is used by most health professions to define and enforce educational expectations. At times, these expectations may be laid out in detail down to the level of square footage per student for laboratory space and the number of hours devoted to specific subjects. In other health professions, educational subject areas may be outlined and institutions left to judge how to best implement the curriculum.

Credentialing implies that the individual, rather than the institution, is evaluated. Credentialing is a generic term indicating a process of verifying that an individual has the desirable or required qualifications to practice a profession. Credentialing often takes the form of **certification**. Certification is generally a profession-led process in which applicants who have completed the required educational process take an examination. Successful completion of formal examinations leads to recognition in the form of certification.

Certification also has come to define specialties and even subspecialties within a profession. Successful completion of a specialty or subspecialty examination may entitle a health professional to call themselves "board-certified." Certification is often a prerequisite for **licensure**, which is a state governmental function and usually requires more than certification. It may include residency requirements, a legal background check, continuing education requirements, etc. Licensure, when applicable, is usually required for practice of a health profession.

Thus, in order to understand what is meant by a particular health profession, it is important to understand the credentials that are expected or required. Let us take a look at the education required for specific health professions, such as physicians, nurses, and public health professionals.

WHAT IS THE EDUCATION AND TRAINING PROCESS FOR PHYSICIANS?

Physicians are a central part of what is called the practice of medicine. They can be categorized as allopathic and osteopathic physicians. Allopathic physicians graduate with an MD degree, while osteopathic physicians graduate from osteopathic medical schools and receive a DO degree. Graduates of both allopathic and osteopathic medical schools are eligible to apply for the same residency and fellowship programs for their postgraduate medical education. The number of osteopathic medical schools has grown rapidly in recent years and now totals approximately 30 nationwide. Allopathic medical schools number approximately 130 and have only recently begun to again grow in size and number.[a]

Within medicine, specialties and subspecialties continue to emerge. For instance hospice and palliative medicine has recently been added to the list of specialties and others such as hospitalists may be moving in that direction. Table 9-1 outlines many of the current specialties and subspecialties within the field of medicine.[2]

Box 9-1 discusses the process of medical education and the changes that have occurred in recent years and continue to evolve.[3]

Now let us take a brief look at the largest of the health professions—nursing.[4]

WHAT IS THE EDUCATION AND TRAINING PROCESS FOR NURSING?

Nursing as a profession dates from the middle of the 19th century, when it began to be organized as a profession in England. Florence Nightingale is often associated with the founding of nursing as a profession. In the United States, the nursing profession grew out of the Civil War and the essential role played by women in this conflict who performed what we would today call nursing functions. Nursing has long been organized as a distinct profession and is governed by its own set of laws often refer to as the "nursing practice acts."

Today, there are a wide range of health professionals that fall under the legal definition of nursing. Licensed practical nurses (LPNs) provide a range of services often under the direction of registered nurses (RN). An LPN's educational requirements vary widely from state to state, ranging from short-term education after high school to a two-year associate's degree.

Registered nurses are central to the nursing profession and they are usually responsible for hospital-based services. Each state defines its own requirements for RN licensure. Traditionally, many nurses graduated with a diploma which was offered through hospital-based programs. The move toward integrating nursing into the formal degree system has resulted in nurses with associate's degrees, bachelor's of science in nursing (BSN), as well as graduate degrees. Being a registered nurse (RN) requires a state license that, depending on the state, may or may not require a BSN degree.

Advanced nursing degrees are offered as masters of science in nursing, or as an academic research-based degree, the PhD and a clinical doctorate, the doctor in nursing practice (DNP).

Until recent years, there was little formal specialization within nursing, at least compared to physicians and other health professions. Nurse midwives and nurse anesthetists, however, are two traditional specializations within nursing. Graduate-level education and training of nurses has expanded rapidly in recent years. Nursing has added a series of advanced practice degrees including nurse practitioners, as well as specialists such as pediatric, geriatric, and intensive care nurses. The Doctor of Nursing Practice (DNP) degree is becoming recognized for a range of specialty areas within nursing. It is expected to replace many nursing master's degrees over the next decade.

Recent changes in nursing have opened up the option to pursue a bachelor's degree in a range of fields followed by a shorter degree program leading to a BSN or a nurse practitioner degree. As we will see later in the chapter, the shortage of nurses is often seen as the most critical workforce issue in the health field. Now, let us take a look public health professionals.[5, 6]

WHAT IS THE EDUCATION AND TRAINING PROCESS FOR PUBLIC HEALTH PROFESSIONALS?

In the United States, education in public health began as part of medicine in the late 19th century. Shortly before and after World War I, with the support of the Rockefeller Foundation, separate schools of public health were established. The aim of the initial schools of public health was to train physicians, nurses, and other professionals who sought to play lead roles in local and state health departments. Thus, for many years public health education was often combined with other professions. Box 9-2 discusses the roles of clinicians in public health.

Public health professionals today include those who specialize in a wide range of disciplines and work in a variety of settings from governmental public health to not-for-profit and for-profit institutions, as well as in educational and healthcare institutions. There are approximately 500,000 public health professionals in the United States and it is estimated that in coming years there will be a substantial shortage, especially in federal and state health departments.[5]

Public health is one of the last health fields to formalize educational and professional requirements. Today, many public health professionals are trained exclusively in public health and the process of formal credentialing is underway. The

---

[a] Osteopathic and allopathic medical education curricula are quite similar today. The prerequisite for admission are similar and both types of medical schools generally require the Medical School Admissions Test (MCAT). However, osteopathic medical education retains its focus on manipulation of the muscular skeletal system and sees itself as providing a holistic approach to medicine, including a greater focus on prevention. A substantially higher percentage of DOs go into primary care as compared to MDs.

TABLE 9-1 Selected Specialities and Subspecialities of Medicine

Example of specialty area	Example of subspecialty area	Example of specialty area	Example of subspecialty area
Anesthesiology	Critical Care Medicine Hospice and Palliative Medicine Pain Medicine	Otolaryngology	Neurotology Pediatric Otolaryngology Plastic Surgery within the Head and Neck Sleep Medicine
Emergency Medicine	Hospice and Palliative Medicine Medical Toxicology Pediatric Emergency Medicine Sports Medicine Undersea and Hyperbaric Medicine	PATHOLOGY Anatomic Pathology and Clinical Pathology Pathology—Anatomic Pathology—Clinical	Blood Banking/Transfusion Medicine Chemical Pathology Cytopathology Dermatopathology Forensic Pathology Hematology Medical Microbiology Molecular Genetic Pathology Neuropathology Pediatric Pathology
Family Medicine	Adolescent Medicine Geriatric Medicine Hospice and Palliative Medicine Sleep Medicine Sports Medicine		
Internal Medicine	Adolescent Medicine Cardiovascular Disease Clinical Cardiac Electrophysiology Critical Care Medicine Endocrinology, Diabetes, and Metabolism Gastroenterology Geriatric Medicine Hematology Hospice and Palliative Medicine Infectious Disease Interventional Cardiology Medical Oncology Nephrology Pulmonary Disease Rheumatology Sleep Medicine Sports Medicine Transplant Hepatology	Pediatrics	Adolescent Medicine Child Abuse Pediatrics Developmental-Behavioral Pediatrics Hospice and Palliative Medicine Medical Toxicology Neonatal-Perinatal Medicine Neurodevelopmental Disabilities Pediatric Cardiology Pediatric Critical Care Medicine Pediatric Emergency Medicine Pediatric Endocrinology Pediatric Gastroenterology Pediatric Hematology-Oncology Pediatric Infectious Diseases Pediatric Nephrology Pediatric Pulmonology Pediatric Rheumatology Pediatric Transplant Hepatology Sleep Medicine Sports Medicine
Obstetrics and Gynecology	Critical Care Medicine Gynecologic Oncology Hospice and Palliative Medicine[1] Maternal and Fetal Medicine Reproductive Endocrinology/Infertility	Physical Medicine and Rehabilitation	Hospice and Palliative Medicine Pain Medicine Neuromuscular Medicine Pediatric Rehabilitation Medicine Spinal Cord Injury Medicine Sports Medicine
Orthopaedic Surgery	Orthopaedic Sports Medicine Surgery of the Hand		

continues

TABLE 9-1 Selected Specialities and Subspecialities of Medicine (continued)

Example of specialty area	Example of subspecialty area	Example of specialty area	Example of subspecialty area
Plastic Surgery	Plastic Surgery within the Head and Neck	RADIOLOGY	Diagnostic Radiological Physics
	Surgery of the Hand	Diagnostic Radiology	Hospice and Palliative Medicine
		Radiation Oncology	Medical Nuclear Physics
PREVENTIVE MEDICINE-	Medical Toxicology	Radiologic Physics	Neuroradiology
Aerospace Medicine	Undersea and Hyperbaric		Nuclear Radiology
Occupational Medicine	Medicine		Pediatric Radiology
Public Health and General			Therapeutic Radiological Physics
Preventive Medicine			Vascular and Interventional Radiology
Psychiatry	Addiction Psychiatry		
Neurology	Child and Adolescent Psychiatry	Surgery	Hospice and Palliative Medicine
Neurology with Special	Clinical Neurophysiology	Vascular Surgery	Pediatric Surgery
Qualifications in	Forensic Psychiatry		Surgery of the Hand
Child Neurology	Geriatric Psychiatry		Surgical Critical Care
	Hospice and Palliative Medicine	Urology	Pediatric Urology
	Neurodevelopmental Disabilities		
	Neuromuscular Medicine		
	Pain Medicine		
	Psychosomatic Medicine		
	Sleep Medicine		
	Vascular Neurology		

Source: Data from American Board of Medical Specialties http://www.abms.org/Who_We_Help/Physicians/specialties.aspx. Accessed December 15, 2008.

recognition of public health as a distinct professional field with its own educational process has been formalized through accreditation of public health schools and programs by the Council on Education for Public Health (CEPH). CEPH requires five areas of knowledge basic to public health: biostatistics; epidemiology; environmental health sciences; social and behavioral sciences; and health services management. Specific disciplines within public health, such as epidemiology and social and behavioral sciences, have provided recognition for specialized training through advanced degrees, such as the academically-oriented Doctor of Philosophy (PhD) degree and the practice-oriented Doctor of Public Health (DrPH) degree.

Specific technical areas have existed within public health for many years and have included competency examinations, especially in fields such as occupational and environmental health. Health educators in recent decades have formalized and standardized their education and increasingly taken on the structure of a profession including examinations, certifications, and continuing education requirements.

Formal certification as a public health specialist has only been available since 2008, when the first certifying examination was given. The examination covers the five areas expected for a professional master's degree, such as a Master's of Public Health (MPH). These are biostatistics, epidemiology, environmental health sciences, social and behavioral sciences, and health policy and management. In addition, new cross-cutting competencies have been defined and are being incorporated into the examination. These include: communications and informatics, diversity and culture, leadership, professionalism, program planning, systems thinking, and public health biology.

The certifying examination tests core competencies, rather than more advanced competencies that students frequently achieve as part of their education in a public health specialty. Certification is a voluntary process, though it is expected that many employers will look for certification as an important credential. Licensure of public health professionals is not yet an issue. Thus, public health, along with health care, has increasingly formalized its educational requirements, formal credentialing, and competencies.[5,6] This process is likely to continue.

BOX 9-1   Medical Education.

Medical education in 19th and early 20th century America was built upon the apprentice system. Future physicians, nearly all men, worked under and learned from practicing physicians. Medical schools were often moneymaking enterprises and primarily used lectures without patient contact or laboratory experiences. That changed with the introduction of the European model of science-based medical education, hospital-based clinical rotations, and a four-year education model. The 1910 Flexner Report formalized these standards, which soon became universal for medical education in the United States, in what came to be called the Flexner era of American medicine. This era extended into the 1980s, and at some institutions into the 21st century. It led to the growth and dominance of specialties and specialists within particular medical fields.

Hospital-based residency programs and fellowships leading to specialty and subspecialty training became the dominant form of clinical training. Emphasizing this trend, medical school education came to be called **undergraduate medical education**. Medical school was traditionally formally or informally divided into two years of basic science or preclinical training, followed by two years of hospital-based clinical rotations in specialty areas including surgery, internal medicine, obstetrics and gynecology, and psychiatry. This division of medical education is reflected in the examinations of the National Board of Medical Examiners, which traditionally included Part 1 after the second year of medical school, Part 2 prior to graduation, and Part 3 after the first year residency often called the "internship." Additional specialty and subspecialty board examinations were linked to completion of training that occurs after medical school.

Change began to accelerate in medical education during the mid-1980s with the increasing movement of health care outside of hospitals, the increased medical school enrollment of women and minorities, a broader view of what should be included in medical education, and a better understanding of how learning takes place. Specific changes have occurred in the last two decades at all stages of medical education and new proposals for change continue to be formally reviewed and implemented. These can be outlined as follows, starting with the pre-med college years and continuing through residency and fellowship training:

- Premedical training in the Flexner era was largely restricted to majors in the physical and biological sciences, plus specific social sciences such as psychology. Beginning in the early 1990s, medical schools encouraged a wider range of majors, while usually retaining biology, chemistry, and physics courses as prerequisites. Medical schools are increasingly receptive to a wide range of preparation for medical education, encouraging completion of courses in behavioral and social sciences including public health, and epidemiology. A comprehensive review of the Medical College Admissions Test (MCAT) is now underway and may greatly broaden the examination to cover disciplines beyond the natural sciences.
- Admission to medical school was dominated by white males throughout the Flexner era. In the last 20–30 years, the percentage of women applicants has increased steadily. Today, the majority of medical students at many institutions are females. Likewise, the increase in minority applicants has paralleled the changes occurring in other aspects of American education and society.
- The first two years of medical school in the Flexner era were dominated by lectures and laboratories. Basic sciences were the focus with little or no patient contact. An important change in the last two decades includes widespread use of Problem Based Learning (PBL). PBL is characterized by small-group, student-initiated learning centered on "cases" or patient-oriented problems. New curricula in medical education, including evidence-based medicine, interviewing skills, and ethics, have become a standard part of coursework. A new simulated patient interview and physical examination are now part of the examination process.
- Changes in the third and fourth years of medical school began in the 1960s, the era of student activism. Since then, the fourth year of medical school has been dominated by electives. Fourth-year students may choose formal courses, elective clinical experiences, or a wide array of other options. These usually include: options for laboratory or clinical research, international experiences, and clinical rotations at other institutions, often called "audition" rotations, designed to increase a graduate's potential for selection as a resident.
- The growing trend of patient treatment outside of the traditional hospital setting has increased the range of types and locations of clinical experiences available. Most medical schools now require primary care experiences, along with traditional specialty rotations.
- Residency training has paralleled the changes in medical school with greater outpatient and less inpatient, or hospital-based education. Fellowship training beyond residency is now a routine part of the process of specialization. The general move toward more and more specialization has led to longer postgraduate training. The rigors of residency training remain, but limits have now been placed on it by the Residency Review Committees (RRCs), which govern graduate medical education. An average of 80 hours per week and 30 hours at one time are now the maximum standards for residents.

(continues)

BOX 9-1 continued.

Further changes in medical education and residency programs can be expected in the near future. The increasing recognition that health care is a group, and not an individual enterprise, is leading to a focus on interprofessional education and practice. An appreciation that evidence is central to improving quality and controlling costs should continue to encourage the critical reading of clinical research as part of evidence-based medicine in medical school and in journal clubs as part of postgraduate education. The use of computer-based information systems should increase the sharing and coordination of information; the ability to monitor and control health care; and the ways that physicians communicate with colleagues and patients. Technology is also likely to have continued unexpected impacts on the ways that medicine is taught, learned, and practiced.

BOX 9-2 Roles of Clinicians in Public Health.

Public health is often distinguished from the clinical health profession by its focus on populations rather than individuals; public service rather than individual service; disease prevention and health promotion rather than disease diagnosis and treatment; and its broad perspective on the determinants of disease. However, at the professional level individuals have commonly combined the two approaches or moved from one to the other.

Clinicians have always played key roles in public health. From the early years of formal public health training nearly a century ago, until the 1960s and 1970s, the Master of Public Health (MPH) degree was aimed primarily at physicians and nurses who were expected to take up leadership roles in health departments. Today, public health professionals come from much more diverse backgrounds, many entering masters programs directly after receiving a bachelor's degree. The role of clinicians in public health is also far more varied. For instance, today's pharmacists—now educated as doctors of pharmacy or PharmDs—play an increasingly important public health role in providing education about drugs for patients and practitioners and controlling prescription drug abuse. Prevention of dental and gum disease and early detection of oral cancers have much improved due to the careful attention of dentists and dental assistants. The dental profession has been a long-standing advocate of fluoridation of public water systems and other population health interventions.

Primary care specialists, including allopathic and osteopathic physicians, nurse practitioners, and physician assistants, are on the front lines of clinical prevention. Their involvement in screening, behavioral counseling, immunization, and the use of preventive medication, is key to the success of these efforts. Primary care clinicians, as well as specialty care clinicians, also have important roles to play in being alert to new diseases or changes in well-known diseases; reporting adverse effects of drugs, vaccines, and medical devices; and coordinating case-finding efforts with public health agencies.

Within medicine, the field of preventive medicine has a long history. Formal specializations exist in public health and general preventive medicine, occupational medicine, as well as aerospace medicine.

Finally, all clinicians have the right and often the responsibility to advocate for improvements in patient care and of the health system as a whole. A few clinical specialties, such as pediatrics, regard advocacy as a core responsibility of the profession. Their work has had major impacts on child health policies ranging from the use of child car restraints, to advocacy for pediatric HIV/AIDS care, to universal coverage of childhood vaccinations, as well as provision of comprehensive insurance coverage for children.

Joint clinical and public health degrees are now widely available. Many schools in the fields of nursing, physician assistants, dentistry, social work, and the law, offer options to pursue both degrees simultaneously. The roles of clinicians in public health are likely to become every more varied in coming years as public health and health care systems and institutions become more closely coordinated.

Remember that we have only touched on three basic types of health professionals: physicians, nurses, and public health professionals. There are several hundred other types of professions in the healthcare realm. As you think about a career in health, you should take a look at a range of health professions using the concepts of education, training, and certification that we have discussed.

To understand the connections between the large number of diverse health professions, we need to look at how clinical care is organized into primary, secondary, and tertiary care.

WHAT IS MEANT BY PRIMARY, SECONDARY, AND TERTIARY CARE?

Primary, secondary, and tertiary care are traditional ways to categorize services delivered within the healthcare system.[7] **Primary care** traditionally refers to the first contact providers of care who are prepared to handle the great majority of common problems for which patients seek care. **Secondary care** often refers to specialty care provided by clinicians who focus on one or a small number of organ systems or on a specific type of service, such as obstetrics and gynecology or anesthesiology. **Tertiary care**, or subspecialty care, is usually defined in terms of the type of institution in which it is delivered, often academic or specialized health centers. Tertiary care may also be defined in terms of the type of problem that is addressed, such as trauma centers, burn centers, or neonatal intensive care units.

Primary care is widely seen as the foundation of a healthcare system and a strong primary care system is viewed as a prerequisite for maximizing the potential benefits of health care. Traditionally, primary care was considered the domain of physicians. Today, a range of health professionals are involved in primary, as well as secondary and tertiary care. In fact, the term "**medical home**" is becoming widely used, suggesting that primary care is increasingly viewed as a team effort.

Today, only about one-third of physicians in the United States practice primary care. Increasingly, primary care is being delivered by physician assistants (PAs) and nurse practitioners (NPs), who in most states have authority to diagnose disease and prescribe medication either under the supervision of a physician (in the case of PAs) or under a nursing practice act (as in the case of NPs). A team approach to primary care is becoming standard practice.

It is important to understand the ideals of primary care, as well as today's realities.[7] Primary care is key to the healthcare system because it is where most care is delivered and it is often the entry point for subsequent specialty care. In addition, primary care is critical to the delivery of clinical preventive services and to the connections between health care and public health. Ideal primary care has been described using 6 Cs: contact, comprehensive, coordinated, continuity, caring, and community.

- Contact implies first contact with patients as they present for health care.
- Comprehensive refers to the ability of primary care practitioners or primary care teams to completely or at least initially address most health issues.
- Coordinated relates to the concept that primary care teams should have the responsibility to ensure that the parts of the healthcare system work together for the good of patients.
- Continuity is the role that primary care teams see themselves playing to hold together the components of the system.
- Caring implies a personalized relationship with each patient.
- Community implies that primary care provides the link with the broader community, including with public health institutions and services.

Despite the fact that many primary care practitioners continue to see this model of primary care as a highly desirable way to deliver clinical care, the realities of today's healthcare system deviate substantially from this model. Table 9-2 outlines the 6 Cs and indicates ways that the current healthcare system differs from this primary care ideal.[7, b]

Thus, there is a large gulf between the ideals of primary care and their execution in practice. Part of the reason for this and other realities of health care can be better understood by looking at how health professionals are rewarded and compensated.

HOW ARE CLINICAL HEALTH PROFESSIONALS REWARDED AND COMPENSATED FOR THEIR SERVICES?

Physicians—and increasingly other health professionals—are compensated through a variety of mechanisms. Compensation levels depend on the site where care is delivered, the nature of the patient's insurance, and the type of institution in which the professional works or is employed.

---

[b] A new approach, often called **concierge practice**, is attempting to provide primary care based upon many of these principles. Concierge practices often limit the number of patients they serve, provide longer time for appointments and guarantee same or next-day access to appointments. However, to provide these services, concierge practices often charge several thousand dollars per patient as a yearly charge, which is not covered by insurance. Thus, concierge practices have been limited to those who can afford to pay for these services.

TABLE 9-2 Ideals and Realities of Primary Care—the 6 Cs

	Primary care ideals	Realities
Contact	The point of first contact with the healthcare system—the entry point	Patients enter the healthcare systems through many disconnected points including: ER, specialists, urgent care centers, nontraditional practitioners, etc.
Comprehensive	Primary care intends to be able to diagnose and treat the great majority of problems	Rapid increase in possible treatments and high-volume practices increase proportion of patient problems that are referred to specialists
Coordinated	Primary care intends to be the focal point for diagnosis and treatment with coordination through referral to specialists for consultation and feedback	Primary care physicians increasingly being replaced by "hospitalists," who are full time in the hospital and provide care for inpatients and direct patient access to specialists
Continuity	Patient followed over many years—continuous care provision	Patients increasingly required or encouraged to change physicians/providers for insurance purposes
Caring	Individualized care based on individual relationships	Primary care increasingly becoming an administrative entity without long-term individual relationships
Community	Primary care designed to connect the individual patient with community resources and community requirements (required examinations, reportable diseases, vaccinations, driver's licenses, etc.)	Healthcare professionals and public health have a long history of distant and—at times—contentious relationships

Source: Data from Institute of Medicine. *Defining Primary Care: An Interim Report.* Washington, DC: National Academies Press; 1994.

Complicating the issues of coordination of services and continuity of care is the fact that patients can and are often encouraged to change insurance coverage on a yearly basis. Thus, clinicians now live in a complex, changing, and often confusing world in which issues of compensation can get in the way of quality care. Despite the best of intentions, many clinicians find themselves having to address compensation as another "C." Table 9-3 outlines a number of methods of financial compensation to providers of health services and examines some of their advantages and disadvantages.

In addition to the mechanism of payment for services, another key factor that affects health professionals is the number of people in the profession. Let us look at how the right number makes a difference.

HOW CAN WE ENSURE THE SYSTEM HAS THE RIGHT NUMBER OF HEALTHCARE PROFESSIONALS?

Financial compensation is the fundamental market mechanism for regulating the supply of most professionals. This mechanism has not generally worked well in the health professions. The demand for positions in medical schools, for instance, far exceeds the supply. Thus, much of the control over the number of professionals that are trained has been made by the profession itself through policies that control the number and size of accredited degree-granting institutions. This control has had limited success. For instance, in the 1980s, dentists determined that there was an oversupply of dentists. A number of dental schools were closed and new dental schools were limited. Today, there is an undersupply of dentists. Balancing the supply and demand for health professionals is a complex undertaking, as illustrated by the current shortage of nurses.[8] The nursing shortage is discussed in Box 9-3.

We have now taken a look at the complex world of health care and public health professions, including the creation of health professions through education, training, and credentialing. We have also looked at issues of compensation and how we can try to ensure the right numbers of health professionals. Now, let us turn our attention to Chapter 10, which examines institutions in which health care is delivered.

TABLE 9-3 Method of Financial Compensation to Providers of Health Services

Compensation method	Meaning	Examples	Advantages	Disadvantages
Fee-for-service	Clinician paid for each covered service	Physicians often paid for medical visits and procedure, but may not be paid for counseling for prevention	Reward linked directly to work performed Encourages efficiency of delivery of services	May encourage delivery of unnecessary, as well as necessary services
Capitation	Clinician is paid a set amount per time period for each patient for whom they are responsible, regardless of level of use of services	Primary care physicians in health plans may be paid a set amount per patient per month and are expected to provide all primary care services	Discourages unnecessary care, may encourage preventive care, allows for predictable budgeting	May discourage necessary care, may encourage referral to specialists unless specialty care is financially discouraged
Episode of care	Institution or clinician is paid a set amount for providing comprehensive services, such as hospital treatment based on the patient's diagnosis	Medicare pays for hospital care based on Diagnosis Related Groups (DRGs) allowing defined number of days per condition	Encourages rapid and efficient delivery of care	May encourage discharge prior to ability to provide self-care
Salary	Set amount per time period	Governmental facilities generally pay clinicians on a seniority-based salary	May allow focus on quality	May discourage efficiency
Pay for Performance "P4P"	Compensation adjusted based on measures of the quality of care delivered	Additional compensation for adherence to evidence-based guidelines	Links income with quality providing strong incentive for quality	Difficult to measure quality, outcomes may be related to factors outside clinician's control

BOX 9-3 The Nursing Shortage and What Can Be Done About It?

The number of U.S.-trained registered nurses (RNs) has not kept up with demand. The shortage of nurses, especially those who work in the increasingly technical hospital environment, continues to grow. The projected size of the shortage is controversial, but estimates of a 20–30 percent shortage of RNs are commonly quoted. Everyone agrees that nursing is one of the most rapidly growing professions in terms of available job positions. The shortage is made worse by the fact that the average age of nurses is increasing because until very recently there was a decline in the number of newly-trained nurses. Why is there such a large and growing shortage? A number of factors contribute to this problem reflecting changes in nursing and American society. There is both a greater demand for nursing services and a supply that is not growing fast enough. Among the factors are:

- **Technology**—The increased availability and use of technology has increased the need for skilled nurses. Most of those who qualify for these technologically-oriented jobs are recent graduates and the number of recent graduates is very small compared to the demand.
- **More patients**—The aging baby boomer generation is expected to have a major impact on the need for nursing services. The large number of baby boomers born between 1946 and 1964 will need and expect increased nursing services.
- **Reduced supply**—Nursing has been viewed as a woman's profession, which has historically limited its attractiveness to men. In addition, many women leave the profession or practice part time, which may be accelerated by the increasingly stressful nature of the work.
- **Restrictions on entry**—Until recently, nursing education was self-contained—to become a nurse you needed to complete an undergraduate nursing degree and the only way to pursue a graduate nursing degree was to already have a bachelor's degree in nursing.
- **Shortage of nursing faculty**—A shortage of nursing faculty and teaching facilities has also contributed to the shortage of nurses and the ability to rapidly expand the size of Colleges of Nursing.

A national effort is now underway to increase the number of nurses in training. The approaches being used include:

- **Better compensation**—higher salaries and more flexible work schedules
- **Increased educational opportunities**—scholarships to encourage admissions to nursing schools and more flexibility in entering nursing after bachelor's degree training in other fields
- **Increase applicant pool**—encouraging male and underrepresented minority group enrollment
- **Raising status of nursing**—greater independence and recognition

Enrollment in Colleges of Nursing is now increasing. However, it will take many years before the supply of nurses meets the demand.

Key Words

- Accreditation
- Credentialing
- Certification
- Licensure
- Primary care
- Secondary care
- Tertiary care
- Medical home

Discussion Questions

Take a look at the questions posed in the following scenarios which were presented at the beginning of this chapter. See now whether you can answer them.

1. *Upon arrival at the hospital, the nurse specialist examines you and consults with the radiologists, the gastroenterologist, and the general surgeon. Your medication is reviewed by the PharmD, and your meals by the clinical nutritionist. Throughout the hospitalization you are followed by a hospitalist. Once you get back home, the home care team comes to see you regularly for the first two weeks and the physician assistant and registered nurse see you in the office. You realize that health care is no longer just about doctors and nurses. You ask yourself: what roles do all of these health professionals play in the healthcare system?*

2. *Jenna decides that after college she wants to become a doctor and practice medicine. "I thought there was only one kind of doctor who could diagnose disease and prescribe medicine," she mentions at a career counseling meeting. "Not so, anymore," says her advisor. "There are allopathic and osteopathic physicians. In addition, there are nurse practitioners who are authorized to diagnose and prescribe medications, and there are physician assistants who do the same under a physician's supervision. The universe of "doctors" now includes doctors of nursing practice, as well as other doctoral degree professionals, such as pharmacists and physical therapists." Understanding careers in health care can be as difficult for students as it is for patients, Jenna thinks to herself. Now she understands why her advisor asked: "what do you mean by 'practice'? What do you mean by 'doctor'?"*

3. *Sarah was about to begin medical school and was expecting two years of "preclinical" classroom lectures focusing on the basic sciences, followed by the study of*

clinical diseases. Then, as she'd heard from her physician father, she expected two years of clinical hospital "rotations" and electives investigating specialties. She is surprised to find that medical school has changed. There are small group problem-based learning sessions where she needs to be able to locate and read the research literature. There is contact with patients and their problems right from the beginning. There is increasingly a four-year approach instead of a preclinical and clinical approach to medical education. She wonders: are these changes for the better? What else needs to be done to improve medical education?

4. *You are interested in clinical care, as well as public health. "I need to make a choice," you think to yourself. "Not necessarily," your advisor says. "There are many ways to combine clinical care with public health." After a little investigation, you find out that undergraduate public health education is increasingly seen as preparation for clinical education and clinical prevention and population health are increasingly becoming part of clinical care. In addition, many careers from health administration, to health policy, to clinical research, combine the individual orientation of clinical care with the population perspective of public health. So what's the best pathway to a public health career for you?*

REFERENCES

1. Shi L, Singh D. *Essentials of the US Health Care System.* Sudbury, MA: Jones and Bartlett Publishers; 2005.

2. American Board of Medical Specialties. Specialties and Subspecialties. Available at: http://www.abms.org/Who_We_Help/Physicians/specialties.aspx. Accessed March 19, 2009.

3. Ludmerer KM. *Time to Heal: American Medical Education from the Turn of the Century to the Era of Managed Care.* New York: Oxford University Press; 2005.

4. American Board of Nursing Specialties. Accredited Certification Programs. Available at: http://www.nursingcertification.org/exam_programs.htm. Accessed March 19, 2009.

5. Association of Schools of Public Health. Public Health Workforce Crisis—What Can Be Done? Available at: http://www.asph.org/document.cfm?page=1039. Accessed March 19, 2009.

6. Gebbie K, Rosenstock L, Hernandez LM, eds. *Who Will Keep the Public Healthy? Educating Public Health Professionals for the 21st Century.* Washington, DC: National Academy Press; 2003.

7. Institute of Medicine. *Defining Primary Care: An Interim Report.* Washington, DC: National Academy Press; 1994.

8. American Association of Colleges of Nursing. Nursing Shortage Fact Sheet. Available at: http://www.aacn.nche.edu/Media/FactSheets/Nursing Shortage.htm. Accessed March 19, 2009.

Healthcare Institutions

George didn't have health insurance and went to the emergency room whenever he needed care. They always treated him there, but then tried to get him connected to a primary care facility. He wasn't eligible for care at the Veterans Administration facilities. So, they sent him to the local community health center, which they called the "safety net" provider. George did go there and they tried to treat his problems and get him his medicines despite his not having insurance. When he got sick, however, George went back to the emergency department. Even George agreed that it wasn't the best way to get care, but he wondered: what is needed to make the system work better?

Laura had breast cancer and it had spread. Her medical records were on file at the hospital, at four doctor's offices, in two emergency rooms, and at an outpatient imaging facility. No one seemed to know how to put the system together. Whenever her old records were essential, they asked her to go get a copy of them and bring them to her next appointment. That worked for a while, but when she ended up in the emergency room her records just weren't available. There must be a better way, Laura thought to herself. Hasn't the healthcare system discovered the Internet yet?

Fred ended his walk one day at the emergency room. He seemed confused about how to get home. "It looks like we are dealing with Alzheimer's," his doctor told Fred's wife, Sonya, at their next appointment. Taking care of Fred at home was not easy. Home health aides and occasional weekend relief called "respite care" eased the burden for a while. The new assisted-living facilities looked attractive, but Fred's family just couldn't afford one. When Fred fell and broke his hip, he required hospitalization for surgery. The hospital discharge planner arranged for a skilled nursing home for rehabilitation services paid for by Medicaid. After a few weeks there, the only alternative was long-term or custodial care in a nursing home. The care at the nursing home was not what the family had expected. The staff did clean Fred up before the announced family visits, but once when the family arrived unannounced, they were shocked to see Fred lying half-naked in his wheelchair. The end came almost two years from the day they moved him to the nursing home. Looking back, the family asked: can the healthcare system do better at addressing the needs of Alzheimer's patients?

These are the types of situations faced by many patients as they try to navigate through the institutions that provide health care in the United States. Let us take a look at these different institutions.

WHAT INSTITUTIONS MAKE UP THE HEALTHCARE SYSTEM?

The number and types of healthcare institutions are almost as diverse and complicated as the number and types of healthcare professionals. In recent years, the complexity has grown as a range of facilities have developed to serve new needs and new financial reimbursement approaches.[1,2] Nonetheless, it is possible to understand the scope of healthcare institutions by categorizing them as **inpatient facilities** and **outpatient facilities**, with inpatient facilities implying that patients remain in the facility for at least 24 hours.

Inpatient facilities include hospitals, skilled nursing and rehabilitation facilities, nursing homes, and institutional hospices. Outpatient facilities include those providing clinical services by one or more clinicians and those providing diagnostic testing or treatment. We will provide an overview of inpatient and outpatient facilities and then ask: do these facilities together provide a coordinated system of care? Let us begin by looking at inpatient facilities.

What Types of Inpatient Facilities Exist in the United States?

We can classify inpatient facilities as: 1) hospitals generally designed for short-term stays by patients; and 2) long-term care facilities. Let us first take a look at hospitals.

The history of hospitals in the United States goes back to the colonial period. However, prior to the middle of the 19th century, hospitals were generally institutions for those without other sources of care, which included the poor, the military, and those with communicable diseases. Hospitals generally provided little more than shelter and food and separated the sick—especially those with communicable diseases—from the healthy.[1]

Today, the American hospital is usually a modern high-tech enterprise that lies at the center of the healthcare system educationally, structurally, and psychologically. You can often identify the hospital from far away because it is frequently the largest and most modern facility in town. The psychological hold that the hospital has on American health care is symbolized by the term "house" and the concept of "housestaff," or residents who practically live full time in the hospital during their training.[3,a]

Hospitals share some common features including:

- Hospitals are licensed by the state and usually accredited by a national organization, such as The Joint Commission (formally called The Joint Commission on the Accreditation of Healthcare Organizations (JCAHO)).
- Hospitals have an organized physician staff and provide 24-hour-a-day nursing services.
- The hospital is governed by a governing board separate from the medical and nursing staff that has overall responsibility for the operation of the hospital consistent with state and federal laws.

The several types of hospitals in the United States differ in their purposes and organizational structures. Hospitals can be categorized as general hospitals and specialty hospitals. General hospitals attempt to serve a wide spectrum of patients and problems, though they may concentrate on serving only children or only those who qualify for services, such as a Veterans Administration (VA) hospital. In the past, specialty hospitals sought to serve the needs of patients who could not be accommodated in general hospitals, such as those with tuberculosis or severe mental illness. Today, these conditions are usually addressed in general hospitals. Today's specialty hospitals are more a result of the specialization of medical services. Institutions focused on cancer, heart disease, psychiatric illness, ophthalmology, and orthopedics, for instance, are rapidly developing.

Hospitals are often categorized today by their funding source and financial arrangements. They can be divided into nonprofit and for-profit, or investor-owned hospitals. Nearly 90 percent of the approximately 5000 hospitals in the United States are nonprofits. These include the broad category of private nonprofit hospitals, hospitals run by state or federal government, and hospitals run by institutions, such as universities.[b]

Approximately half of these 5000 hospitals are private nonprofit hospitals, many of which have affiliations with religious denominations, but accept patients of all faiths. State and local governments run nearly 20 percent of hospitals, many of which are described—along with private nonprofit hospitals—as community hospitals. Federal medical institutions include the Veterans Administration hospitals and the military hospital system. For-profit or investor-owned hospitals make up over 10 percent of all hospitals, many of which are owned by several large corporations specializing in providing healthcare services.

Hospitals today are often more than an inpatient facility. The most rapidly growing component of most hospitals is the

---

[a] The book *The House of God*, written in the 1960s, captured the mentality of the housestaff of the era and has been unofficial required reading by subsequent generations of residents. It portrays housestaff as having their own culture and portrays patients, as well as community physicians, in often disparaging ways.

[b] Hospitals are also categorized as teaching and nonteaching hospitals. A teaching hospital is one that has one or more accredited residency programs. Today, many community hospitals, as well as federal and state hospitals, have residency programs. The designation **academic health center** implies a medical school, one or more other health professions schools, and an affiliated hospital.

spectrum of outpatient services they provide. In addition to emergency departments, hospitals usually also provide outpatient surgical and medical services including diagnostic and treatment services and may provide facilities for routine office-type visits.

The hospital should no longer be viewed as one building. Hospital networks or systems are increasingly being created, some of which provide a range of services including skilled nursing and rehabilitative services, as well as long-term care.

We have classified inpatient facilities as including hospitals and long-term care facilities. Today, there are a range of long-term care facilities, some of which are not primarily operated as healthcare facilities.[1,2] These facilities may include skilled nursing facilities, nursing homes, assisted living and dementia care, and at times, hospice care. To fully understand the provision of long-term care, you also need to appreciate the types of services that are increasingly being provided in an individual's home.

It is important to distinguish between skilled nursing and rehabilitative services in contrast to nursing home services. Skilled nursing and rehabilitative services, like hospital services, are generally short term and aimed at accomplishing specific objectives, such as recovery from a stroke or injury. Though these services may continue for many months, they are not designed to provide long-term care beyond the point at which improvement can no longer be expected.

Nursing homes, on the other hand, are designed for long-term or custodial care while also providing a limited amount of healthcare services. Individuals in nursing homes usually require care because of their inability to perform the activities of daily living, such as dressing, feeding, and bathing themselves. Nursing homes may provide routine medical care and some acute care, but this type of facility is not primarily designed to improve the medical status of its residents.[c]

Nursing homes are generally operated according to a specific set of nursing home regulations determined by and enforced by the states. Federal minimal standards are set as part of the requirements to receive payment through the Medicare and Medicaid systems. Most nursing homes, like most hospitals, are run as private nonprofit institutions. However, for-profit or investor-owned nursing homes provide approximately 15 percent of the beds nationally. There are over 16,000 nursing homes in the United States with over 1.5 million residents.

Most, but not all residents are elderly and over 80 percent need help with mobility, nearly two-thirds are considered incontinent, and nearly half require assistance with eating. Alzheimer's patients are the most rapidly growing population in the nursing home system of care.[1,2]

Although not strictly inpatient healthcare facilities, assisted-living facilities and home health care increasingly provide long-term care for those who have less severe impairments. Assisted-living facilities are not organized as healthcare facilities, but may provide or coordinate health care as part of their services. New concepts, such as continuing care retirement communities, attempt to provide a range of options including independent-living, assisted-living and nursing home facilities.

Most elderly and disabled individuals are not residents in long-term care institutions, rather they live on their own or with family members. Thus, much attention in recent years has been paid to providing and financing home healthcare services including home health aides, healthcare delivered at home, and respite care. Respite care provides short-term time away for primary caregivers such as family members.

The hospice movement today can be viewed as part of the long-term care system. It is care provided to those with a life expectancy of six months or fewer as determined by a physician. The goal of hospice care is to provide comfort, emotional support, and palliation—not to increase longevity. In some cases, hospice care may occur in a separate institution, but today it is more often provided in the patient's place of residence.

What Types of Outpatient Facilities Exist in the United States?

The variety of types of outpatient facilities is even more diverse and complicated than those of inpatient facilities. The basic distinction between clinical facilities and diagnostic testing or therapeutic facilities helps define the types of services provided.

Clinical services were traditionally viewed as being provided in "the doctor's office." None of these words—the/doctor's/office—does a good job of describing the current organization of clinical services. "The" implies one. Today, clinical services are rarely organized around one doctor or clinician. Group practice and multispecialty practices have become the rule. "Doctors" (or physicians) are by no means the only health professionals to organize and provide clinical services. Physical therapists, nurse practitioners, audiologists, optometrists, clinical psychologists, and a long list of other health professionals often provide their own office services. Rather than "doctor," the term **provider** is increasingly used

[c] Some states, such as California, have developed an additional long-term care model which is not part of the "medical model." That is, limited or no nursing care is provided and the facility is not obliged to provide services if the individual's health status changes substantially.

to encompass this growing array of health professionals. Even the term "office" is no longer appropriate. In addition to the traditional office setting, many clinicians now provide services in shopping centers, work places, and even make house calls.

The average American has over three visits for clinical services per year. An increasing number of these visits are provided outside of "the doctor's office" in the traditional sense. These sites now include a growing network of community health centers designed to provide what is called the "safety net" services for those who cannot or do not wish to seek other types of clinical services. Box 10-1 provides an overview of community health centers.[4]

A key issue in the organization of health care is the delivery of quality services. Let us take a look at what we mean by quality and what mechanisms are being used to ensure the quality of healthcare services.

WHAT DO WE MEAN BY THE QUALITY OF HEALTHCARE SERVICES?

The quality of healthcare services may mean different things to different people. Administrators may focus on the structures, such as the availability of operating rooms or laboratory services. Clinicians may focus on the process, such as the technical competence of the practitioners. Patients may focus on different types of processes like the personal relationships and their personal satisfaction. External reviewers may focus on the outcome—lives saved or disabilities prevented.

Quality can be assessed using what are called **structure**, **process**, and **outcome measures**. Structure focuses on the physical and organizational infrastructure in which care is delivered. Process concentrates on the procedures and formal processes that go into delivering care—for example, systems for ensuring credentialing of health professionals and procedures to ensure timely response to complaints. Outcome measures implies a focus on the result of care from rates of infection to readmissions with complications.

Defining and measuring quality remains a controversial subject. However, the National Committee for Quality Assurance (NCQA) has developed a widely-recognized framework to assist with this challenge.[5] Table 10-1 outlines this framework.[d]

The complexity of inpatient and outpatient services in the United States has made the delivery of quality healthcare ser-

---

[d] Note that NCQA's framework emphasizes structure and process measures. These have little emphasis on the actual outcomes of care.

BOX 10-1 Community Health Centers.

Initially named neighborhood health centers, community health centers were established in 1965 as part of the Johnson administration's War on Poverty. The centers were designed based on a community empowerment philosophy that encouraged the flow of funds directly to nonprofit, community-level organizations, often bypassing state governments.

The Health Centers Consolidation Act of 1996 combined community health centers with healthcare services for migrants, the homeless population, and residents of public housing to create the consolidated health centers program under Section 330 of the Public Health Service Act. These centers are often called 330 grantees. To receive a 330 grant, a clinic must meet certain statutory requirements. It must:

- Be located in a federally-designated medically-underserved area (MUA) or serve a federally-designated medically-underserved population (MUP).
- Have nonprofit, public, or tax exempt status.
- Provide comprehensive primary healthcare services, referrals, and other services needed to facilitate access to care, such as case management, translation, and transportation.
- Have a governing board, the majority of whose members are patients of the health center.
- Provide services to all in the service area regardless of ability to pay and offer a sliding fee schedule that adjusts according to family income.

Community health centers have undergone rapid expansion in recent years and now serve over 15 million individuals annually at more than 4000 sites in all 50 states and the District of Columbia. Nearly half of the patients are uninsured and nearly the same number is eligible for Medicaid. Only a small number have private insurance. According to a recent review, "[h]ealth centers have proven to be an effective investment of federal funds, have garnered sustained goodwill and advocacy in the communities they serve, and, as a result, generally have enjoyed broad, bipartisan support."[4]

TABLE 10-1 Characteristics of Healthcare Quality—National Committee for Quality Assurance

Characteristic	Meaning	Examples	How measured?
Access and service	Access to needed care and good customer service	Enough primary care physicians and specialists Satisfaction of patients in terms of problems obtaining care	Patient satisfaction surveys, patient grievances and follow-up, interviews with staff
Qualified providers	Personnel licensed and trained and patients satisfied with services	System for checking credentials, sanctions Patient satisfaction with providers of care	Presence of system for checking credentials Patient satisfaction surveys
Staying healthy	Quality of services that help people maintain good health and avoid illness	Presence of guidelines for appropriate clinical preventive services Evidence that patients are receiving appropriate screening tests	Review of independently-verified clinical records Review of responses from patients
Getting better	Quality of services that help people recover from illness	Presence of method for evaluating new procedures, drugs, and devices to ensure that patients have assess to the most up-to-date care Providing specific services, such as smoking cessation	Review of independently-verified clinical records Interviews with staff
Living with illness	Quality of services that help people manage chronic illness	Programs to assist patients to manage chronic conditions like asthma Provision of specific services, such as eye examinations for diabetics	Review of independently-verified clinical records Interviews with staff

Source: Data from NCQA Health Plan Report Care. Available at: http://www.ncqa.org/. Accessed November 9, 2008.

vices very challenging. The complexity of the system raises two closely connected questions:

- How can the pieces of the system be coordinated to provide integrated care?
- How can we improve and ensure the quality of health care?

The coordination and integration of healthcare delivery is often considered key to both the efficiency and the quality of health care. Let us begin by taking a look at how healthcare delivery can be coordinated between institutions.

HOW CAN HEALTH CARE BE COORDINATED AMONG THE MULTIPLE INSTITUTIONS THAT PROVIDE HEALTHCARE SERVICES?

The types of institutions that deliver health care in the United States have continued to proliferate in recent years. Each type differs in its governance, finance, accreditation, and organizational structure. It is not surprising that most patients, policy makers, and even clinicians do not have a good overview of the system. Connecting the institutions to achieve an organized system has become a major challenge.

Healthcare delivery systems aim to connect inpatient and outpatient services, as well as short-term and long-term clinical services to provide a coordinated system of care. The desire for an integrated healthcare delivery system is not a new idea. For many years, the concept of "the patient's doctor" was seen as the mechanism to hold together the system. The doctor provided all care or coordinated the care with other clinicians. The doctor "followed" the patient into the inpatient facility and provided their "follow-up" care after they left.

Like the concept of "the doctor's office," the concept of "the patient's doctor" is no longer a reflection of reality. Once again "the" rarely reflects the reality of multiple providers of care. Primary care physicians are now far less likely to follow the patient into the hospital or the nursing home and far less likely to be aware of the patient's multiple sources of and approaches to care.

Efforts to integrate the system are underway. We will look at two basic approaches that are being used: the development of integrated healthcare delivery systems and the use of integrated electronic medical records. These approaches are likely to be used together and form the basis for a future integrated system of healthcare delivery. In order to understand the uses and potential of these two approaches, we first need to think about the types of coordination of care that we want to see occur and the purposes they serve.

WHAT TYPES OF COORDINATION OF CARE ARE NEEDED AND WHAT PURPOSES DO THEY SERVE?

As we have discussed, the traditional approach to coordination of care revolved around the clinician-patient or doctor-patient relationship. Traditionally, the concepts of continuity of care and coordination of care have been almost synonymous. This approach assumed that the relationship between one doctor and one patient would provide the individualized knowledge, trust, and commitment that would ensure the coordination of care by ensuring the continuity of care. The concepts of primary care that we have discussed were built in large part upon this concept of one-to-one continuity.

Today, there is an increasing emphasis on ensuring coordination rather than one-to-one continuity. Coordination is sought between institutions and settings where care is delivered. The approach that leaves continuity of information and continuity of responsibility for care to individual clinicians alone has often failed to produce the desired results. As we will see, efforts are underway to formally link institutions, services, and information between the various healthcare delivery sites and institutions.

Institutional coordination often relies on financial coordination. If services are covered by insurance in one setting but not another, the system is not likely to function efficiently or effectively. When services are not covered at all, patients may receive excellent care in one setting only to lose the benefits of that care when necessary preparation or follow-up is not paid for and not accomplished in another setting.

Coordination is not just an issue within the healthcare delivery system, it is also an issue that straddles healthcare delivery and public health functions. Communicable disease control and environmental protections, such as controlling antibiotic resistance and lead exposure, cannot be successful without effective and efficient coordination between healthcare and public health professionals and institutions. Table 10-2 outlines these types of coordination, their intended function, and the types of challenges that commonly occur with their implementation.

Let us take a look at the development of healthcare delivery systems as one approach to ensuring coordination of health care.

WHAT TYPES OF HEALTHCARE DELIVERY SYSTEMS ARE BEING DEVELOPED AND HOW CAN THEY HELP ENSURE COORDINATION OF HEALTH CARE?

We will use the term **healthcare delivery system** to imply a linkage of institutions and healthcare professionals that together take on the responsibility of delivering coordinated care.[e]

In a nation such as the United States, in which health care is provided by a range of providers and institutions, holding together one delivery system is not easy. A wide range of efforts are under way to connect the pieces. Let us take a look at some successful examples.

Care coordination challenges have been quite successfully met in the emergency response system. Today, there is a network of institutions, including government agencies and private emergency medical services providers, that cooperate with hospital emergency departments to facilitate and expedite the care of the seriously ill and injured. The emergency response system helps to quickly respond to emergencies, provide onsite assistance and information, and identify the healthcare institution that is best prepared to handle the emergency based on location, staffing, and capabilities. This system, while not perfect, demonstrates that coordination of care—at least urgent care—is possible.

Coordination of routine health care has proven to be a more difficult challenge. Healthcare systems are beginning to be developed often based on common ownership or governance. These integrated systems are designed to provide a wide range of services from outpatient clinical care, diagnostic testing and treatment services, to inpatient, home health, skilled nursing, nursing home and even hospice care.

Two of the longest standing and most developed healthcare systems are the Kaiser Permanente and Veterans Administration systems.[6, 7] These are discussed in Box 10-2. Many more healthcare systems are being formed by caregivers, such as multispecialty group practices, and by institutions, such as

---

[e] We will distinguish **healthcare delivery systems**, **healthcare system**, and **health systems**. Healthcare delivery systems include the delivery of healthcare services to a defined population. A healthcare system also includes the financial arrangements needed to pay for the care. A health system, the broadest of the three terms, includes the public health system, as well as the health care system.

TABLE 10-2 Type of Coordination of Care, Intended Functions, and Challenges with Implementation

Type of coordination	Intended function	Challenges with implementation
Clinician-patient relationship	Continuity as a mechanism for ensuring coordination Development of one-to-one relationships built on knowledge and trust over extended periods of time	Multiple clinicians involved in care Team rather than individual concept of primary care Frequent changes in insurance coverage require change in health professionals
Institutional coordination	Coordination of individual's information between institutions needed to inform individual clinical and administrative decision making	Different structures and governance often lead to lack of coordination between inpatient facilities and between inpatient and outpatient facilities
Financial coordination	Implies that a patient has comprehensive coverage for services provided by the full range of institutions Maximize the efficiency of the care received and minimize the administrative effort required to manage the payment system	Lack of comprehensive insurance coverage often means that essential services cannot be delivered or cannot be delivered at the most efficient or effective institutional site
Coordination between health care and public health	Coordination of services between clinical care and public heath requires communication to ensure follow-up and to protect the health of others	Lack of coordination of services between public health services and clinical care is often based on lack of communications

university medical centers. The coming years are likely to produce a number of successful models that will become examples that others will try to copy.

HOW CAN ELECTRONIC MEDICAL RECORDS BE USED TO FACILITATE COORDINATION OF CARE AND IMPROVE QUALITY?

There is widespread agreement that an electronic health record system could improve coordination of care, as well as achieve a number of other quality objectives. The Institute of Medicine (IOM) outlined the following potential roles for an electronic health information system. These roles aim in large part to provide the cornerstone for coordination of healthcare delivery.

- *Health information and data*—laboratory and pharmacy data, as well as records of a patient's history and findings on examination including past medical records

- *Results management*—integration of findings from multiple providers at multiple sites
- *Order entry/management*—electronic ordering of tests and prescriptions to maximize accuracy and speed implementation
- *Decision support management*—computer reminders and prompts to encourage timely follow-up and adherence to evidence-based guidelines
- *Electronic communication and connectivity*—facilitation of communications between providers and between providers and patients
- *Patient support*—tools for patient education and patient involvement in decision making
- *Administrative processes*—facilitation of scheduling, billing, and other administrative services to increase efficiency and reduce costs
- *Reporting and population health*—improvements in the efficiency and completeness of required reporting

BOX 10-2   Healthcare Delivery Systems: Kaiser Permanente and the Veterans Administration.

The Kaiser Permanente and the Veteran's Administration healthcare systems are two of the largest organized healthcare systems in the United States. They have very different histories, philosophies, and serve quite different populations. Nonetheless, they have both moved in the direction of developing an integrated set of healthcare delivery institutions linked together by an electronic health record and fostering evidence-based interventions. They share a common advantage in that they are financed by single sources, the Kaiser Permanente health plan and the federal government, respectively.

Kaiser helped introduce the concept of the health maintenance organization by offering a comprehensive package of preventive and curative services at a fixed monthly fee. The Kaiser Permanente health system has its roots in World War II when employers offered health benefits when they were prohibited from raising wages. In the subsequent decades, Kaiser Permanente grew from its California base, enrolling over 8 million individuals. It was created as a staff model prepaid health plan, enrolling patients who would receive all of their services directly from clinicians and institutions that were part of the plan. This allowed Kaiser Permanente to develop an integrated approach to healthcare delivery.

Kaiser, the management component, owns or contracts with hospitals, skilled nursing facilities, home healthcare systems, and a range of other institutions that provide care under their management. Permanente, the physician component, aims to provide an integrated set of inpatient and outpatient services. Kaiser Permanente competes actively in the market for healthcare services and often limits the amount and types of care that can be provided. Nonetheless, it has been able to develop an integrated healthcare delivery system, promote evidence-based interventions, and introduce an integrated electronic health record system.

The Veterans Administration healthcare system began as an outgrowth of World War I, though its roots go back to the Revolutionary War. After World War II, the Veterans Administration hospital system rapidly increased in size and developed strong relationships with medical schools and other health professional training schools for education and research. Today, the VA heath care system is part of the Cabinet-level Department of Veterans Affairs and serves over six million patients each year.

For many years, the VA system was accused of poor quality care and lack of coordination of care because it emphasized inpatient services and patients often went back and forth between the VA and other healthcare delivery sites. In the mid-1990s, the VA health system underwent a major "systems reengineering," designed to improve quality. The changes included the development of an integrated electronic health record and an emphasis on evidence-based interventions for preventive, acute, and chronic care.

In recent years, the VA health system has been organized into a series of networks, including inpatient and outpatient facilities. Many of the networks aim to provide comprehensive outpatient and inpatient services including skilled nursing and nursing home services, as well as outpatient and hospital services. Survey data collected a decade after the systems reengineering initiative began suggests that the VA health system provides an increasing quality of integrated care based upon evidence-based interventions.

The VA and Kaiser Permanente systems represent two of the largest healthcare systems in the United States. Both aim to serve a large number of patients and provide coordinated care utilizing evidence-based interventions and integrated healthcare records. The success of these two quite different healthcare systems suggests that an integrated system of care, patient information, and financing is possible and can be widely applied to improve the quality of health care.

and the speed and completeness of public health surveillance

The IOM also concluded that electronic record systems have the potential for helping achieve quality and efficiency objectives as outlined in Box 10-3.[8]

Efforts to implement a national system of electronic health records are underway. Nearly $20 billion has been allocated to this effort as part of the 2009–2010 stimulus plan. A federal plan envisions the widespread adoption of an integrated electronic record by 2014. Recent efforts to include patients as direct users of their health information may spur more rapid acceptance of the electronic records. The need for security of data and control by patients over who has access and for what purposes is critical to acceptance and use of an electronic system such as this. Assuming that security issues can be adequately addressed, you should expect to see widespread use of electronic records and an increased role for patients in accessing and managing their own medical records.[f]

---

[f] Despite the national commitment to implement electronic health records, the usage by physicians in their offices has remained low and far behind that of other developed countries. This is expected to change rapidly with the infusion of new funding.

BOX 10-3   Use of Electronic Health Records to Improve Quality and Efficiency of Healthcare Delivery.

The IOM report indicates that the electronic health record has the potential to improve quality and efficiency of patient care in the following ways:

- *Improve patient safety.* Safety is the prevention of harm to patients. Each year in the United States, tens of thousands of people die as a result of preventable adverse events due to health care. Electronic records containing information on prescribed drugs and other treatments are expected to improve patient safety.
- *Support the delivery of effective patient care.* Effectiveness is providing services based on scientific knowledge to those who could benefit and at the same time refraining from providing services to those not likely to benefit. Only about one-half (55 percent) of Americans receive recommended medical care that is consistent with evidence-based guidelines. Reminder systems that require clinicians to accept or reject the recommendations of a clinical guideline are expected to increase the use of evidence-based guidelines.
- *Facilitate management of chronic conditions.* More than half of those with chronic conditions have three or more different providers and report that they often receive conflicting information from those providers; moreover, many undergo duplicate tests and procedures, but still do not receive recommended care. Physicians also report difficulty in coordinating care for their patients with chronic conditions and believe that this lack of coordination produces poor outcomes. Electronic records can help inform clinicians of other care being given to their patients.
- *Improve efficiency.* Efficiency is the avoidance of waste, in particular, waste of equipment, supplies, ideas, and energy. Methods must be found to enhance the efficiency of healthcare professionals and reduce the administrative and labor costs associated with healthcare delivery and financing. Electronic records, if consistently and widely implemented in the healthcare arena, can be expected to reduce costs as they have in many other fields.

Electronic health records are only one of the many ways that technology is changing the delivery and quality of healthcare services in the United States.

HOW IS TECHNOLOGY BEING USED TO IMPROVE THE QUALITY OF CARE?

The United States is among the leaders in adoption of new healthcare technologies, especially those that allow for technological approaches to disease diagnosis and treatment. In comparison with most other nations, the United States has more rapidly developed and accepted the use of medical technologies ranging from magnetic resonance imaging (MRI), to invasive cardiac procedures, to surgery for weight loss.

This country has generally relied on market mechanisms to develop, introduce, and disseminate or diffuse technology. This has resulted in extremely rapid innovation in areas with high levels of financial compensation and slower innovation in areas with less financial support. For instance, high-tech procedures ranging from heart surgery to hip replacements have been well compensated and have seen rapid innovation and diffusion. Well-compensated preventive procedures, such as mammography, have likewise seen widespread use. Other tech-

nologies like telemedicine are likely to have widespread applications only after financial reimbursement is provided.

Longer term innovations in technology have been fueled by the long-term U.S. investment in basic and applied research through the National Institutes of Health (NIH). The budget for the NIH was doubled during the 1990s, but has been relatively flat in recent years when adjusted for inflation. New stimulus funding has again at least temporarily increased funding. The innovations in care and in technology pioneered by NIH have often led to new approaches and new health-related industries. In recent years, the NIH has begun to focus on translational research or efforts to bring the benefits of new knowledge and new technologies to individual patients and whole communities.

Increased knowledge of the human genome has laid the groundwork for new diagnostic and therapeutic approaches, as well as a better understanding of the causes of disease. Better understanding of brain function and better technology for measuring changes in the brain are leading to new strategies for dealing with diseases ranging from Alzheimer's to depression. Advances in technology continue to provide hope and new challenges to improving health care.

We have now looked at how the development of integrated healthcare delivery systems and electronic health records and other technologies are being used to try to improve the quality and efficiency of healthcare delivery. Now, let us take a look at mechanisms that are being developed to monitor and ensure quality of care.

WHAT MECHANISMS ARE BEING USED TO MONITOR AND ENSURE THE QUALITY OF HEALTH CARE IN THE UNITED STATES?

In Chapter 9, we looked at a variety of methods, such as academic accreditation and individual credentialing, to help monitor and attempt to ensure that health professionals are well educated and prepared for clinical practice. Increasing requirements for continuing education and often recertification are being used to help ensure maintenance of competence. Integrating financial compensation with quality of care through the use of pay-for-performance approaches is gaining momentum as an approach to ensuring quality.

In addition, we have discussed the development and use of evidence-based recommendations and guidelines. Today, these recommendations are often available to clinicians in the form of protocols or step-by-step advice on approaches to diagnosis and treatment of specific conditions. The complexity of clinical practice and the limits of current research, however, mean that evidence-based recommendations are available for only a small percentage of the problems that clinicians face on a daily basis.

In addition to these approaches, a series of other mechanisms attempts to address issues of quality. They include:

- hospital privileges and approval to perform specific procedures,
- accreditation of additional healthcare organizations including clinical practices,
- malpractice liability, not only for physicians, but increasingly for other health professionals, and
- disclosure of medical errors.

Hospital privileges imply that hospitals may set criteria for allowing clinicians to practice in their facility. The criteria may include specialty and/or subspecialty boards. Approval to perform specific procedures implies the need to demonstrate competence either by training or experience or both.

Accreditation of hospitals and long-term care facilities have been long-standing efforts. It is often linked to reimbursement, and thus essential to the survival of these institutions. Accreditation of clinical practices, especially large group practices, is a growing trend. The NCQA and the Joint Commission are encouraging this process and providing quality criteria that need to be met. While still a voluntary process, these new forms of accreditation are becoming a sign of quality that is useful when recruiting patients and dealing with insurance companies.

BOX 10-4 Medical Malpractice.

Medical malpractice is a body of state law, therefore it differs from state to state. It is part of the civil law, as opposed to criminal law, which means that a case may be decided by a jury based upon what is called the **preponderance of the evidence**. This implies that malpractice was more likely than not. Despite the differences that exist from state to state, malpractice law builds upon a tradition known as **negligence law**, which is intended to protect the individual from harm.

The occurrence of harm or a bad outcome resulting from health care is not the same as negligence or malpractice. Errors in judgment and unsuccessful efforts are only considered medical malpractice if the patient can establish all four of the following: 1) a duty was owed; 2) a duty was breached; 3) the breach caused an injury; and 4) damages occurred. Let us look at each of these requirements.[g]

1. A duty was owed—This implies that a healthcare provider undertook the care or treatment of a patient. This duty may stem from services provided ranging from a long-term relationship, a single visit, or a telephone call to a contractual relationship based upon an insurance agreement.
2. A duty was breached—This implies a failure of the healthcare provider to meet a relevant standard of care. The standard of care is defined in terms of the clinician's specialty. A healthcare provider is generally expected to possess the knowledge and skill and exercise the care and judgment expected of a reasonably competent clinician of the same specialty.
3. The breach caused the injury—The legal concept of causation is based on what is called proximal cause. In medical malpractice, responsibility for an injury lies with the last negligent act. Proximal cause asks whether the injury or other event would have occurred if the negligent act had not occurred. Causation can be divided between different "parties," including clinicians and institutions.

(continues)

BOX 10-4 continued.

4. Damages occurred—Damages can be divided into direct, indirect, and punitive categories. Direct damages include lost earnings, as well as current and future medical expenses. Indirect damages may include pain and emotional distress. Punitive damages may be awarded when conduct is intentionally harmful or grossly negligent.[h]

Instructions to a jury in a medial malpractice case include efforts to convey the meaning of each of these components of malpractice law. However, juries have a great deal of latitude when interpreting their meaning. For example, the concept of proximal causation used in the law may not conform to the jurors' understanding of causation. Assume a clinician refused to continue to provide prenatal care after the first 13 weeks. The jury may decide based upon their own understanding of causation that the clinician's refusal was the cause of a subsequent birth defect.

Medical malpractice is a complex and changing field. Many factors affect whether or not a malpractice suit is brought. These include the extent of damages, the relationship between the patient and the healthcare provider, and the standards of practice of both medicine and law in the community.

[g] Physicians are not the only providers of health care that can be sued under malpractice laws. Other clinicians such as pharmacists may be sued, especially those that do not work directly under the authority of physicians. In addition, healthcare facilities as institutions may be sued and are often included as additional defendants in malpractice cases. In this section, we will refer to the defendant in a malpractice suit as a healthcare provider.

[h] Indirect damages may include what has been called a "loss of consortium," which includes services provided by a domestic partner including companionship, homemaking, etc., and future reproductive capabilities of either sex. Gross negligence includes the intentional or wanton omission of care that would be proper to provide or alternatively doing of that which would be improper to do. Punitive damages are often justified as a method of deterring such conduct by other providers of care.

The United States healthcare delivery system has a unique body of law called **medical malpractice**. Medical malpractice is hailed by its supporters as the ultimate guarantor of quality. It is attacked by its detractor as leading to defensive medicine, increased costs, and shortages in vulnerable professions, such as obstetrics. Regardless of your view of malpractice, it has come to have a major impact on the relationship between clinicians and patients. Box 10-4 examines the criteria for malpractice so you can understand what it means.[9]

Malpractice is an inherently adversarial process. Increasingly, patients, clinicians, and healthcare institutions are looking for alternatives. One recent approach is the disclosure of medical errors.

CAN DISCLOSING MEDICAL ERRORS CONTRIBUTE TO QUALITY OF CARE AND SERVE AS AN ALTERNATIVE TO MALPRACTICE?

In its report, *To Error is Human*, the IOM documented the extent to which medical errors produce harm to patients—they estimated over 40,000 deaths per year.[10] This makes medical errors a slightly more common cause of death than either breast cancer or motor vehicles. Errors may be due to deficiencies in the diagnostic or therapeutic process on the part of clinician(s). They may also be due to what are called **system errors**, problems resulting from deficiencies in the system for delivering health care.

As we discussed in Chapter 3, clinicians in the not-too-distant past often withheld key information from patients, including a diagnosis of cancer and the potential harms of recommended treatment. Today, disclosure of these types of information is an expected part of clinical practice. However, until recently, disclosure of medical errors had not been an expected part of clinical practice.

Beginning in 2001, the Joint Commission requires that patients be informed of all outcomes of care including "unanticipated outcomes." Recent efforts to develop a system of disclosure have included a far more specific set of expectations including conveying to the patient:

- facts about the event
- presence of error or systems failure
- expression of regret
- a formal apology

In addition, institutions are expected to integrate the disclosure process with other aspects of patient safety and risk management activities, provide support for the process including educating clinicians, and keeping track of the use of disclosure at their institutions. Such formal efforts to disclose errors are becoming increasingly common in clinical care. It is still too early to determine the impact of these efforts on quality and their ability to reduce malpractice suits. However, there has already been an a growing acceptance of disclosure as a way of addressing medical errors.[11]

We have examined the structure of the U.S. healthcare delivery system, including the types of services that are provided in the inpatient and the outpatient settings. We have seen the need for and difficulty in developing a coordinated system to provide continuity of care. We have also seen how the U.S. system is developing models of coordination linking institutions and providers in new ways. The use of technology is a major strategy used by the U.S. healthcare delivery system to hold itself together through electronic medical records and innovative approaches to diagnosis and treatment. The development of the healthcare delivery system is closely tied to the way that health care is financed and services are paid for. Therefore, let us turn our attention directly to the issue of paying for health care in Chapter 11.

Key Words

- Inpatient facilities
- Outpatient facilities
- Academic health center
- Provider
- Structure, process, and outcome measures
- Healthcare delivery system
- Healthcare system
- Health systems
- Preponderance of the evidence
- Negligence law
- Proximal cause
- System errors

Discussion Questions

Take a look at the questions posed in the following scenarios which were presented at the beginning of this chapter. See now whether you can answer them.

1. *George didn't have health insurance and went to the emergency room whenever he needed care. They always treated him there, but then tried to get him connected to a primary care facility. He wasn't eligible for care at the Veterans Administration facilities. So, they sent him to the local community health center, which they called the "safety net" provider. George did go there and they tried to treat his problems and get him his medicines despite his not having insurance. When he got sick, however, George went back to the emergency department. Even George agreed that it wasn't the best way to get care, but he wondered: what is needed to make the system work better?*

2. *Laura had breast cancer and it had spread. Her medical records were on file at the hospital, at four doctor's offices, in two emergency rooms, and at an outpatient imaging facility. No one seemed to know how to put the system together. Whenever her old records were essential, they asked her to go get a copy of them and bring them to her next appointment. That worked for a while, but when she ended up in the emergency room her records just weren't available. There must be a better way, Laura thought to herself. Hasn't the healthcare system discovered the Internet yet?*

3. *Fred ended his walk one day at the emergency room. He seemed confused about how to get home. "It looks like we are dealing with Alzheimer's," his doctor told Fred's wife, Sonya, at their next appointment. Taking care of Fred at home was not easy. Home health aides and occasional weekend relief called "respite care" eased the burden for a while. The new assisted-living facilities looked attrac-*tive, but Fred's family just couldn't afford one. When Fred fell and broke his hip, he required hospitalization for surgery. The hospital discharge planner arranged for a skilled nursing home for rehabilitation services paid for by Medicaid. After a few weeks there, the only alternative was long-term or custodial care in a nursing home. The care at the nursing home was not what the family had expected. The staff did clean Fred up before the announced family visits, but once when the family arrived unannounced, they were shocked to see Fred lying half-naked in his wheelchair. The end came almost two years from the day they moved him to the nursing home. Looking back, the family asked: can the healthcare system do better at addressing the needs of Alzheimer's patients?*

REFERENCES

1. Shi L, Singh D. *Delivering Health Care in America: A Systems Approach.* 4th ed. Sudbury, MA: Jones and Bartlett Publishers; 2008.

2. Sultz HA, Young KM. *Health Care USA: Understanding Its Organization and Delivery.* 6th ed. Sudbury, MA: Jones and Bartlett Publishers; 2009.

3. Shem S. *The House of God: The Classic Novel of Life and Death in an American Hospital.* New York: Delta Trade Paperbacks; 2003.

4. Taylor J. *The Fundamentals of Community Health Centers, National Health Policy Forum.* Washington, DC: The George Washington University; 2004: 23.

5. National Committee for Quality Assurance. Report Cards. Available at: http://www.ncqa.org/. Accessed April 3, 2009.

6. Kaiser Permanente. Kaiser Permanente—More than 60 Years of Quality. Available at: http://xnet.kp.org/newscenter/aboutkp/historyofkp.html. Accessed April 3, 2009.

7. United States Department of Veterans Affairs. History of the Department of Veterans Affairs. Available at: http://www1.va.gov/opa/feature/history/index.asp. Accessed April 3, 2009.

8. Institute of Medicine Committee on Data Standards for Patient Safety. *Key Capabilities of an Electronic Health Record System: Letter Report.* Washington, DC: National Academies Press; 2004.

9. Louisville Law Kentucky Legal Resources on the Internet. Elements of Proof—Medical Malpractice. Available at: http://www.louisvillelaw.com/medical/malpractice/elements.htm. Accessed April 3, 2009.

10. Institute of Medicine. *To Error is Human: Building a Better Health Care System.* Washington, DC: National Academies Press; 1999.

11. The Joint Commission. Medical Errors Disclosure—Selected Bibliography. Available at: http://www.jointcommission.org/patientsafety/me_bibliography.htm. Accessed April 3, 2009.

CHAPTER 11

Healthcare Systems

LEARNING OBJECTIVES

By the end of this chapter, the student will be able to:

- identify the largest insurance systems in the United States and explain the basic principles of their financing.
- identify the basic types of managed healthcare organizations and explain the principles of how they differ.
- illustrate how individual circumstances affect the most favorable type of employment-based insurance.
- describe the extent and consequences of being uninsured or underinsured in the United States.
- describe the basic structure and financing aspects of the healthcare systems in Canada and the United Kingdom and compare them to those of the United States.
- identify options for addressing the cost of health care in the United States.

The politicians seem to agree that health care is too expensive. However, some argue for greater regulation, while others argue for less. You ask yourself: what are the options for controlling costs and what are the consequences?

You take a job right out of college and need to select from among your company's healthcare options or alternatively choose not to be insured. The choices appear to be quite complicated and none of them seems just right for you. How can you go about choosing between health insurance options?

You decide to take your chances and refuse the expensive health insurance offered by your employer. What are the consequences of not having insurance?

Members of the Smith family live in the United States, Canada, and the United Kingdom. They have the same inherited disease. The recommended treatment is quite similar in the three countries and can be delivered as part of primary care. How might the delivery of care and the payment for care differ among the three countries?

You wonder how the United States ranks globally in terms of the performance of its healthcare system. You're surprised when you find out that its ranking is not #1 or even near the top. Why is that? you ask yourself.

These are the types of questions we are faced with when trying to understand and evaluate healthcare systems. Understanding healthcare systems requires us to understand the workforce and institutions that make up the system. It also requires us to examine the central measures of success: the issues of cost, quality, and access to health care.

We have already examined issues of the quality of health care. In this chapter, we will take a look at questions of access to and the costs of health care. Both of these issues are closely tied to issues of healthcare finance or paying for health care. As we will see, in the United States the ability to access health care is very much dependent on having health insurance. Thus, to better understand the U.S. healthcare system, we will begin by taking a look at the finances. We need to know how much money is spent and how it is spent. This will require us to look at health insurance—including insurance provided by government, employers, and issues of the uninsured and underinsured. Then, we will look at the overall features of the U.S. healthcare system and compare them to features of the systems in Canada and the United Kingdom.

Equipped with this understanding, we will see how health systems can be scored or graded and how the United States compares with other nations. Finally, we will examine the issue of controlling costs while maintaining or improving care quality—a major challenge facing the U.S. health system today. Let us start by looking at how much we currently spend on health care.

HOW MUCH MONEY DOES THE UNITED STATES SPEND ON HEALTH CARE?

The United States spends well over $2 trillion per year on health care. That represents over 16 percent of the gross domestic product or over $7000 per person per year. Dollars spent have been growing faster than inflation for over 40 years. At the current rate of growth, the United States is estimated to spend 20 percent of its gross domestic product on health care by the year 2020.

Continuing that rate of growth takes money away from other activities, which makes it more difficult for the United States to compete globally. Other developed countries, such as Canada, the United Kingdom, France, Germany, Japan, and Australia, spend about half as much per person and generally spend 10 percent or less of their gross domestic product on health care.

To understand how we spend so much of our money on health care, it is critical to know more about the U.S. health insurance system.[1, 2] Much of the money spent on health care pays for insurance coverage with the majority of the remaining funds being spent to fill the holes in insurance coverage through direct payments by patients called out-of-pocket expenses.

Let us look at the basic types of insurance available in the United States. We start by examining government-financed insurance. We'll then take a look at employment-based insurance, and finally we'll examine the issue of having no insurance or being underinsured. Before getting started, however, it is important to understand the language of health insurance. Box 11-1 defines some important insurance terms.

WHAT TYPES OF GOVERNMENT-SUPPORTED HEALTH INSURANCE ARE AVAILABLE?

The two largest government programs of insurance are **Medicare** and **Medicaid**.[1, 2] Both programs began in the mid

---

BOX 11-1   Important Insurance Definitions.

Cap—A limit on the total amount that the insurance will pay for a service per year, per benefit period, or per lifetime.

Copayment—An amount that the insured is responsible for paying even when the service is covered by the insurance. **Coinsurance**, in contrast, is the percentage of the charges that the insured is responsible for paying.

Covered service—A service for which health insurance will provide payment or coverage if the individual is eligible, i.e., any deductible has already been paid.

Customary, prevailing, and reasonable—These standards are used by many insurance plans to determine the amount that will be paid to the provider of services. Under many employer-based plans, the provider may bill patients above and beyond this amount. This is known as **balance billing**.

Deductible—The amount that an individual or family is responsible for paying before being eligible for insurance coverage.

Eligible—An individual may need to meet certain criteria to be eligible for enrollment in a health insurance plan. These may include: an income level for Medicaid, age and enrollment in the Social Security system for Medicare, or specific employment requirements for employer-based insurance. Health status is not generally a factor in eligibility or premium costs for these types of group insurance, but often is when applying for an individual policy.

Medical loss ratio—The ratio of benefit payments paid to premiums collected—indicating the proportion of the premiums spent on medical services. Lower medical loss ratios imply that a larger amount of the premium is retained by the insurance company for administrative costs, marketing and/or profit.

Out-of-pocket cost—The cost of health care that is not covered by insurance and is the responsibility of the insured. These costs may be due to caps on insurance, deductibles, copayments, and/or balance billing.

Portability—The ability to continue employer-based health insurance after leaving a job—usually by paying the full cost of the insurance. A federal law, known as COBRA, generally ensures employees 18 months of portability.

Premium—The price paid by the purchaser for the insurance policy on a monthly or yearly basis.

1960s, but have very different funding sources, coverage, and populations served.[a]

Medicare began as a program for persons 65 and older. It was expanded to include disabled persons eligible for social security benefits and those with end-stage renal disease. Today, over 40 million Americans are eligible for Medicare and the number is expected to increase to 60 million by 2020.

When Medicare began it was designed primarily to cover hospital services and doctors' services. It did not cover drugs, most preventive services, or nursing home care. Drugs are now partially covered by Part D of Medicare. Preventive services are covered only when specifically approved by Congress or when it can be shown that they actually save the Medicare system money. Skilled nursing or rehabilitative care, but not nursing home or custodial care is covered by Medicare. Hearing aids and eyeglasses, perhaps the two most important medical devices for the elderly, are not covered by Medicare.

Medicare is a federal government program which means that eligibility and benefits are consistent throughout the United States. It is funded by a payroll tax of 1.45 percent from employees and 1.45 percent from employers. There is no income limit on this tax. That is, all income from employment is taxed. Self-employed individuals pay the employer, as well as the employee share. Medicare is a complicated program because there are four different parts: A, B, C, and D. The following describes the current basic costs and coverage of Medicare. The details are expected to change in coming years.

Part A covers hospital care, as well as follow-up skilled nursing care, home health care after a hospitalization, and hospice care. It is paid for primarily by the payroll tax and no premium is required. Currently, the annual deducible is approximately $1000.

Part B is a voluntary supplementary insurance that covers a wide range of diagnostic and therapeutic services provided by physicians, emergency departments, and other outpatient services. Seventy-five percent of Part B is funded by general tax revenues and 25 percent by a monthly premium, which is approximately $100 per month with additional payments by those with higher incomes. Copayments of 20 percent apply to most services, as well as a relatively small deductible. Health in-surance policies called **Medigap policies** offered by private insurance companies are often obtained by individuals to cover all or most of the 20 percent copayment.

Part C is a special program designed to encourage Medicare beneficiaries to enroll in prepaid health plans.

Part D is a relatively new prescription drug coverage plan. It is a complicated plan that is open to those who are enrolled in Parts A and B of Medicare. It requires a monthly premium of approximately $30 per month and an annual deductible of approximately $300. The exact terms depend on contracts through private plans which compete by offering lower costs or greater coverage. Standard coverage includes 75 percent of the costs of covered drugs once the deductible is satisfied up to approximately $2500 in drug costs. A gap or "doughnut hole" occurs above the $2500 limit. No coverage is provided for drug costs within the doughnut hole. Once an enrolled individual reaches a "catastrophic level" of total annual drug costs of about $5000, Medicare pays 95 percent of the additional cost of drugs.

Medicaid is a federal plus state program designed to pay for health services for specific categories of poor people and other designated categories of individuals. The federal government pays a variable amount of the cost ranging from 50–83 percent, depending on the per capita income of the state. All states have chosen to be part of the program and therefore must provide benefits for such groups as the disabled and children and pregnant women with a family income of less than 133 percent of the federal poverty level. The federal poverty level for a family of four is currently slightly more that $20,000 per year. Thus, there are a substantial number of poor and near-poor individuals, especially men, who are not eligible for Medicaid.

States at their discretion may include other categories of "medically needy" and may increase the eligible income level up to 185 percent of the federal poverty level. Most states cover custodial care in nursing homes for eligible individuals who have limited financial resources. As a result, Medicaid has become the largest source of insurance funds for nursing homes.[b]

In order to obtain federal funding through Medicaid, states which administer the program must provide basic services that include most inpatient and outpatient services, including preventive services. States may choose to offer these services and the federal government will provide matching funds for a wide range of services including drugs, eyeglasses, and transportation services. Thus, for those who are eligible

---

[a] The federal government also provides health care through the Veterans Administration, military health systems, and the Indian Health Service. The Veterans Administration is required to provide health care for military service-related conditions, but may—contingent upon resources—also provide care to veterans for nonservice-related conditions. The military health-care system provides care directly or contracts for care through the TriCare system for all active duty military and their families. American Indian and Alaskan Native members of federally-recognized tribes are eligible for comprehensive health services, as well as public health services provided or funded through the Indian Health Service.

---

[b] Medicaid requires that eligible individuals have very limited financial resources. Those with financial resources are generally expected to utilize most of these resources before becoming eligible. This process is known as "spending down." Complicated rules govern this process, including efforts to transfer the funds as gifts to others, including family members.

for Medicaid the coverage is usually quite comprehensive. However, the reimbursement rates to clinicians are often comparatively low and clinicians may choose not to participate in the Medicaid program.

A program begun in the late 1990s called the **State Child Health Insurance Program (SCHIP)** provides additional funds that states may use to enhance the Medicaid program for children. This may include raising the income level for eligibility, starting eligibility more rapidly, and ensuring longer periods of eligibility. In 2009 Congress expanded and made this program more flexible utilizing funds from an increase in the tax on cigarettes.

Medicaid now covers approximately 50 million individuals, about half of whom are children. Funds spent on the elderly, who constitute less than ten percent of Medicaid beneficiaries, exceeds that spent on children. The rising costs and increasing number of individuals eligible for the Medicaid program has led many states to require that Medicaid enrollees become members of a Medicaid managed care organization in an effort to reduce costs and improve continuity of care.

WHAT TYPES OF EMPLOYMENT-BASED HEALTH INSURANCE ARE AVAILABLE?

Employment-based insurance is the largest single category of insurance coverage in the United States. Over 50 percent of all Americans have the option to purchase some form of this type of insurance.

Employment-based insurance is in large part an accident of history. During World War II, employers were prohibited from raising wages. Instead, they offered healthcare benefits. Employment-based insurance grew rapidly in the 1950s and 1960s based on a principle known as **community rating**. Community ratings implied that the cost of insurance was the same regardless of the health status of a particular group of employees. Community rating has since been replaced by what is called **experience rating**. This concept means that employers and employees pay based on their groups' use of services in previous years.[c]

In the 1950s and 1960s and in many parts of the country well into the 1990s, employment-based insurance provided payments to clinicians and hospitals based almost entirely on **fee-for-service** payments. Fee-for-service, as its name implies, consists of charges paid for specific services provided and as a

payment system, it encourages provision of as many services as possible. Thus, this system has been accused of increasing healthcare costs through overuse of services.

In 1973, the federal government began to encourage an alternative approach to employment-based insurance called Health Maintenance Organizations (HMOs). HMOs charged patients a monthly fee designed to cover a comprehensive package of services. Clinicians or their organizations were paid based upon the number of individuals that enrolled in their practice. Their compensation was based on what is called **capitation**, which is a fixed number of dollars per month to provide services to an enrolled member regardless of the number of services provided. Classic HMOs were traditionally "staff model" HMOs, like Kaiser Permanente, that directly or indirectly provided the entire package of services.

Capitation, as opposed to fee-for-service, has the potential for underuse of services in an effort to reduce costs. HMOs, in contrast to a fee-for-service system, generally covered preventive services and thus argue that they do a better job of keeping people healthy.[d]

Classic fee-for-service systems and staff model HMOs represent the two traditional models of employment-based health insurance in the United States. Beginning in the 1990s, both these systems began to change in ways that brought them closer together.

Fee-for-service systems often evolved into what are called **Preferred Provider Plans** or **PPOs**. Staff model HMOs developed options for what are called **Point of Service Plans (POSs)**. PPOs imply that the insurance system decides to work with only a limited number of clinicians called preferred providers. These providers agree to a set of conditions that usually includes reduced payments and other conditions. Patients may choose to use other clinicians, but if they do so, they typically will pay more out-of-pocket.

Point of Service Plans imply that patients in an HMO may choose to receive their care outside the system provided by the health plan. Like a PPO, patients who choose the POS option must expect to pay more out-of-pocket. PPOs and POSs are today the most common forms of employment-based insurance. They now come in a variety of forms and together can be called mixed models. An employer may offer its employees a number of complicated mixed model choices, as well as ones that are closer to the classic fee-for-service and HMO staff model, or HMO classic. To better understand the types of options faced by employees take a look at Box 11-2.

---

[c] It has been argued that community rating is a form of health insurance that is closer to the social justice approach to health care because individuals and groups with better health subsidize those with poorer health and greater expenses. This implies that experience rating has moved the system toward a market justice approach. Note that mental health services are now treated the same as services directed at physical health under all types of health insurance plans.

---

[d] It has been argued that the reason HMOs provided preventive services is related to the increased interest and use of these services by healthy individuals. Enrolling predominately healthy individuals has been called **skimming**. By enrolling these individuals, HMOs can reduce their overall costs because healthy individuals are far less likely to require large amounts of health care.

BOX 11-2 Prototype Health Insurance Options.

Let us imagine that you go to work for a large employer that offers a full range of health insurance options. The options fall into three basic categories: fee-for-service classic, mixed-model HMO, and HMO classic. Your employer offers the following chart (Table 11-1) comparing the benefits and costs of each of these three options. Employers often subsidize the cost of insurance for the employee but not for the rest of the family.

TABLE 11-1 Prototype Health Insurance Options

	Fee-for-Service Classic	Mixed Model	HMO Classic
Monthly cost to employee	$200 for employee $1200 Family of 4 $1000 yearly deductible per person	$100 for employee $600 Family of 4 $500 yearly deductible per person	$50 for employee $300 Family of 4 No yearly deductible
Choice of physician	No restrictions–full coverage Physicians paid "prevailing fee"	No restrictions, 20% copayment for out of network Physicians paid lower discounted fee for service	Staff physicians only Full coverage Physicians paid through capitation
Access to specialists including OB-GYN	Access without referral–full coverage	Access with referral–full coverage Access without referral–20% copayment	Access with referral only
Drugs	Full coverage as ordered	$20 copayment for generic or approved/formulary drugs	$10 copayment for generic or approved/formulary drugs
Hospital	Full coverage as authorized by physician	80% coverage if preauthorized by plan	100% coverage if preauthorized by plan
Skilled nursing	Full coverage if ordered by physicians	80% coverage if found necessary by plan	100% coverage if found necessary by plan
Hospice	100% coverage based on physician authorization	80% coverage based on plan authorization	100% coverage based on plan authorization
Preventive services	Not covered	100% coverage in network 20% copayment out of network	100% coverage in network
Emergency Department and out-of-area services	100% coverage	Requires prior authorization except in emergencies as defined by "reasonable person"	Requires prior authorization except in emergencies as defined by "reasonable person"

(continues)

BOX 11-2 *continued.*

Now, let us put ourselves in the position of those who might need to choose among these options and think about which option they might choose. Remember—there is a fourth option—to not to enroll in any of the heath insurance plans.

- *A healthy, single, 22–year-old male right out of college with an income of $30,000*—This person might choose not to be covered if they consider themselves at low risk of needing health care and are willing to take their chances in exchange for cost savings. However, they would need to be willing to take the substantial risks associated with being uninsured.
- *A healthy 30-year-old recently married professional who intends to start a family in the next year. Their family income is $60,000*—This person might choose the plan with the most comprehensive and flexible coverage for pregnancy—their most pressing health issue. Thus, they might choose a classic fee-for-service plan with the knowledge that they will receive full choice of services for the additional cost of coverage.
- *A 40-year-old married employee with a family of four with a family income of $80,000. Both husband and wife require ongoing treatments to prevent illness, including regular preventive care and expensive medications. They want to choose which clinicians to use while controlling the costs of care.*—This person might choose the mixed-model plan because it provides greater choice than the HMO classic model, while reducing the cost compared to the fee-for-service model.
- *A 35-year-old single parent of two young children and an income of $30,000. The mother and children need preventive care and the mother needs regular mental health care*—This person might favor the HMO classic model because it minimizes costs and maximizes benefits. However, they would need to be willing to accept the restriction on access to care built into the plan.
- *A 55-year-old single professional with an income of $250,000 and no current major medical problems*—This person might choose the fee-for-service model if they were concerned about future healthcare needs. However, they may choose not to enroll in any of these plans and to accept the risk of paying for health care out of pocket. They might be attracted to healthcare savings accounts, which allow them to put aside pretax earnings to pay for current and future health care. Despite their high income, they might become one of the uninsured.

Today these types of choices face most employees of large organizations. No one plan is likely to be the best plan for everyone. In reality, there are often far more choices and the best choice for each employee can be very difficult to determine. The classic models are rapidly disappearing and a wide range of mixed models are now the usual options facing employees.

In addition to those people with government and employment-based insurance, the other large category of individuals in the United States are those who are called uninsured or underinsured. Let's look at the extent and consequences of being uninsured and underinsured.

WHAT ARE THE EXTENT AND CONSEQUENCES OF BEING UNINSURED AND UNDERINSURED IN THE UNITED STATES?

Over 15 percent of all Americans do not have any form of health insurance. This percentage has increased in recent years even in years of economic growth and continues to grow. A national debate is now underway to address the issue of the uninsured and underinsured.

It is important to understand what types of people are uninsured and underinsured and to think about the consequences. Let us look first at the issue of the uninsured. The uninsured can be classified into the following quite different groups:

- Healthy, often young, individuals who choose not to purchase insurance through their employer
- Poor or near-poor individuals who do not qualify for Medicaid
- Self-employed persons or employees of small companies that despite substantial incomes decide not to purchase insurance because they must pay much higher premiums than those usually offered through large organizations

Approximately 20 percent of employed persons do not have health insurance. It may surprise you to learn that nearly 40 percent of the uninsured population comes from families that can be considered to have middle-class or higher incomes. The largest number of uninsured are in the 18–24 year-old age group with approximately 30 percent of this age group being uninsured.

In addition to the issue of the uninsured, we need to recognize the additional issue of underinsurance. A large number of individuals and families have health insurance that does not adequately cover expected or potential healthcare costs. The three models of health insurance discussed in Box 11-2 are representative of those offered by large employers. Despite their deductibles, copayments and caps on these insurance options are considered comprehensive coverage. It is estimated that for every two individuals who are uninsured, there is another American who has health insurance, but their coverage is not considered comprehensive. They are categorized as underinsured and often have large out-of-pocket expenses if they require extensive medical care.

Who are the underinsured? They are primarily individuals and families who have obtained health insurance through employment, especially employment at smaller firms, that often is not as comprehensive as those described. In addition, individuals may purchase less than comprehensive plans on their own.

The consequences of being uninsured and underinsured can be very great. The Institute of Medicine (IOM)[3] and the Henry J. Kaiser Family Foundation[4] have identified a series of consequences. Being uninsured, and to a lesser extent underinsured, harms individuals and families in at least the following ways:

- They receive less preventive care, are diagnosed at more advanced stages of disease, and receive less treatment once diagnosed.
- They are much less likely to have a usual source of health care and more likely to use the emergency department for routine care.
- They have an increased mortality rate—an estimated nearly 20,000 excess deaths per year.

Those without insurance can and often do use an emergency department to obtain care. Emergency departments are required to provide routine care, as well as life-threatening emergency care. However, after stabilizing an individual with a life-threatening emergency, they may transfer them to an institution that provides care for those without insurance. For other conditions, the uninsured and underinsured may delay care until it is too late to fully benefit. The Institute of Medicine has described the care of the uninsured as too little and too late.[3]

When the uninsured and underinsured do seek health care, clinicians and healthcare institutions often bill the individual undiscounted prices for the healthcare services provided. When these individuals require substantial amounts of outpatient or inpatient health care, they often find themselves faced with large debts and in some cases declare bankruptcy. When these individuals fail to pay their medical bills, the costs are often picked up by other patients with insurance, thus raising the costs of health care for all who purchase health insurance.

A number of approaches for addressing these issues have been put forward and extensive experimentation is underway. Box 11-3 outlines some of the approaches that have been suggested.

We have described the basic components of the U.S. healthcare system, including the health professionals and institutions that provide health care, and addressed issues of quality, cost, and access. We are now ready to compare the U.S. healthcare system to that of other developed countries. First, let us look at a framework that we can use to describe and compare healthcare systems.

HOW CAN WE DESCRIBE HEATHCARE SYSTEMS IN GENERAL AND THE U.S. HEALTHCARE SYSTEM IN PARTICULAR?

One approach to describing healthcare systems is to define their characteristics using the following categories:

- Method of financing
- Method of insurance and reimbursement
- Methods for delivering services
- Comprehensiveness of insurance
- Cost and cost containment
- Degree of patient choice
- Administrative costs

Table 11-2 uses these categories to describe the complex U.S. healthcare system.

The U.S. system is often compared to those of Canada and the United Kingdom. Despite the fact that these countries have much in common, their healthcare systems have evolved in very different ways.

HOW CAN WE DESCRIBE THE HEALTHCARE SYSTEMS IN CANADA AND THE UNITED KINGDOM?

Let us use the same chart we used to describe the U.S. system to outline the features of the Canadian[5] and United Kingdom[6] healthcare systems. Table 11-3 describes the Canadian healthcare system.

Now, take a look at Table 11-4 describing the healthcare system in the United Kingdom.

WHAT CONCLUSIONS CAN WE REACH FROM THESE DESCRIPTIONS OF THE U.S., CANADIAN, AND U.K. HEALTHCARE SYSTEMS?

These charts highlight key features of the three systems, while demonstrating substantial differences. When describing these characteristics we can ask: on the spectrum of market justice versus social justice, where do the United States, Canada, and the United Kingdom lie?

It can be argued that the United States relies most heavily on market justice, while the United Kingdom places the greater

BOX 11-3 Potential Approaches to Providing Health Insurance to the Uninsured and Underinsured.

A large number of approaches to providing at least basic coverage for all Americans have been put forth. A growing majority favors insuring all or the vast majority of individuals, which is called **universal coverage**. Considerable disagreement exists on the best way to accomplish this goal. Most of the approaches being advocated fall into one of the following categories.

- **Employer mandate**—Employers are required to provide comprehensive insurance coverage for all their employees. A number of variations on this approach have been put forward, some of which provide subsidies for small employers. Another option, called "play-or-pay," requires payments by employers who fail to provide comprehensive coverage.
- **Individual mandate**—Individuals are required to purchase individual health insurance policies which include at least standardized minimum coverage. Those with limited income may receive subsidies to allow them to pay for the insurance. Variations on this approach have been discussed including allowing individuals to refuse to purchase insurance, but then requiring them to pay when receiving services. Another variation encourages individuals to put aside funds in tax-free accounts referred to as "health savings accounts" to pay for health services.
- **Single-payer**—This approach is characterized by a single source of payment for all basic healthcare services usually provided by the government at the state or federal level. Funding may come entirely from taxes or premiums may be charged to individuals or employers.

For over half a century, employer-based health insurance has been the most common method for financing health care. These options above imply that the choice is either to expand this system or to move to a new system. The option of individual mandates retains the basic insurance structure, but puts the burden on individuals rather than employers. The single-payer system envisions a single entity, most likely the government, which directly or indirectly will pay all the bills. This system might be similar to the current Medicare system or to the health insurance system for federal employees including members of Congress.

The United States is in the process of healthcare reform. It is expected that one or more of the above approaches will form the basis for the emerging system. For updates on healthcare reform in the United Sates, see www.publichealth101.org.

emphasis on social justice. Canada lies somewhere in between. In describing these systems, it can also be useful to identify areas in which the United States has unique approaches and unique results. The following distinguish the U.S. healthcare system not only from that of Canada and the United Kingdom, but from the healthcare systems of most other developed countries:

- The United States spends considerably more per person and as a percentage of gross domestic product (GDP).
- The United States has far more uninsured and underinsured individuals.
- The U.S. healthcare system is more complex for patients and providers of care and costs far more to administer.
- The U.S. healthcare system places more emphasis on specialized physicians and on nurse practitioners and physician assistants to provide primary care.
- The United States encourages rapid adoption of technology, especially for diagnosis and treatment.
- The United States places greater emphasis on giving patients a wider choice of clinicians.
- The United States has a more complex system for ensuring quality and a unique system of malpractice law.

Equipped with all this information, we will now see if it is possible to grade or score the performance of the U.S. healthcare system compared to those of other developed countries.

HOW CAN A HEALTHCARE SYSTEM BE SCORED?

The Commonwealth Fund's Commission on a High Performance Health System (The Commission) has developed The National Scorecard on the U.S. Health System (National Scorecard).[7] The national scorecard uses a standardized set of measurements to try to objectively measure performance in 19 developed countries.[e] Box 11-4 outlines the criteria used to score these healthcare systems and the types of measurements that are used.

---

[e] The Commonwealth Fund describes itself as "a private foundation working toward a high performance health system." The national scorecard on U.S. Health Systems Performance was developed by a Commission appointed by the Commonwealth Fund made up of individuals who, according to the Commonwealth Fund, are "…a distinguished group of experts and leaders representing every sector of health care, as well as the state and federal policy arena, the business sector, professional societies, and academia…."

TABLE 11-2 Describing the U.S. Healthcare System

Category	Description
Financing	Cost over 16% of GDP and rising rapidly Complicated mix of federal, state, employer and self-pay
Type(s) of insurance and reimbursement	Employment-based insurance plus government insurance through Medicare and Medicaid provide most insurance Mix of fee-for-service, capitation, and salary with incentives are the most commonly used methods
Delivery of care	Mix of practice types with private practice dominant Physicians: $\frac{1}{3}$ Primary Care; $\frac{2}{3}$ Specialists Primary care increasingly based upon nurse practitioners and physician assistants Hospitalists increasingly coordinate inpatient care Need for better continuity of care between institutions and between clinicians
Comprehensiveness of insurance	15% uninsured plus half again as many underinsured Drug benefits included for elderly and those with comprehensive insurance Preventive services increasing, but not comprehensive
Cost and cost containment	Emphasis on competition as means of controlling costs, plus cost sharing by patients
Patient choice	Considerable choice of primary care and often direct access to specialty care Greatly increased access for those with comprehensive insurance
Administrative costs	High: 25–30% of total costs including administrative costs of health insurance, clinicians and institutions, but this does not include administrative time spent by patients and their families

Let us take a look at how the United States scores in comparison with other developed countries based upon the national scorecard.

USING THE NATIONAL SCORECARD, HOW DOES THE UNITED STATES' HEALTHCARE SYSTEM PERFORM COMPARED TO THOSE OF OTHER DEVELOPED COUNTRIES?

The Commission scored the performance of 19 developed countries, including the United States, 14 European nations, Canada, Japan, New Zealand, and Australia. It set benchmarks high, but established realistic levels of performance for each area using the score of the top three countries as the highest standard. Thus, high but realistic performance is given a score of 100.[f]

Table 11-5 summarizes the performance of the United States on each of the criteria as well as the overall score.

These scores for the United States in 2008 were actually slightly lower than the scores for 2006 with a substantial reduction of the access score from 67 in 2006 to 58 in 2008.

The scorecard leaves us with some fundamental questions including: how can access be improved, quality be increased, and costs be controlled. We have looked at the issues of quality in Chapter 10 and reviewed a series of current and proposed mechanisms for improving quality. In this chapter, we have looked at issues of access and outlined the options for obtaining universal or near-universal coverage. Perhaps the greatest negative aspect of the U.S. healthcare system is the issue of high and escalating costs. Let's complete our look at the U.S. healthcare system by examining the options for controlling costs.

---

[f] The Commission also used the performance of the top ten percent of states in the United States to make comparisons within the United States.

TABLE 11-3 Describing the Canadian Healthcare System

Category	Description
Financing	National policy to keep expenditures under 10% of GDP Combination of Provincial and Federal ~70% government through taxes ~30% private insurance payments by individuals
Type(s) of insurance and reimbursement	Government insurance for basic services, individual policies with subsidies for the poor for most other services Negotiated fee-for-service reimbursement with single payer for basic services
Delivery of care	Mix of practice types with private practice dominant—emphasis on physicians in primary care Physicians ~50% primary care and ~50% specialists Primary care physicians generally admit to the hospital and are responsible for continuity of care Concerns about access to high tech procedures
Comprehensiveness of insurance	Three-tiered: 1. Medically necessary basic services—Universal coverage. Government funded and guaranteed to all without any cost-sharing, including preventive services. No private insurance allowed for medically necessary services 2. Private insurance and government subsidized insurance for other medical services including drugs, long-term care, home care with government payment for needy. Negotiated bulk purchasing of drugs on formulary 3. Private insurance or self-pay for dental, vision, and many nonphysician services
Cost and cost containment	Capital purchases, such as of high-tech diagnostic equipment, are regulated Concern about waiting time for access Negotiated fees between providers and government with government as single payer having considerable negotiating power
Patient choice	Choice of primary care physician Referral often needed to see specialists
Administrative costs	Low—approximately 15% or less of total costs

HOW CAN THE COSTS OF HEALTH CARE BE CONTROLLED IN THE UNITED STATES?

To understand the options for controlling costs, it is important to first understand the reasons that costs are increasing. The United States is not alone in facing increased costs for health care. There are a number of forces at work in most developed countries that increase and most likely will continue to increase the costs of health care, including the following:

- *The aging of the population:* The success of public health and healthcare efforts over the last century has produced a population that is living longer. Longer life is strongly associated with the development of chronic diseases, many of which require expensive care over many years or decades.
- *Technological innovations have greatly expanded treatment options:* A wide range of interventions are now possible, some of which can have dramatic impacts on longevity and the quality of life. However, many

TABLE 11-4 Describing the United Kingdom's Healthcare System

Category	Description
Financing	Budget about 7–8% of GDP has been rising
	Tax-supported comprehensive and universal coverage through National Health Service
	Private insurance system with overlapping coverage purchased as additional coverage by ~15% of the population with perception of easier access and higher quality
Type(s) of insurance and reimbursement	National Health Service is single payer with capitation, plus incentives for General Practitioners, i.e., physicians responsible for panel of patients
	Specialists generally salaried in National Health Service often earn substantial additional income through private insurance
Delivery of care	Governmental system of healthcare delivery in National Health Service including government-owned and administered hospitals
	Emphasis on physicians
	Primary care general practitioners ~$^2/_3$
	Specialist physicians ~$^1/_3$
	General practitioners generally do not admit to hospital
Comprehensiveness of insurance	National Health Service comprehensive with little cost sharing plus may cover transportation costs
	Incentives to provide preventive services and home care
Cost and cost containment	Overall limit on national spending ("Global budgeting")
	Negotiated rates of capitation and salary with government as single payer within National Health Service having considerable negotiating power
Patient choice	National Health Service provides limited choice of general practitioners
	Waiting lines for services in National Health Service especially specialists and high-tech procedures
	Referral to specialists generally needed
	Greater choice with private insurance
Administrative costs	Greater than Canada, less than U.S.

others produce very modest improvements at high costs. It may be difficult to distinguish these different types of results.

- *The successes of medical care over the last half century have raised the expectations of patients:* Greater expectations for access to technology, preventive interventions, individualized care, rapid access to care, privacy and protection of confidentiality, are now all possible, but often quite expensive.

Nearly all developed countries face these forces to a greater or lesser extent. Many countries in Europe, as well as Japan, face an even more rapidly aging population than the United States. How the healthcare systems respond to these challenges will determine in large part the overall costs of health care in each country.

The United States, however, also faces some issues to a far greater extent than other developed countries. The United States has a far more complex and changing structure. The sheer complexity of the system has led to a need for multiple levels of administration, which are not required in most other countries. In addition, patients are often expected to fill out and process complex insurance applications and claim forms. Clinicians are often required to bill for each service provided,

BOX 11-4 Criteria and Measurements Used in the Commonwealth Fund's Commission on a High Performance Health System

The Commission's scorecard measures the following five areas of health system performance:
- *Healthy lives:* National health outcomes using such measures as: life expectancy, infant mortality, HALEs at age 60, limitations in activities among adults under 65, and missed school days by children due to illness or injury
- *Quality:* Quality of preventive, curative, and rehabilitative health care using such measures as: adults and children receiving recommended preventive services; control of chronic diseases; availability of services (including mental health) after hours and on an urgent basis; hospital quality of care including the ratio of observed to expected mortality; and preventive measures in nursing homes
- *Access:* Availability of care using such measures as insurance coverage including the percentage of uninsured and underinsured, as well as the impact of the cost of insurance
- *Efficiency:* Inappropriate, wasteful, or fragmented care using such measures as: emergency departments use for routine care, hospital admissions for preventable conditions, short-term readmission rates, and costs of administration
- *Equity:* Disparities in health services and health outcomes by racial/minority status and income using such measures as: access to preventive and acute services, control of chronic diseases, insurance coverage, and measures of healthy lives

The scores from each of these areas are added together to produce overall scores.

TABLE 11-5 Performance of U.S. Compared to Best Performing Countries

Area of performance	U.S. score (out of 100)
Healthy lives	72
Quality	71
Access	58
Efficiency	53
Equity	71
Overall score	65

Source: The Commonwealth Fund. Commission on a High Performance Health System. Available at: http://www.commonwealthfund.org/programs/programs_list.htm?attrib_id=11932. Accessed November 9, 2008.

justify the services provided, and in many cases obtain approval for payments prior to treating patients. Today, a clinician's office usually has far more individuals involved in administering the system compared to those directly delivering care to patients.

The United States also has a far more complex and changing system of quality control. As we have seen, healthcare quality is monitored and maintained via a system that includes accreditation, certification, licensure, and malpractice, to name a few. The direct and indirect costs of this system may themselves contribute to the large and escalating cost of health care. A variety of efforts have been and are being made to reduce costs in the United States. These include:

- *Cost control through reimbursement incentives:* The concept of capitation has been widely used as a mechanism for controlling or reducing costs. A special form of capitation, diagnosis-related groups (DRGs), have been successfully used to reduce the length of stay in hospitals. DRGs pay hospitals a set amount for a particular diagnosis regardless of the length of hospital stay. However, reimbursement systems at times have moved the costs from one part of the system to another. Restrictions on payment for procedures may increase the number of procedures performed. Restriction on inpatient reimbursement may encourage an increase in outpatient or home care services.
- *Cost sharing:* This involves efforts to shift the costs of health care to individuals on the assumption that individuals will spend less when the costs are coming out of their pockets. Measures, such as deductibles, copayments, and caps are all intended to reduce costs by shifting them to individual patients.
- *Regulation:* At times, efforts have been made to reduce costs by placing limits on how much care can be provided or how much compensation can be provided. Government-controlled health insurance, such as

Medicare and Medicaid, is targeted for regulation. National issue of rates of compensation for clinicians and hospitals have become part of the political process.

- *Restrictions on malpractice:* It has been argued that the U.S. malpractice system encourages clinicians to practice "defensive medicine," that is, to perform unnecessary tests to protect themselves against lawsuits. The extent of the problem and the impact of changes in malpractice are controversial, but efforts are being made to reduce the number of lawsuits that reach the court system and to restrict the amount of compensation that can be awarded beyond actual damages.

A more general approach to reducing costs favored by many in the United States is to increase competition between providers of health services including institutions and individual clinicians and groups of clinicians. To better understand the potential for competition to succeed and the changes that are occurring to encourage competition, take a look at Box 11-5.[8]

Understanding healthcare systems is a challenge for patients, as well as those who work in the system. Understanding the roles of healthcare professionals, institutions, and the issues of quality, access, and cost help us understand the system as a whole. **The United States is undergoing a major review and reform of the healthcare system. For an update on the United States healthcare system, see the student Web site for Public Health 101: Healthy People-Healthy Populations at www.publichealth101.org.**

A well-functioning healthcare system is essential to the public's health. An efficient system that works in concert with organized public health efforts and leaves adequate financial resources to invest in programs directed at the health of the entire population is a key goal. The population health approach thus needs to pay considerable attention to the workings of the public and private healthcare system, as well as that of the public health system. In Chapter 12, we will seek to better understand what we mean by public health institutions and the public health system.

BOX 11-5   Using Competition to Control Costs.

The healthcare system in the United States is perhaps the most market-oriented system of any major nation. To successfully control costs through market mechanisms, a number of characteristics of a well-functioning market need to be in place. It has been argued that, until recently, the U.S. healthcare system has not reflected most of these characteristics. Advocates of a market approach often share these concerns, but argue that it is possible to modify the U.S. healthcare system so that it functions as a better market system.

Let us take a brief look at key features of a well-functioning market, examine the extent to which the U.S. healthcare systems fulfills these conditions, and examine changes that are being made or considered to move the United States toward a more effective market-based system.

- **Informed purchaser:** An informed purchaser is a key requirement for a well-functioning healthcare market. In the U.S. healthcare system, the employer often serves an intermediary role in selecting the health plans from which their employees may choose. Until recent years employers paid little attention to the details of the health plans that they offered. However, that habit is changing rapidly. Cost information is now widely available to both employees and employers, and quality measures are also becoming available. Employers often rely on accreditation standards, such as those of the National Committee on Quality Assurance, which now accredits a range of types of health plans and group practices. In addition, data on outcomes for surgical and medical procedures are increasingly available at the level of the hospital and group practice.
- **Purchasing power:** The second requirement of a well-functioning market is the ability of those who need the product to have the purchasing power to obtain it. In the United States, approximately 15 percent of the population is uninsured and many more are underinsured. Thus, many cannot afford the available product. Any effort to make the U.S. healthcare market work better needs to ensure adequate purchasing power for those who need it to pay for health insurance and thereby participate in the system.
- **Multiple competing providers:** Well-functioning markets give purchasers a choice of service providers. Consumers' choices then generally favor providers who offer the services at reduced costs and/or increased quality. The availability of choices for employed individuals has increased in recent years, especially for those whose employers pay a substantial portion of the premiums. Employees of large firms and organizations typically have a range of choices and can choose their health plan based on

(continues)

BOX 11-5 *continued.*

criteria including cost, quality, and convenience. Many other consumers, however, have limited or no choice in healthcare coverage.

- **Negotiation:** Negotiation is the key to putting information, purchasing power, and competition together. These negotiations increasingly take place through the employer. However, labor unions are becoming more involved in issues related to health benefits as well because health insurance constitutes an increasing percentage of their current, as well as future, benefits. The individual employee often has little negotiating power and needs to rely on their employee representatives and/or their employers.

If the U.S. healthcare system continues to move in the direction of becoming a competitive healthcare market, it will need to ensure that these conditions are fulfilled as much as possible.

Key Words

- Medicare
- Medicaid
- Medigap
- State Child Health Insurance Program (SCHIP)
- Community rating
- Experience rating
- Fee-for-service
- Capitation
- Skimming
- Preferred Provider Organization (PPO)
- Point-of-Service Plan (POS)
- Universal coverage
- Employer mandates
- Individual mandates
- Single payer

Discussion Questions

Take a look at the questions posed in the following scenarios which were presented at the beginning of this chapter. See now whether you can answer them.

1. *The politicians seem to agree that health care is too expensive. However, some argue for greater regulation, while others argue for less. You ask yourself: what are the options for controlling costs and what are the consequences?*

2. *You take a job right out of college and need to select from among your company's healthcare options or alternatively choose not to be insured. The choices appear to be quite complicated and none of them seems just right for you. How can you go about choosing between health insurance options?*

3. *You decide to take your chances and refuse the expensive health insurance offered by your employer. What are the consequences of not having insurance?*

4. *Members of the Smith family live in the United States, Canada, and the United Kingdom. They have the same inherited disease. The recommended treatment is quite similar in the three countries and can be delivered as part of primary care. How might the delivery of care and the payment for care differ among the three countries?*

5. *You wonder how the United States ranks globally in terms of the performance of its healthcare system. You're surprised when you find out that its ranking is not #1 or even near the top. Why is that? you ask yourself.*

REFERENCES

1. Shi L, Singh D. *Delivering Health Care in America: A Systems Approach.* 4th ed. Sudbury, MA: Jones and Bartlett Publishers; 2008.
2. Sultz HA, Young KM. *Health Care USA: Understanding Its Organization and Delivery.* 6th ed. Sudbury, MA: Jones and Bartlett Publishers; 2009.
3. Institute of Medicine. Hidden Costs, Value Lost: Uninsurance in America. Washington, DC: National Academies Press; 2003.
4. The Henry J. Kaiser Family Foundation. Health Coverage and the Uninsured. Available at: http://www.kff.org/uninsured/index.cfm. Accessed April 3, 2009.
5. Health Canada. Health Care System. Available at: http://www.hc-sc.gc.ca/hcs-sss/index-eng.php. Accessed April 3, 2009.
6. National Health Service History. Chapter from "From Cradle to Grave: 50 Years of the NHS." Available at: http://www.nhshistory.net/envoi1.html. Accessed April 3, 2009.
7. The Commonwealth Fund. Commission on a High Performance Health System, Available at: http://www.commonwealthfund.org/programs/programs_list.htm?attrib_id=11932. Accessed April 3, 2009.
8. CATO Institute. Health Care Needs a Dose of Competition. Available at: http://www.cato.org/pub_display.php?pub_id=5070. Accessed April 3, 2009.

Section IV:
Cases and Discussion Questions

When Nursing Meets Medicine

Maureen felt she had no other choice but to let the hospital administrator know when a physician had repeatedly prescribed the wrong dose of medication. How many times could she double-check with Dr. George Ludwig just to be sure that she had understood his orders. "Orders, they still call them," she thought to herself, "that is certainly what they want them to be."

The days of obeying orders were over for Maureen. She had been through nursing school and after five years working in the hospital she went back to get her master's as a nurse specialist so she could work in an intensive care unit. Now she was doing the weekend 12-hour nursing shift to make ends meet and finish her degree. Nurses were in short supply so she could now for the first time speak her mind without fear of losing her job. Nursing, she realized, was by its very name designed to nurture and take care of patients, but that did not apply to physicians. Their arrogance was so deep she didn't think they saw it.

Hospital policy required nurses to follow the orders after first checking with the head nurse and then double-checking with a physician. Complaints could be filed with the hospital quality assurance committee, but the process took months and the nurse who initiated the process could be reprimanded if the committee found their complaints to be unfounded or trivial. Trivial, this wasn't, but when she confronted the hospital administrator, he confided, "Don't put me in the middle of this." The pharmacist finally agreed to call the doctor and check on whether he preferred the "standard dose" of medication or the "unusual dose" he had first ordered. Dr. Ludwig agreed that the standard dose was "worth a try," so Maureen went ahead and followed the doctor's new orders.

Not too many months later, Maureen found herself confronted with new decisions in her first job as a nurse specialist in the intensive care unit. She now worked under "standing orders," which allowed her to make many a decision on her own. For the first time, she felt like she was calling the shots and making the decisions that made a difference for patients.

On one shift, late in her middle of the night, she was running from bed to bed covering the intensive care unit when she realized that she had given a patient the wrong medication. Fortunately, it was not a life-threatening mistake. She sighed with relief. Checking the chart carefully, however, she winced when her eyes fell upon the name of the attending physician, Dr. George Ludwig.

1. How is Maureen's situation affected by the structure of the nursing profession?
2. How is Maureen's situation affected by the changes in roles of women that have occurred in the United States in the last 30 years?
3. How is Maureen's situation affected by the changes that have occurred in the delivery of health care over the last 10–20 years?
4. What changes do you think are needed in the healthcare system to prevent the types of mistakes illustrated in this case?

Jack and Continuity of Care

Jack was told that he had high blood pressure and high cholesterol when he was in the army. Because the conditions didn't bother him, Jack paid little attention to them. His job did not provide health insurance, so he decided to take his chances. Anyway, he was strong and athletic. Over the years, Jack gained weight, exercised less, and developed a "touch of diabetes."

When the diabetes produced symptoms, he went to the emergency room where they did a good job of diagnosing his problem and sent him off with a prescription and a few pills to get started. The pills seemed to help, but Jack couldn't afford to fill the prescription or follow-up with his "family doctor" because he didn't have one. Jack didn't understand all the terms the doctors and nurses used to describe his condition, but he knew it was serious and could get worse.

It wasn't long before he was sick again, so this time he sought care at a free clinic. He didn't qualify for Medicaid, but the treatment was free. For a couple of months, he followed up and was feeling better, but on the next scheduled visit they told him, "you need to be in the hospital—you're getting worse." They got him to the hospital where he was admitted to the university service and assigned to a young resident who just graduated from a well-known medical school. The resident reviewed his condition, developed a treatment plan, and explained to Jack what needed to be done. He ordered a TB skin test and collected sputum to check for TB because of Jack's chronic cough. Unfortunately, before the treatment could be implemented the resident rotated to another service and Jack's new resident didn't seem to pay much attention to him.

Jack decided to leave the hospital against medical advice and left no forwarding address. His TB skin test was never read. When his positive sputum culture for TB came back, the laboratory alerted the local health department. Not knowing where Jack lived, the health department was not able to follow up.

Before he left, the hospital made sure that Jack had signed all the forms to receive Medicaid payments for the hospitalization. However, Jack didn't complete the forms because he didn't plan to get any more medical care. That changed one day when the pain was more than he could stand. He decided to try another emergency room. This time the place was very crowded and he had to wait hours to be seen. Once he was examined, the physicians and nurses tried to get information from him on his condition and treatment, but Jack couldn't provide much useful information.

He was prescribed pain medicine and sent home. He was told to follow up with a doctor in the next few days. By then it was too late. In the middle of the night, Jack had a terrible headache and lost his speech. He struggled to call 911. Despite the fact that he could not speak, the operator was able to send an ambulance by tracing his telephone location. The EMTs rushed to Jack's home and got him to the nearest hospital. Once again, the emergency room clinicians evaluated him, but this time it was too late to be of much help. Jack was admitted for a stroke.

He stayed in the hospital for a week and made some improvement, but he needed help with the activities of daily living and could only speak a few words. The hospital was able to place him in a rehabilitation center since Jack qualified for skilled nursing care. He was transferred to the facility and received intensive rehabilitation services for the next month until he no longer improved. At that point, Jack was no longer eligible for skilled nursing care. He was transferred to a facility closer to his only relatives. The new facility had a large number of patients needing "custodial care." It provided all the services required by law, but Jack soon realized that he was just another stroke patient.

1. How does this case illustrate the lack of institutional continuity?
2. How does this case illustrate the lack of continuity between the healthcare and public health systems?
3. How does this case illustrate the lack of financial continuity?
4. What role does the lack of information play in this case? How can information technology serve to reduce or eliminate these lapses in continuity? Which lapses require other types of interventions?

Susan and the System

"PAYMENT REJECTED" was stamped in large letters on the bill that Susan received from her health insurance. She didn't find out much more after waiting on the phone and being transferred three times. All she was told was that her assigned doctor had not followed the guidelines distributed by the plan.

Susan had been doing well until a small area of breast cancer was discovered at the site of her original mastectomy. She now wondered if she had made the right decision in deciding not to take the medication she was prescribed. She never admitted to anyone that she just couldn't afford the medication, but after the alimony checks stopped coming she had to make some hard choices. Her doctor told her that he now thought she should be aggressive. After a consultation with her oncologist, he prescribed what he called a "new approach using approved drugs."

When Susan's doctor finally got through the managed care system, he was told "we don't pay for promising new treatments—we only pay for established or proven treatments." The new emphasis on patients' rights had given Susan the right to appeal. But the issue was not whether or not she and her doctor had made a reasonable decision for her. The question was: did her managed care health insurance contract cover this type of promising new treatment?

It didn't look like she had a chance on appeal and she decided to pay for her care herself, or out-of-pocket, as they call it in insurance language. Actually, at first it was out of her modest savings and then when that dried up she began to use her credit cards. "What choice do I have?" she often cried out in frustration. It was death or bankruptcy and at least with bankruptcy she got a second chance.

The treatment worked, but as expected Susan ran out of savings and credit. For follow-up care, Susan ended up on Medicaid, the health insurance system designed for the poor. Her oncologist didn't take Medicaid—she was told she'd have to make other arrangements. That wasn't easy—the only oncologist she could find who accepted Medicaid was across town in an area she was afraid to be in after dark. But, she went ahead anyway and despite the initial fears, she was pleased when the doctor seemed to understand her situation medically and personally.

Susan's cancer finally was under control and she was determined to put herself back on her feet financially. Susan found a new job, but couldn't manage to work full time and thus could not afford her employer-sponsored health insurance. Being on Medicaid made her feel like a second-class citizen. Now, when she finally seemed to be getting back on her feet financially, they were going to take it away. "The safety net is sure full of holes. The only right in health care is the right of the doctors and hospitals to be paid," she thought to herself.

1. How did the structure and operation of her health insurance plan affect the care that Susan received?
2. How did the structure and operation of Medicaid affect the care that Susan received?
3. What other factors influenced the care that Susan received?
4. What changes would you make in healthcare financing to address the issues raised in this case?

Donna's Doctor—To Error Is Human

Donna's heart was racing again and there just didn't seem to be a reason for it. She wasn't upset and hadn't been exercising. She was only 48 and no one seemed to take her seriously when she told everyone that something was wrong with her heart. She knew it was more than her recent divorce and raising a couple of teenagers. Not even the diagnosis of menopause satisfied her.

She decided to change primary care doctors having heard that Dr. Stein actually listened. He did listen and examined her carefully, but didn't find anything. He ordered a 24-hour test to monitor her heart. Donna did her usual activity and the portable device recorded a basic electrocardiogram. She had one brief episode of racing heart. She recorded the time and length of the episode just as requested and sure enough she was having a brief episode of what the doctor called "atrial fibrillation" at the time.

A week later Donna got the results—episodes of atrial fibrillation. The upper chambers of her heart, called the atria, were beating very rapidly. Her lower chambers, called the ventricles which pumps the blood out of the heart, were doing just fine so she was not in immediate danger. "The real danger is blood clots and potentially a stroke," Dr. Stein told her, "and we should thin or anticoagulate your blood." The thought of a stroke was enough to convince Donna to go ahead.

Anticoagulation may require a drug called Warfarin often known by the brand name Coumadin she was told, but it has

to be done carefully. It can cause bleeding if it is not checked often. Taking Coumadin, Donna felt protected. She went back for the tests to adjust the dose. She felt better and now had lots of energy, but she still had some of those episodes of rapid heart rate.

When the hot flashes began, she knew that menopause had in fact arrived, but she felt better than ever and found herself skipping her blood tests because she wanted to be sure that she had time for her exercise routine. She didn't realize that anything was wrong until she fell off her bike one day, hitting her head. Fortunately, she was wearing a helmet so the injury didn't seem too bad. However, she did feel dizzy afterwards. And then a few hours later, her son told her that her speech was slurred. "Have you been drinking, Mom?" he asked. The look of disdain on his mother's face was enough to worry her son who now insisted on taking her to the emergency room.

Dr. Stein met Donna and her son in the emergency room. He arranged an emergency MRI scan that showed evidence of a small bleed and the blood test showed her anticoagulation level was too high. The doctors rapidly reversed the level and over the next few days Donna's mental state returned to normal. "What a relief," she thought, "but there has to be a better answer than going back to anticoagulation." Her doctors in the hospital asked for a consultation. First, the medical student, then the resident, and finally the professor came to look her over, examined her carefully, and then talked about her just outside her door where she could hear bits and pieces of their conversation. "Dr. Stein sure missed the diagnosis,"..."If she had only been compliant, none of this would have happened,"..."An obvious case of hyperthyroidism,"... "No need for Coumadin."

"The blood tests confirm overactivity of your thyroid, which is a condition called hyperthyroidism," the resident told her. "This caused your atrial fibrillation and your increased energy. You need treatment, but we don't do that here—we'll give you a referral." Donna could hardly absorb everything and didn't get a chance to even ask questions.

She went back to Dr. Stein who told her how badly he felt about missing the hyperthyroidism—he too had learned a lesson and he apologized for what had happened. He told her that there was very good treatment for hyperthyroidism and he would be pleased to take care of her after consultation with a specialist. Donna knew that doctors make mistakes, but she didn't know that they admitted them. She knew that Dr. Stein was a good doctor and that he would pay extra attention to her. Donna hoped that things would go well and was confident that she was in good hands with Dr. Stein.

1. Did Dr. Stein's care fulfill the duty, breach, causation, and damages criteria for medical malpractice?
2. What additional aspects of Dr. Stein's care affected whether a malpractice case resulted?
3. What role do you think the disclosure of error played in preventing a malpractice suit?
4. What attitudes toward decision making in health care on the part of Donna influenced the approach she took to her healthcare?

Health Care in America—For Better or Worse?

The final hours came as no surprise to his wife and family, who made daily visits to the hospital where Sam had been treated on and off for the final year of his life. His doctor had spared no expense to give him the most effective treatments available. "But wouldn't it have been nice if he could have died at home," they thought to themselves as they gathered at the funeral. "At least he held out until after the baby was born."

Sam's diagnosis of colon cancer did not shock him. His father died of colon cancer and he had been thinking it was time to be checked. Surgery went well and he and his doctor were optimistic about the future. The surprise came about 18 months later, when during a follow-up examination, he was told that there might be a recurrence.

Chemotherapy seemed to do more harm than good. There didn't seem to be a good answer. Sam's physician sought out the newest treatment, but it didn't seem to help. The final shock to his system came after he received a dose of the wrong medicine administered by a nurse who was new to the unit. She was hired in response to the recent accreditation review, which criticized the hospital for understaffing.

Though his death was no surprise, the bills from the hospital and physician were an unexpected burden in the months and years that followed. The health insurance that was offered through Sam's employer did not pay for screening for the colon cancer that killed him. In addition, its loopholes, caps, and copayments left the family with bills that would require years to repay. It was not just the uncovered expenses that they had to pay out-of-pocket, it was the mountains of paperwork that arrived in the mail.

Nonetheless, the family understood. The doctors had done everything possible and treated Sam and them with respect and responded quickly to their calls and continuous questions. Maybe things weren't ideal, they concluded, but at least they did everything they could.

1. What strengths of the U.S. healthcare system are illustrated in this case?
2. What limitations of the U.S. healthcare system are illustrated in this case?
3. What steps would you recommend to improve the delivery of preventive and curative services to better serve patients like Sam?
4. How might Sam's health care have been different in other developed countries, such as Canada and the United Kingdom? In what ways might it have been better and in what ways might it have been worse?

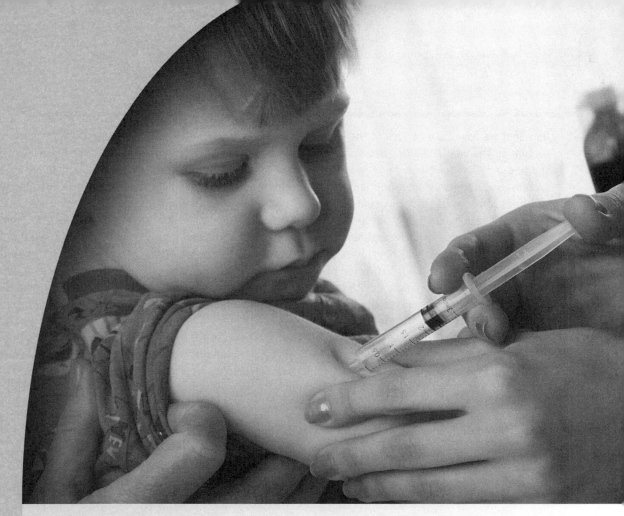

SECTION V

Public Health Institutions and Systems

Now that we have taken a look at the U.S. healthcare institutions and healthcare system, we need to turn our attention to the public health system. Treating healthcare and public health systems as separate systems is artificial because they have many points of overlap and collaboration. However, historically public health institutions and systems have developed from different philosophies, have different goals, and have organizational structures and lines of accountability different from those of the healthcare system.

We will begin by outlining the current goals and roles of public health agencies. Then, we will look at the current system of local/state, federal, and global public health institutions and examine how they are organized. We will explore why public health agencies need to coordinate with each other to achieve the goals of public health.

We will then return to our definition of population health—*the totality of all evidence-based public and private efforts to preserve and promote health and prevent disease, disability and death*. This broad 21st century definition requires public health agencies and professionals to collaborate with a range of government agencies and healthcare professionals and institutions.

In Chapter 13, the final chapter, we will turn our attention to the roles that public health needs to play in planning for the future. We will begin by examining its role in preparing for and responding to disasters. We will then take a look at what we can learn from the past that can help us predict and prepare for the future. Finally, we will examine and illustrate the emerging approach known as systems thinking which can help us see and address the big picture issue of health.

Thus, in this final chapter of *Public Health 101*, we will examine the complex puzzle that we call population health. We will look at frameworks for putting the pieces together to address the health issues that will inevitably be part of your future. Regardless of where your career leads, you will find that public health affects every corner of your lives and every corner of our world.

Let us turn our attention in Chapter 12 to the current public health institutions and public health systems.

CHAPTER 12

Public Health Institutions and Systems

LEARNING OBJECTIVES

By the end of this chapter, the student will be able to:

- identify goals of governmental public health.
- identify the ten essential services of public health.
- describe basic features of local, state, and federal public health agencies in the United States.
- identify global public health organizations and agencies and describe their basic roles.
- identify roles in public health for federal agencies not identified as health agencies.
- illustrate the need for collaboration by governmental public health agencies with other governmental and nongovernmental organizations.
- describe approaches to connecting public health and the health-care system.

A young man in your dormitory is diagnosed with tuberculosis. The health department works with the student health service to test everyone in the dorm, as well as in his classes, with a TB skin test. Those who are positive for the first time are advised to take a course of a medicine called INH. You ask: is this standard operating procedure?

You go to a public health meeting and learn that many of the speakers are not from public health agencies, but from the Departments of Labor, Commerce, Housing, and Education. You ask: what do these departments have to do with health?

You hear that a new childhood vaccine was developed by the NIH, approved by the FDA, endorsed for federal payment by the CDC and recommended for use by the American Academy of Pediatrics. You ask: do all these agencies and organizations always work so well together?

A major flood in Asia leads to disease and starvation. Some say it is due to global warming, others to bad luck. Coordinated efforts by global health agencies, assisted by nongovernmental organizations (NGOs) and outside governmental donors, help get the country back on its feet. You ask: what types of cooperation are needed to make all of this happen?

A local community health center identifies childhood obesity as a problem in their community. They collect data demonstrating that the problem begins as early as elementary school. They develop a plan that includes clinical interventions at the health center and also at the elementary school. They ask the health department to help them organize an educational campaign and assist in evaluating the results. Working together, they are able to reduce the obesity rate among elementary school children by one-half. This seems like a new way to practice public health, you conclude. What type of approach is this?

These cases all reflect the responsibilities of public health agencies at the local, federal, and global levels. They illustrate public health working the way it is supposed to work. Of course, this is not always the case. Let us start by taking a look at the goals and roles of public health agencies.

WHAT ARE THE GOALS AND ROLES OF GOVERNMENTAL PUBLIC HEALTH AGENCIES?

Public health is often equated with the work of governmental agencies. The role of government is only a portion of what we mean by public health, but it is an important component. So important, in fact, that we often define the roles of other components in terms of how they relate to the work of governmental public health agencies.

In 1994, the United States Public Health Service put forth the "Public Health in America Statement," which provided the framework that continues to define the goals and services of governmental public health agencies.[1] These goals should already be familiar to you. They are:

- to prevent epidemics and the spread of disease
- to protect against environmental hazards
- to prevent injuries
- to promote and encourage healthy behaviors
- to respond to disasters and assist communities in recovery
- to ensure the quality and accessibility of health services

These are ambitious and complicated goals to achieve. To be able to successfully achieve them, it is important to further define the roles that governmental public health agencies themselves play, and by implication, the roles that other governmental agencies and nongovernmental organizations need to play.

The Public Health in America Statement built upon the Institute of Medicine's (IOM) 1988 report called The Future of Public Health.[2] The IOM defined three **core public health functions** that governmental public health agencies need to perform. The concept of "core function" implies that the job cannot be delegated to other agencies or to nongovernmental organizations. It also implies that the governmental public health agencies will work together to accomplish these functions because as a group they are responsible for public health as a whole—no one agency at the local, state, or federal level is specifically or exclusively responsible for accomplishing the essential public health services.[a]

The core functions defined by the IOM are: 1) assessment, 2) policy development, and 3) assurance.[2]

- **Assessment** includes obtaining data that defines the health of the overall population and specific groups within the population, including defining the nature of new and persisting health problems.
- **Assurance** includes governmental public health's oversight responsibility for ensuring that key components of an effective health system, including health care and public health, are in place even though the implementation will often be performed by others.

- **Policy development** includes developing evidence-based recommendations and other analyses of options, such as health policy analysis, to guide implementation including efforts to educate and mobilize community partnerships.

The three core functions, while useful in providing a delineation of responsibilities and an intellectual framework for the work of governmental public health agencies, were not tangible enough to provide a clear understanding or definition of the work of public health agencies. Thus, in addition to the goals of public health, the Public Health in America Statement defined a series of **ten essential public health services** that build upon the IOM's core functions, guide day-to-day responsibilities, and provide a mechanism for evaluating whether the core functions are fulfilled. These ten services have come to define the responsibilities of the combined local, state, and federal governmental public health system.

WHAT ARE THE TEN ESSENTIAL PUBLIC HEALTH SERVICES?

Table 12-1 outlines the ten essential public health services and organizes them according to which IOM core function they aim to fulfill.[1] A description of each service is presented in column two and examples of these essential services are listed in column three.

We have now looked at the core public health functions and the ten essential services of public health agencies. Figure 12-1 puts these together to allow you to see the connections.

These public health services are delivered through a complex web of local and federal agencies, as well as via increasing involvement of global organizations. Let us take a look at the work of public health agencies at each of these levels.

Figure 12-2 provides a framework to guide our review of the delivery of public health services. It diagrams the central role of governmental public health agencies and the complicated connections required to accomplish their responsibilities. We will begin by taking at look at the structure and function of governmental public health agencies at the local/state, federal, and global levels. Then, we will examine the key connections with other governmental agencies, community, and private organizations, and finally with the healthcare delivery system as a whole.

WHAT ARE THE ROLES OF LOCAL AND STATE PUBLIC HEALTH AGENCIES?

The United States Constitution does not mention public health. Thus, public health is first and foremost a state responsibility. States may retain the authority, voluntarily request or

---

[a] This does not imply that components of the work cannot be contracted to nongovernmental organizations. This activity is increasingly occurring. The concept of core function, however, implies that public health agencies remain responsible for these functions even when the day-to-day work is conducted through contracts with an outside organization.

TABLE 12-1 Ten Essential Public Health Services

Essential service	Meaning of essential service	Example
ASSESSMENT—Core function		
1. Monitor health status to identify and solve community health problems	This service includes accurate diagnosis of the community's health status; identification of threats to health and assessment of health service needs; timely collection, analysis, and publication of information on access, utilization, costs, and outcomes of personal health services; attention to the vital statistics and health status of specific groups that are at a higher risk than the total population; and collaboration to manage integrated information systems with private providers and health benefit plans.	Vital Statistics Health Surveys Surveillance, including reportable diseases
2. Diagnose and investigate health problems and health hazards in the community	This service includes epidemiologic identification of emerging health threats; public health laboratory capability using modern technology to conduct rapid screening and high-volume testing; active infectious disease epidemiology programs; and technical capacity for epidemiologic investigation of disease outbreaks and patterns of chronic disease and injury.	Epidemic investigations CDC–Epidemiology Intelligence Service State Public Health Laboratories
POLICY DEVELOPMENT—Core function		
3. Inform, educate, and empower people about health issues	This service includes social marketing and media communications; providing accessible health information resources at community levels; active collaboration with personal health care providers to reinforce health promotion messages and programs; and joint health education programs with schools, churches, and worksites.	Health education campaigns, such as comprehensive state tobacco programs
4. Mobilize community partnerships and action to identify and solve health problems	This service includes convening and facilitating community groups and associations, including those not typically considered to be health-related, in undertaking defined preventive, screening, rehabilitation, and support programs; and skilled coalition-building to draw upon the full range of potential human and material resources in the case of community health.	Lead control programs: testing and follow-up of children, reduction of lead exposure, educational follow-up, and addressing underlying causes
5. Develop policies and plans that support individual and community health efforts	This service requires leadership development at all levels of public health; systematic community and state-level planning for health improvement in all jurisdictions; tracking of measurable health objectives as a part of continuous quality improvement strategies; joint evaluation with the medical health care system to define consistent policy regarding prevention and treatment services; and development of codes, regulations, and legislation to guide public health practice.	Newborn screening program for PKU and other genetic and congenital diseases

continues

TABLE 12-1 Ten Essential Public Health Services (continued)

Essential service	Meaning of essential service	Example
ASSURANCE—Core function		
6. Enforce laws and regulations that protect health and ensure safety	This service involves full enforcement of sanitary codes, especially in the food industry; full protection of drinking water supplies; enforcement of clean air standards; timely follow-up of hazards, preventable injuries, and exposure-related diseases identified in occupational and community settings; monitoring quality of medical services (e.g. laboratory, nursing home, and home health care); and timely review of new drug, biological, and medical device applications.	Local: Fluoridation and chlorination of water State: Regulation of nursing homes Federal: FDA drug approval and food safety
7. Link people to needed personal health services and ensure the provision of health care when otherwise unavailable	This service (often referred to as "outreach" or "enabling" service) includes ensuring effective entry for socially disadvantaged people into a coordinated system of clinical care; culturally- and linguistically-appropriate materials and staff to ensure linkage to services for special population groups; ongoing "care management"; and transportation.	Community Health Centers
8. Ensure the provision of a competent public and personal health care workforce	This service includes education and training for personnel to meet the needs for public and personal health services; efficient processes for licensure of professionals and certification of facilities with regular verification and inspection follow-up; adoption of continuous quality improvement and lifelong learning within all licensure and certification programs; active partnerships with professional training programs to ensure community-relevant learning experiences for all students; and continuing education in management and leadership development programs for those charged with administrative/executive roles.	Licensure of physicians, nurses, and other health professionals
9. Evaluate effectiveness, accessibility, and quality of personal and population-based health services	This service calls for ongoing evaluation of health programs, based on analysis of health status and service utilization data, to assess program effectiveness and to provide information necessary for allocating resources and reshaping programs.	Development of evidence-based recommendations
ALL THREE IOM—Core function		
10. Research for new insights and innovative solutions to health problems	This service includes continuous linkage with appropriate institutions of higher learning and research and an internal capacity to mount timely epidemiologic and economic analyses and conduct needed health services research.	NIH, CDC, AHRQ other federal agencies

Source: Data from Public Health in America. Essential Public Health Services. Available at http://www.health.gov/phfunctions/public.htm. Accessed November 8, 2008.

FIGURE 12-1 Essential public health services and IOM core functions

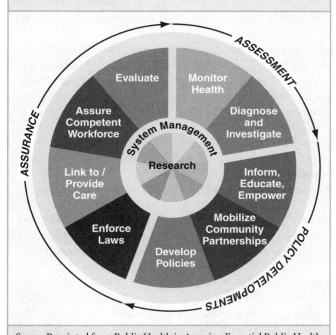

Source: Reprinted from Public Health in America. Essential Public Health Services. Available at http://www.health.gov/phfunctions/public.htm. Accessed November 8, 2008.

FIGURE 12-2 Framework for viewing governmental public health agencies and their complicated connections

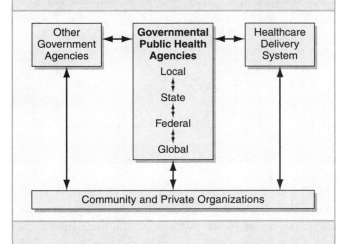

accept help from the federal government, or delegate their responsibility and/or authority to local agencies at the city, county, or other local levels.[b]

Box 12-1 describes a brief history of public health agencies in the United States. It is a complex history and has resulted in more structures than there are states—more because large cities often have their own public health systems.[3] In addition, the District of Columbia and several U.S. territories have their own systems and often have authority to make public health system decisions as if they were states.

To understand the role of local health departments, it is useful to think of two models.[4] In the first model, which we will call the home rule or local autonomy model, authority is delegated from the state to the local health department. The local health department, or the local government, has a great deal of autonomy in setting its own structure and function and often raising its own funding.

In the second model, which we will call the branch office model, the local health department can be viewed as a branch office of the state agency with little or no independent authority or funding. Most health departments lie somewhere in between these two extreme models, however these models provide a framework for understanding the many varieties of department structures. Thus, when we speak of local public health, we may be speaking of a state agency with branch offices or a relatively independent local agency. Regardless of which model a state uses, many public health responsibilities of local public health departments are quite similar and they usually have authority and responsibility for at least the following:[4]

- immunizations for those not covered by the private system
- communicable disease surveillance and initial investigation of outbreaks
- communicable disease control, often including at a minimum tuberculosis and syphilis case finding and treatment
- inspection and licensing of restaurants
- environmental health surveillance
- coordinating public health screening programs, including newborn and lead screenings
- tobacco control programs
- public health preparedness and response to disasters

Health departments in many parts of the United States have also served as the healthcare provider for those without

---

[b] This delegation may occur at the discretion of the state government or it may be included in the state's constitution providing what is called **home rule authority** to local jurisdictions. In general, jurisdictions with home rule authority exercise substantially more autonomy.

BOX 12-1   Brief History of American Public Health Agencies

An understanding of the history of American public health institutions requires an understanding of the response of local, state, and federal governments to public health crises and the complex interactions between these levels of government.

The colonial period in America saw repeated epidemics of smallpox, cholera, and yellow fever focused in the port cities. These epidemics brought fear and disruption of commerce, along with accompanying disease and death. One epidemic in Philadelphia in 1793 in what was then the nation's capital nearly shut down the federal government. These early public health crises brought about the first municipal Boards of Health, made up of respected citizens authorized to act in the community's interest to implement quarantine, evacuation, and other public health interventions of the day. The federal government's early role in combating epidemics led to the establishment in 1798 of what later became known as the U.S. Public Health Service.

Major changes in public health awaited the last half of the 19th century with the great expansion of understanding of disease and the ability to control it through community actions. The Shattuck Commission in Massachusetts in 1850 outlined the roles of state health departments as responsible for: sanitary inspections, communicable disease control, food sanitation, vital statistics, and services for infants and children. Over the next 50 years, the states gradually took the lead in developing public health institutions based upon delivery of these services.

Local health departments outside of the largest cities did not exist until the 20th century. The Rockefeller Foundation stimulated and helped fund early local health departments and campaigns in part to combat specific diseases, such as hookworm. There was no standard model for local health departments. Local health departments developed in at least 50 different ways in the 50 states and were chronically underfunded.

The federal government played a very small role in public health throughout the 1800s and well into the 20th century. An occasional public health crisis stimulated in part by media attention did bring about federal action. The founding of the Food and Drug Administration in 1906 resulted in large part from the journalistic activity known as "muckraking," which exposed the status of food and drug safety. The early years of the 20th century set the stage for expansion of the federal government's role in public health through the passage of the 16th Amendment to the Constitution authorizing federal income tax as a major source of federal government funding.

The Great Depression, in general, and the Social Security Act of 1935, in particular, brought about a new era in which federal funding became a major source of financial resources for state and local public health departments and nongovernmental organizations. The founding of the what was then called the Communicable Disease Centers (CDC) in 1946 led to a national and eventually international leadership role for the CDC which attempts to connect and hold together the complex local, state, and federal public health efforts and integrate them into global public health efforts.

The Johnson Administration's War on Poverty, as well as the Medicare and Medicaid programs, brought about greatly expanded funding for health care services and led many health departments to provide direct healthcare services especially for those without other sources of care. The late 1980s and 1990s saw a redefinition of the roles of governmental public health including the Institute of Medicine's definition of core functions and the development of the 10 Essential Public Health Services. These documents have guided the development of a broad population focus for public health and a move away from the direct provision of healthcare services.

As we will explore in Chapter 13, the terrorism of 9/11 and the subsequent anthrax scare moved public health institutions to the center of efforts to protect the public's health through emergency and disaster preparedness. The development of flexible efforts to respond to expected and unexpected hazards is now a central feature of public health institutions' roles and funding. The success of these efforts requires new levels of coordination of local, state, federal, and global public health agencies utilizing state-of-the-art surveillance, laboratory technology, and communications systems.

other sources of health care. This has been called the **healthcare safety net**. In recent years, many health departments have reduced or discontinued these services often transferring them to the healthcare system or integrating their efforts into community health centers. The concept of core functions holds that while these activities can be performed by other organizations or agencies, the public health agencies still retain responsibility for ensuring access to and the quality of these services.

The work of local public health agencies cannot be viewed in isolation. The State Health Department usually retains important roles even in those states where the local departments have home rule authority. These responsibilities often include: collecting vital statistics, running a public health laboratory, licensing of health professionals, administering nutrition programs, and regulation of health facilities, such as nursing homes. In addition, drinking water regulation, administration of the state Medicaid program, and the office of the medical examiner may also fall under the authority of the State Health Department.

Today, the federal government has a great deal of involvement in national and global issues of public health and often works closely with local agencies. Let us take a look at the structure and role of the federal government in public health.

WHAT ARE THE ROLES OF FEDERAL PUBLIC HEALTH AGENCIES?

As we saw in Chapter 5, the federal government's role in public health does not explicitly appear in the United States Constitution. It has been justified largely by the Interstate Commerce clause, which provides federal government authority to regulate commerce between the states. Federal public health authority often rests on the voluntary acceptance by the states of funding provided by the federal government. This funding may come with requirements for state action in order to qualify for the funding.

The Department of Health and Human Services (HHS) is the central public health agency of the federal government. It includes operating agencies each of which report directly to the cabinet-level Secretary of HHS. Table 12-2 outlines most of these agencies, their roles and authority, and their basic public health structure and activities.[5]

The National Institutes of Health (NIH) is far and away the largest agency within HHS with a budget of over $30 billion—as much as all the other six agencies' budgets combined. However, most of its efforts are devoted to basic science research and the translation of research into clinical practice. Some of the federal agencies, such as the Health Services and Resources Administration (HRSA), Substance Abuse and Mental Health Services Administration (SAMHSA), and the Indian Health Service, provide or fund individually-oriented health services in addition to population-oriented preventive services. The Indian Health Service is unique because it is responsible for both public health and healthcare services for a defined population.

The Centers for Disease Control and Prevention (CDC) is perhaps the agency most closely identified with public health at the federal level. Box 12-2 describes its first 50 years from 1946 to 1996 in a reprint of its official history first published in the *Morbidity and Mortality Weekly Report* (MMWR), a weekly publication of agency.[6]

Today, the CDC's role in connecting federal, state, and local governmental public health efforts is central to the success of the system. Approximately half of the CDC's current approximately $10 billion budget is channeled to state and local health departments. A key function of the CDC is to provide national leadership and to coordinate the efforts of local/state and federal public health agencies.

To understand the local/state and federal public health system, it is important to appreciate that only five percent of all health-related funding goes to public health and of that, less than half goes to population-based prevention as opposed to providing healthcare services as a safety net for individuals. In addition, the role of governmental public health is limited by social attitudes toward government. For instance, we have seen that there are constitutional limitations on the authority of public health and other government agencies to impose actions on individuals. These may limit public health agencies' abilities to address issues ranging from tuberculosis and HIV control to responses to emergencies. The social attitudes of Americans may also limit the authority and resources provided to public health agencies. Americans often favor individual or private efforts over governmental interventions when they believe that individuals and private organizations are capable of success. For instance, some Americans resist active efforts in the schools to provide information and access to contraceptives, while others resist the type of case-finding efforts for HIV/AIDS that have been used successfully in investigating and controlling other communicable diseases.

Today, governmental public health is a global enterprise. Let us take a look at the roles of global health organizations and agencies.

WHAT ARE THE ROLES OF GLOBAL HEALTH ORGANIZATIONS AND AGENCIES?

Public health is increasingly becoming a global enterprise. Global governmental efforts have grown dramatically in recent years. The World Health Organization (WHO) was created in 1948. Its impact has become more prominent in the 21st century with the increasing importance of global health issues. The WHO is a part of the United Nations organizations, which also include the United Nations Infant and Child Emergency Fund (UNICEF) and the Joint United Nations Programme on AIDS/HIV (UNAIDS).[7]

Today, the World Bank and other multilateral financial institutions are the largest funding source for global health efforts.[8] National governmental aid programs, including the United States Agency for International Development (USAID), also play an important role in public health. Table 12-3 outlines the structure/governance, roles, and limitations of global public health agencies.

TABLE 12-2 Key Federal Health Agencies of the Department of Health and Human Services

Agency	Roles/Authority	Examples of Structures/Activities
Centers for Disease Control and Prevention (CDC) and Agency for Toxic Substances and Disease Registry (ATSDR)	CDC is the lead agency for prevention, health data, epidemic investigation, and public health measures aimed at disease control and prevention. The CDC administers ATSDR, which works with the Environmental Protection Agency to provide guidance on health hazards of toxic exposures.	The CDC and ATSDR work extensively with state and local health departments. The CDC's Epidemiology Intelligence Service (EIS) functions domestically and internationally at the request of governments.
National Institutes of Health (NIH)	Lead research agency. Also funds training programs and communication of health information to the professional community and the public.	17 institutes in all—the largest being the National Cancer Institute. The National Library of Medicine is part of NIH Centers. The Centers include the John E. Fogarty International Center for Advanced Study in the Health Sciences. NIH is the world's largest biomedical research enterprise with intramural research at NIH and extramural research grants throughout the world.
Food and Drug Administration (FDA)	Consumer protection agency with authority for safety of foods and safety and efficacy of drugs, vaccines and other medical and public health interventions	Divisions responsible for food safety, medical devices, drug efficacy and safety pre- and post- approval
Health Resources and Services Administration (HRSA)	Seeks to ensure equitable access to comprehensive quality health care	Funds community health centers, HIV/AIDS services, scholarships for health professional students
Agency for Healthcare Research and Quality (AHRQ)	Research agenda to improve the outcomes and quality of health care, including patient safety and access to services	Supports U.S. Preventive Services Task Force, Evidence-based medicine research, and Guidelines Clearinghouse
Substance Abuse and Mental Health Services Administration (SAMHSA)	Works to improve quality and availability of prevention, treatment, and rehabilitation for substance abuse and mental illness	Research, data collection and funding of local services
Indian Health Service (IHS)	Provides direct health care and public health services to federally-recognized tribes	Services provided to 550 federally-recognized tribes in 35 states. Only comprehensive federal responsibility for health care, plus public health services

BOX 12-2   History of the CDC.

The Communicable Disease Center was organized in Atlanta, Georgia on July 1, 1946; its founder, Dr. Joseph W. Mountin, was a visionary public health leader who had high hopes for this small and comparatively insignificant branch of the Public Health Service (PHS). It occupied only one floor of the Volunteer Building on Peachtree Street and had fewer than 400 employees, most of whom were engineers and entomologists. Until the previous day, they had worked for Malaria Control in War Areas, the predecessor of CDC, which had successfully kept the southeastern states malaria-free during World War II and, for approximately 1 year, from murine typhus fever. The new institution would expand its interests to include all communicable diseases and would be the servant of the states, providing practical help whenever called.

Distinguished scientists soon filled CDC's laboratories, and many states and foreign countries sent their public health staffs to Atlanta for training....Medical epidemiologists were scarce, and it was not until 1949 that Dr. Alexander Langmuir arrived to head the epidemiology branch. Within months, he launched the first-ever disease surveillance program, which confirmed his suspicion that malaria, on which CDC spent the largest portion of its budget, had long since disappeared. Subsequently, disease surveillance became the cornerstone on which CDC's mission of service to the states was built and, in time, changed the practice of public health.

The outbreak of the Korean War in 1950 was the impetus for creating CDC's Epidemiological Intelligence Service (EIS). The threat of biological warfare loomed, and Dr. Langmuir, the most knowledgeable person in PHS about this arcane subject, saw an opportunity to train epidemiologists who would guard against ordinary threats to public health while watching out for alien germs. The first class of EIS officers arrived in Atlanta for training in 1951 and pledged to go wherever they were called for the next 2 years. These "disease detectives" quickly gained fame for "shoe-leather epidemiology" through which they ferreted out the cause of disease outbreaks.

The survival of CDC as an institution was not at all certain in the 1950s. In 1947, Emory University gave land on Clifton Road for a headquarters, but construction did not begin for more than a decade. PHS was so intent on research and the rapid growth of the National Institutes of Health that it showed little interest in what happened in Atlanta. Congress, despite the long delay in appropriating money for new buildings, was much more receptive to CDC's pleas for support than either PHS or the Bureau of the Budget.

Two major health crises in the mid-1950s established CDC's credibility and ensured its survival. In 1955, when poliomyelitis appeared in children who had received the recently approved Salk vaccine, the national inoculation program was stopped. The cases were traced to contaminated vaccine from a laboratory in California; the problem was corrected, and the inoculation program, at least for first and second graders, was resumed. The resistance of these 6- and 7-year-olds to polio, compared with that of older children, proved the effectiveness of the vaccine. Two years later, surveillance was used again to trace the course of a massive influenza epidemic. From the data gathered in 1957 and subsequent years, the national guidelines for influenza vaccine were developed.

CDC grew by acquisition....When CDC joined the international malaria-eradication program and accepted responsibility for protecting the earth from moon germs and vice versa, CDC's mission stretched overseas and into space.

CDC played a key role in one of the greatest triumphs of public health, the eradication of smallpox. In 1962 it established a smallpox surveillance unit, and a year later tested a newly developed jet gun and vaccine in the Pacific island nation of Tonga....CDC also achieved notable success at home tracking new and mysterious disease outbreaks. In the mid-1970s and early 1980s, it found the cause of Legionnaires disease and toxic-shock syndrome. A fatal disease, subsequently named acquired immunodeficiency syndrome (AIDS), was first mentioned in the June 5, 1981, issue of *MMWR*.

Although CDC succeeded more often than it failed, it did not escape criticism. For example, television and press reports about the Tuskegee study on long-term effects of untreated syphilis in black men created a storm of protest in 1972. This study had been initiated by PHS and other organizations in 1932 and was transferred to CDC in 1957. Although the effectiveness of penicillin as a therapy for syphilis had been established during the late 1940s, participants in this study remained untreated until the study was brought to public attention. CDC was also criticized because of the 1976 effort to vaccinate the U.S. population against swine flu, the infamous killer of 1918–1919. When some vaccinees developed Guillain-Barre syndrome, the campaign was stopped immediately; the epidemic never occurred.

As the scope of CDC's activities expanded far beyond communicable diseases, its name had to be changed. In 1970 it became the Center for Disease Control and in 1981, after extensive reorganization, Center became Centers. The words "and Prevention" were added in 1992, but, by law, the well-known three-letter acronym was retained. In health emergencies CDC means an answer to SOS calls from anywhere in the world, such as the recent one from Zaire where Ebola fever raged.

Fifty years ago CDC's agenda was non-controversial (hardly anyone objected to the pursuit of germs), and Atlanta was a backwater. In 1996, CDC's programs are often tied to economic, political, and social issues, and Atlanta is as near Washington as the tap of a keyboard.

Source: Reprinted from Centers for Disease Control and Prevention, MMWR 1996;45: 526–528.

TABLE 12-3 Global Public Health Organizations

Type of agency	Structure/Governance	Role(s)	Limitations
World Health Organization	United Nations Organization Seven "regional" semi-independent components, e.g., Pan American Health Organization covers North and South America	Policy development, e.g., tobacco treaty, epidemic control policies Coordination of services, e.g., SARS control, vaccine development Data collection and standardization, e.g., measures of health care quality, measures of health status	Limited ability to enforce global recommendations, limited funding and complex international administration
International organizations with focused agenda	UNICEF UNAIDS	Focus on childhood vaccinations Focus on AIDS	Limited agendas and limited financing
International financing organizations	The World Bank Other multilateral regional banks, e.g., InterAmerican and Asian Development Banks	World Bank is largest international funder. Increasingly supports "human capital" projects and reform of health care delivery systems and population and nutrition efforts Provides funding and technical assistance primarily as loans	Criticized for standardized approach with few local modifications
Bilateral governmental aid organizations	USAID Many other developed countries have their own organizations and contribute a higher percentage of their gross domestic product to those agencies than does the United States	Often focused on specific countries and specific types of programs, such as the United States' focus on HIV/AIDS, and maternal and child health	May be tied to domestic politics and global economic, political, or military agendas

The complexity of local, state, federal, and global public health agencies raises the question of whether or not these agencies can and do work together. It should not surprise you that close collaboration, while the goal, is often difficult to achieve with so many organizations involved. Thus, it is important to ask: how can public health agencies work together?

HOW CAN PUBLIC HEALTH AGENCIES WORK TOGETHER?

Coordination among public health agencies has been a major challenge that is built into our local, state, and federal system of governance. Increasingly, coordination also requires a global aspect as well. Efforts on all levels have a long way to go. There are signs of hope with the recent progress in such fields as tobacco control, food safety, and most notably, the response to SARS. Box 12-3 discusses the dramatic events of the 2003 SARS epidemic, providing an example of what can be done and what needs to be done to address future public health emergencies.[9]

Collaboration needs to be an everyday effort, and not just a requirement for emergencies or epidemics. Let us look at the relationships and needed collaboration among governmental

BOX 12-3　SARS and the Public Health Response.

The SARS epidemic of 2003 began with little notice, most likely somewhere in the heartland of China and then spread to other areas of Asia. The world took notice after television screens filled with reports of public health researchers sent to Asia to investigate the illness subsequently contracting and dying from the disease. Not an easily transmissible disease except for those in very close contact, such as investigators, family members, and healthcare providers, the disease spread slowly but steadily through areas of China. Among those infected, the case-fatality rate was very high especially without the benefits of modern intensive care facilities.

The disease did not respond to antibiotics and was thought to be a viral disease by its epidemiological pattern of spread and transmission, but at first no cause was known. The outside world soon felt the impact of the brewing epidemic when cases appeared in Hong Kong that could be traced to a traveler from mainland China. Fear spread when cases were recognized that could not be explained by close personal contact with a SARS victim.

The epidemic continued to spread jumping thousands of miles to Toronto, Canada, where the second greatest concentration of disease appeared. Soon, the whole world was on high alert, if not quite on the verge of panic. At least 8000 people worldwide became sick and almost 10 percent of them died. Fortunately, progress came quite quickly. Researchers coordinated by the World Health Organization (WHO) were able to put together the epidemiological information and laboratory data and establish a presumed cause, a new form of the coronavirus never before seen in humans leading to the rapid introduction of testing.

The WHO and the CDC put forth recommendations for isolation, travel restrictions, and intensive monitoring that rapidly controlled the disease even in the absence of an effective treatment aimed at a cure. SARS disappeared as rapidly as it emerged, especially after systematic efforts to control spread were put in place in China. Not eliminated, but no longer a worldwide threat, SARS left a lasting global impact. The WHO established new approaches for reporting and responding to epidemics—these now have the widespread formal acceptance of most governments.

Once the world could step back and evaluate what happened, it was recognized that the potential burden of disease posed by the SARS epidemic had worldwide implications and raised the threat of interruption of travel and trade. Local, national, and global public health agencies collaborated quickly and effectively. Infection control recommendations made at the global level were rapidly translated into efforts to identify disease at the local level and manage individual patients in hospitals throughout the world. It is a model of communicable disease control that will be needed in the future.

public health and other governemental agencies, nongovernmental organizations, and the healthcare delivery system.

WHAT OTHER GOVERNMENT AGENCIES ARE INVOLVED IN HEALTH ISSUES?

To address health issues, it is important to recognize the important roles that government agencies not designated as health agencies play in public health. Such agencies exist at the local/state, federal, and global levels. To illustrate the involvement of these agencies in health issues, let's begin with the roles of nonhealth agencies at the federal level.

A number of federal agencies serve public health functions even though they are not defined as health agencies. The roles they play are important especially when we take the population health perspective that includes the totality of efforts to promote and protect health and prevent disease, disability, and death.

Environmental health issues are an important part of the role of the Environmental Protection Agency (EPA). Reducing injury and hazardous exposures in the workplace are key goals of the Occupational Safety and Health Administration (OSHA), which is part of the Department of Labor.

Protecting health as part of preparation and response to disasters and terrorism is central to the role of the Department of Homeland Security. The Department of Agriculture shares with the FDA the role of protecting the nation's food supply. The Department of Housing and Urban Development influences the built environment and its impacts on health. The Department of Energy plays important roles in setting radiation safety standards for nuclear power plants and other sources of energy.

The multiple federal agencies involved in health-related matters often means that coordination and collaboration are required across agencies. This is certainly the case with food safety and disaster planning and response. It is true as well for efforts to address problems that cut across agencies, such as lead exposure or efforts to reduce the environmental causes of asthma.

WHAT ROLES DO NONGOVERNMENTAL ORGANIZATIONS PLAY IN PUBLIC HEALTH?

Nongovernmental organizations play increasingly important roles in public health in the United States and around the world. The United States has a long tradition of private groups organizing to advocate for public health causes, delivering public health services, and providing funding to support public health efforts. In recent years, these efforts have been expanding globally as well.

The American Red Cross and its network of international affiliates represent a major international effort to provide public health services. The organization plays a central role in obtaining volunteers for blood donations and ensuring the safety and effectiveness of the U.S. and world supply of blood products in collaboration with the U.S. Food and Drug Administration. The ability of the Red Cross to obtain donations, mobilize volunteers, and publicize the need for disaster assistance has allowed it to play a central role in providing lifesaving public health services.

Many private organizations provide public health education, support research, develop evidence-based recommendations, and provide other public health services. Many of these are organized around specific diseases or types of disease, such as the American Cancer Association, the American Heart Association, the American Lung Association and the March of Dimes, which focuses on birth defects. Other private organizations focus primarily on advocacy for individuals with specific diseases, but these organizations also may advocate for specific public health interventions. For instance, Mothers Against Drunk Driving (MADD) has had a major impact on the passage and enforcement of drunk driving laws. HIV/AIDS advocacy groups have influenced policies on confidentiality, funding, and public education.

Globally, nongovernmental organizations (NGOs) increasingly play a key role in providing services and advocating for public health policies. CARE and OXFAM are examples of the types of organizations involved in global health-related crises. Physician groups, including Physicians for Social Responsibility and Doctors without Borders, have been active in advocating for public health efforts, seeking funding for public health needs, and addressing the ethical implementation of public health programs.

New combinations of governmental and nongovernmental organizations are increasingly developing to fill in the gaps. At the global level, the Global Fund to Fight AIDS, Tuberculosis and Malaria, a public-private effort, provides funding for evidence-based interventions to address these diseases. It is funded not only by governments, but also by private foundations, such as the Bill and Melinda Gates Foundation.

Private foundations have played major roles in funding public health efforts and also stimulating governmental funding. The Rockefeller Foundation's efforts were instrumental in developing local health departments and initiating Schools of Public Health in the United States during the early years of the 20th century. The Kellogg Foundation, the Robert Wood Johnson Foundation, and most recently the Gates Foundation have all played key roles in advancing public health efforts in areas ranging from nutrition to tobacco control to advancing new public health technologies.

Foundation funding has been the catalyst in initiating new funding efforts and sustaining those that are not adequately funded by governments. They cannot be expected, however, to provide long-term support for basic public health services. Thus, additional strategies are required. One key strategy is to link public health efforts with the efforts of healthcare professionals and the healthcare system.

HOW CAN PUBLIC HEALTH AGENCIES PARTNER WITH HEALTH CARE TO IMPROVE THE RESPONSE TO HEALTH PROBLEMS?

We have already seen a number of traditional connections between public health and health care. Clinicians and public health professionals increasingly share a common commitment to evidence-based thinking, cost-effective delivery of services, and computerized and confidential data systems. They also increasingly share a commitment to provide quality services to the entire population and eliminate health disparities. The potential for successful collaboration between public health and health care is illustrated by the National Vaccine Plan, which is discussed in Box 12-4.[10]

In the mid-1990s, a Medicine-Public Health Initiative was initiated to investigate better ways to connect public health with medicine, in particular, and health care, in general. Connecting these two fields has not always had easy or successful results. Additional structures are needed to formalize effective and efficient bonds. Models do exist and new ideas are being put forth to connect clinical care and public health. Box 12-5 discusses one such model called **community-oriented primary care (COPC)**.[11]

Despite efforts in the healthcare system to reach out to the community and address public health issues (such as COPC), it remains the primary responsibility of public health to organize and mobilize community-based efforts. Working with nongovernmental organizations and healthcare professionals and organizations is imperative to effectively and efficiently accomplish the goals of public health. But, how exactly can public health agencies accomplish these goals?

BOX 12-4 National Vaccine Plan.

In 1994, a National Vaccine Plan was developed as part of a coordinated effort to accomplish the following goals:
1. Develop new and improved vaccines.
2. Ensure the optimal safety and effectiveness of vaccines and immunizations.
3. Better educate the public and members of the health profession on the benefits and risks of immunizations.

A recent Institute of Medicine (IOM) report evaluated progress since 1994 on achieving the above goals and made recommendations for the development of a revised National Vaccine Plan.[10] The IOM highlighted a number of successes since 1994 in achieving each of the goals of the Plan. These successes illustrate the potential for improved collaboration between public health systems and healthcare systems.

In terms of the development of new and improved vaccines since 1994, over 20 new vaccine products resulting from the collaborative efforts of the National Institutes of Health (NIH), academic, and industry researchers were approved by the Food and Drug Administration (FDA). Novel vaccines introduced include vaccines against pediatric pneumococcal disease, meningococcal disease, and the human papillomavirus (HPV)—a cause of cervical cancer.

In terms of safety, vaccines and vaccination approaches with improved safety have been developed since 1994, including those directed against rotavirus, pertussis (whooping cough), and polio. The FDA Center for Biologics Evaluation and Research (CBER), which regulates vaccines, now has an expanded array of regulatory tools to facilitate the review and approval of safe and efficacious vaccines. The FDA and the Centers for Disease Control and Prevention (CDC) have collaborated on surveillance for and evaluation of adverse events. Efforts have also been made to increase collaboration with the Centers for Medicare and Medicaid, the Department of Defense, and the Department of Veterans Affairs to improve surveillance and reporting of adverse events following immunization in the adult populations these agencies serve.

In terms of better education of health professionals and the public, progress has also been made. The American Academy of Pediatrics (AAP) collaborates with the CDC for its Childhood Immunization Support. The American Medical Association (AMA) cosponsors the annual National Influenza Vaccine Summit, a group that represents 100 public and private organizations interested in preventing influenza.

Despite the growing collaboration and success in vaccine development and use, new issues have appeared in recent years. Vaccines are now correctly viewed by the health professionals and the public as having both benefits and harms. In recent years, the public has grown more concerned about the safety of vaccines, including the issue of the use of large numbers of vaccines in children. The limitations of vaccines to address problems, such as HIV/AIDS, have also been increasingly recognized. Hopefully, the new National Vaccine Plan will build upon these recent successes and address the new realities and opportunities.

HOW CAN PUBLIC HEALTH TAKE THE LEAD IN MOBILIZING COMMUNITY PARTNERSHIPS TO IDENTIFY AND SOLVE HEALTH PROBLEMS?

An essential service of public health is the mobilization of community partnerships and action to identify and solve health problems. These efforts by public health agencies are critical to putting the pieces of the health system together to protect and promote health and prevent disability and death.

Examples of successful collaboration include state tobacco control programs that have been led by public health agencies, but rely heavily on nongovernmental organizations, healthcare professionals and other governmental agencies. These efforts have been able to substantially reduce statewide cigarette smoking rates.

Efforts to organize coordinated programs for lead control have also met with some success. Collaborative efforts between public health and health care have identified and treated children with elevated lead levels. Cooperation with other agencies has provided for the removal of lead paint from homes and testing and control of lead in playgrounds, water, and most recently, toys.

It is possible to view the coordinated mobilization of public and private efforts as **community-oriented public health (COPH)**. We can see this as a parallel to COPC. In COPC, healthcare efforts are expanded to take on additional public health roles. In COPH, public health efforts are expanded to collaborate with healthcare delivery institutions, as well as other community and governmental efforts. Child oral health, an example of COPH, is illustrated in Box 12-6.[12]

BOX 12-5   Community Oriented Primary Care (COPC).

Community-oriented primary care (COPC) is a structured effort to expand the delivery of health services from a focus on the individual to also include an additional focus on the needs of communities. Serving the needs of communities brings healthcare and public health efforts together. COPC can be seen as an effort on the part of healthcare delivery sites, such as community health centers, to reach out to their community and to governmental public health institutions.

Table 12–4 outlines the six steps in the COPC process and presents a question to ask when addressing each of these steps. Notice the parallels between COPC and the evidence-based approach that we have outlined. In both cases, the process is actually circular because evaluation efforts often lead to recycling to move the process ahead.

TABLE 12-4 The Six Sequential Steps of Community-Oriented Primary Care (COPC)

Steps in the COPC process	Questions to ask
1. Community definition	How is the community defined based upon geography, institutional affiliation, or other common characteristics, e.g., use of an Internet site?
2. Community characterization	What are the demographic and health characteristics of the community and what are its health issues?
3. Prioritization	What are the most important health issues facing the community and how should they be prioritized based upon objective data and perceived need?
4. Detailed assessment of the selected health problem	What are the most effective and efficient interventions for addressing the selected health problem based upon an evidence-based assessment?
5. Intervention	What strategies will be used to implement the intervention?
6. Evaluation	How can the success of the intervention be evaluated?

Source: Data from District of Columbia Area Health Education Center. The Conceptual Framework for COPC. Available at: http://dcahec.gwumc.edu/education/session4/index.html. Accessed November 8, 2008.

A series of principles underlies COPC including:
- Healthcare needs are defined by examining the community as a whole, not just those who seek care.
- Needed healthcare services are provided to everyone within a defined population or community.
- Preventive, curative, and rehabilitative care are integrated within a coordinated delivery system.
- Members of the community directly participate in all stages of the COPC process.

The concept of COPC, if not the specific structure, has been widely accepted as an approach for connecting the organized delivery of primary health care with public health. It implies that public health issues can and should be addressed when possible at the level of the community with the involvement of healthcare providers and the community members themselves.

Developing community partnerships is a time-consuming and highly political process that requires great leadership and diplomatic skills. Central authority and command and control approaches are generally not effective in the complex organizational structures of the United States. New approaches and new strategies are needed to bring together the organizations and individuals who can get the job done.

We have now looked at the organization of the public health system and the challenges it faces in accomplishing its core functions and providing its essential services. The role of

BOX 12-6 Child Oral Health and Community Oriented Public Health (COPH).

The problem of childhood dental disease illustrates the potential for community-oriented public health (COPH). A lack of regular dental care remains a major problem for children in developed, as well as developing countries. The need for this type of care is often high on the agenda of parents, teachers, and even the children themselves.

Public health efforts to improve oral health go back to the late 19th- and early 20th centuries when toothbrushing and toothpaste were new and improved technologies. The public health campaigns of the early 20th century were very instrumental in making toothbrushing a routine part of American life. The history of public health interventions in childhood oral health is a story of great hope and partial success. The benefits of the fluoridation of drinking water were well grounded in evidence. The American Dental Association and the American Medical Association have supported this intervention for over half a century. Resistance from those who view it as an intrusion of governmental authority, however, has prevented universal use of fluoridation in the United States. After over a half century of effort, fluoridation has reached less than two-thirds of Americans through the water supply.

Today, new technologies from dental sealants to more cost-effective methods for treating cavities have again made oral health a public health priority. However, the number of dentists has not grown in recent years to keep up with the growing population. In addition, dental care for those without the resources to pay for it is often inadequate and inaccessible. Thus, a new approach is needed to bringing dental care to those in need. Perhaps a new strategy of COPH can make this happen.

Community-oriented public health can reach beyond the institutional and geographical constraints that COPC faces when based in a community health center or other institutions serving a geographically defined population or community. COPH as a governmentally led effort allows a greater range of options for intervention includes those that require changes in laws, incentives and governmental procedures. These might include: authorizing new types of clinicians, providing services in nontraditional settings such as schools, funding innovations to put new technologies into practice, and addressing the regulatory barriers to rapid and cost-effective delivery of services.

public health cannot be viewed only in its current form. Understanding public health also requires considering its future and how we can plan for the expected and the unexpected. Let us take a look at the role of public health in planning for the future in Chapter 13.

Key Words

- Core public health functions
- Assessment
- Assurance
- Policy development
- Ten essential public health services
- Home rule authority
- Healthcare safety net
- Community-oriented primary care (COPC)
- Community-oriented public health (COPH)

Discussion Questions

Take a look at the questions posed in the following scenarios which were presented at the beginning of this chapter. See now whether you can answer them.

1. *A young man in your dormitory is diagnosed with tuberculosis. The health department works with the student health service to test everyone in the dorm, as well as in his classes, with a TB skin test. Those who are positive for the first time are advised to take a course of a medicine called INH. You ask: is this standard operating procedure?*

2. *You go to a public health meeting and learn that many of the speakers are not from public health agencies, but from the Departments of Labor, Commerce, Housing, and Education. You ask: what do these departments have to do with health?*

3. *You hear that a new childhood vaccine was developed by the NIH, approved by the FDA, endorsed for federal payment by the CDC and recommended for use by the American Academy of Pediatrics. You ask: do all these agencies and organizations always work so well together?*

4. *A major flood in Asia leads to disease and starvation. Some say it is due to global warming, others to bad luck. Coordinated efforts by global health agencies, assisted by nongovernmental organizations (NGOs) and outside governmental donors, help get the country back on its feet. You ask: what types of cooperation are needed to make all of this happen?*

5. *A local community health center identifies childhood obesity as a problem in their community. They collect data demonstrating that the problem begins as early as elementary school. They develop a plan that includes clinical interventions at the health center and also at the elementary school. They ask the health department to*

help them organize an educational campaign and assist in evaluating the results. Working together, they are able to reduce the obesity rate among elementary school children by one-half. This seems like a new way to practice public health, you conclude. What type of approach is this?

REFERENCES

1. Public Health in America. Essential Public Health Services. Available at: http://www.health.gov/phfunctions/public.htm. Accessed April 3, 2009.

2. Institute of Medicine. *The Future of Public Health.* Washington, DC: National Academies Press; 1988.

3. Turnock BJ. *Public Health: What It Is and How It Works.* 4th ed. Sudbury, MA: Jones and Bartlett Publishers; 2009.

4. Turnock BJ. *Essentials of Public Health.* Sudbury, MA: Jones and Bartlett Publishers; 2007.

5. United States Department of Health and Human Services. Organizational Chart. Available at: http://www.hhs.gov/about/orgchart/. Accessed April 3, 2009.

6. Centers for Disease Control and Prevention. History of CDC. *Morbidity and Mortality Weekly Report.* 1996;45: 526–528.

7. World Health Organization. About WHO. Available at: http://www.who.int/about/en/. Accessed April 3, 2009.

8. The World Bank. Health, Nutrition and Population. Available at: http://web.worldbank.org/WBSITE/EXTERNAL/TOPICS/EXTHEALTH NUTRITIONANDPOPULATION/0,,menuPK:282516~pagePK:149018~piPK :149093~theSitePK:282511,00.html. Accessed April 3, 2009.

9. Duffin J, Sweetman A. *SARS in Context: Memory, History, Policy.* Montreal: McGill-Queen's University Press; 2006.

10. Institute of Medicine. Initial Guidance for an Update of the National Vaccine Plan: A Letter Report to the National Vaccine Program Office. Available at: http://www.nap.edu/catalog/12257.html. Accessed April 3, 2009.

11. District of Columbia Area Health Education Center. The Conceptual Framework for COPC. Available at: http://dcahec.gwumc.edu/education/session4/index.html. Accessed April 3, 2009.

12. Pfizer Global Pharmaceuticals. *Milestones in Public Health: Accomplishments in Public Health over the Last 100 Years.* New York: Pfizer Global Pharmaceuticals; 2006.

CHAPTER **13**

The Future of Population Health

LEARNING OBJECTIVES

By the end of this chapter, the student will be able to:

- explain the basic uses of outbreak investigations.
- identify public health roles in disaster prevention and management.
- explain the basic public health roles in preventing and responding to bioterrorism.
- identify lessons for the future that can be learned from past public health mistakes.
- identify trends in public health that may have implications for the future.
- identify possible impacts of climate change.
- explain how principles of systems thinking can be used to address complex problems.
- explain the importance of an educated citizenry to the future of public health.

It is 2015 and you are working at a large organization with its own cafeteria where most employees eat lunch. An outbreak of an acute diarrhea occurs among your coworkers who eat there. The company calls in the local health department. To your surprise, they cannot identify a known cause and request help from the CDC's Epidemic Intelligence Service (EIS). You are quite impressed when the EIS detects a never-before-recognized strain of toxin-producing E.coli and sends out a worldwide alert. You wonder: could this be a bioterrorism attack or just a routine outbreak? The "all-hazards" team assures you that this is just routine and that we're making progress. Now that a systems approach is in place, only 10 percent of Americans suffers foodborne illnesses each year. Back in the early 21st century, it was closer to 25 percent.

It is 2025 and the worst predictions about infectious disease have come true. It seems like every day there is a new outbreak of drug-resistant infections. New technology has allowed us to get the word out instantly and mount rapid campaigns to control infections and develop vaccines to protect those at greatest risk. Clean water is increasingly scarce and infectious disease outbreaks are emerging throughout the world as nations compete for the remaining sources of clean water. You worry about your child who is about to be born into a new world of emerging infections.

It is 2035 and you are now middle-aged. The epidemic of obesity has reached your waistline—on top of that, you have high cholesterol, high blood sugar, and high blood pressure. Fortunately, cigarettes are history, but heart disease and strokes are making a comeback as the number one killers. It seems like everyone is having surgery to treat their obesity and look better, but you wonder if there just might be a better approach. In other ways, the world is beginning to come to grips with problems including the pressures of population growth and environmental deterioration. You begin to see hope for the future.

It is 2055 and at this point in your life, you thought you'd be getting ready for retirement. Now, you look ahead to working until you are 75 or maybe 80. Life expectancy at birth is now approaching 90, so the retirement age is going up, too. You're delighted that people are living longer, but you still hope that a cure for Alzheimer's will come along soon. It seems like people are living longer, but are they living better? The world has agreed to put a limit on what it spends for medical care on those over 85 and instead invests in new technology to deal with climate change.

It is 2076 and you are about to celebrate the 300th birthday of the United States. There is a lot to celebrate. Economic progress has spread throughout the world and the population health approach has greatly improved the quality, as well as the quantity, of life. Technology has produced a cure for Alzheimer's and many other diseases. Climate change turned out to be a real challenge, but the global cooperation that it produced has had positive side effects. HIV/AIDS is still with us, but we have learned how to effectively prevent its spread and it no longer needs to shorten how long people live. New challenges continue to face you as you look ahead. However, now that there is a health system that uses a systems thinking approach and an educated citizenry that understands public health problems and approaches, you are confident about the future.

All of these issues illustrate the roles of public health in preparing for and planning for the future. Let us start by taking a look at current and emerging efforts to deal with outbreaks of disease, as well as crises and disasters. Then we will examine how we can learn from the past to help us plan for the future. Finally, we will take a look at some approaches that should help us address the inevitable health crises we will face in coming years.

WHAT IS PUBLIC HEALTH'S ROLE IN ADDRESSING OUTBREAKS OF DISEASE?

Public health's role in emergencies and disasters has roots in responses to epidemics of infectious disease. In recent decades, perhaps the most visible role of public health agencies has been in outbreak investigations. The image of public health professionals, sometimes called "disease detectives," working in the field in big cities, as well as remote areas of the United States and around the world, has become a positive image often featured on television and in films. Box 13-1 discusses some of the successes health departments and the CDC have had in outbreak investigations.[1]

HOW ARE PUBLIC HEALTH AGENCIES INVOLVED IN PROTECTING AGAINST TERRORISM AND BIOTERRORISM?

Public health surveillance and investigation of outbreaks were well established as key public health functions well before the September 11, 2001 terrorism attacks and the subsequent anthrax bioterrorism episode. These events, however, had a major impact on the role of public health in society. Box 13-2 reviews the anthrax case and describes its impact on public health.[2]

BOX 13-1 Outbreak Investigations.

Outbreak investigations have been a key component of public health's effort to respond to epidemics and clusters of acute disease. These investigations are often successfully handled by local and state health agencies. The Centers for Disease Control (CDC), however, may be called in to assist with them. The CDC is involved in hundreds of outbreak investigations each year.

Famous investigations include the 1976 outbreak of what came to be called Legionnaires' disease. Hundred of military veterans, called Legionnaires, gathering in Philadelphia in July to celebrate the nation's bicentennial, were infected and many died from pneumonia. The CDC identified the cause as a previously-unrecognized bacteria—now called Legionella—that can grow in hot water and can be spread through the air. In the early 1980s, an outbreak of life-threatening cardiovascular shock, known as toxic shock syndrome (TSS), was traced to a new type of absorbent tampon. It brought to light the need for surveillance of new products, even those not suspected of causing disease. The most important outbreak of the late 20th century was investigated and brought to professional and public attention in 1981 by the CDC. It came to be called acquired immunodeficiency syndrome (AIDS).

Outbreak investigations are not limited to communicable diseases. In fact, the illnesses may originate, for example, from an environmental toxin, a food additive or supplement, or a drug reaction. For instance, eosinophilia-myalgia syndrome (EMS) is an incurable and sometimes fatal neurological condition that often presents with vague flu-like symptoms. It was traced by the CDC to poorly-produced L-trytophan, an amino acid widely used as a food supplement. Reye's syndrome, an often fatal acute liver disease of children, was traced to the use of "baby aspirin" for healthy children during acute viral infections.

Over 1000 outbreak investigations are conducted in the United States each year and are mostly handled by state and local health departments. These types of investigations can take months or even years to complete. Often the outbreak is over before the investigation can be completed. Outbreak investigations will remain an important part of public health. However, new technologies, new tracking systems, and better communications systems, will hopefully make these critical investigations more rapid and efficient. In addition, new forms of investigation are being developed to address the issues of terrorism and bioterrorism.

BOX 13-2 Bioterrorism.

Shortly after the terrorism attack on the United States on September 11, 2001, a second attack occurred which greatly altered the course of public health in the country. The attack occurred in the form of letters containing a powdered form of anthrax bacteria delivered through the U.S. mail to Congress and national news networks.

Anthrax is a bacteria long known for its occasional spread from cattle to humans by close contact and its potential to cause a life-threatening pneumonia. It is considered a particularly deadly agent for bioterrorism with the potential to kill tens of thousand of people. When prepared in the form of a weapon and delivered in quantity, it has the potential to widely disperse over an entire city or region. Early detection of the substance and treatment of its effects are key to controlling such an attack, including preventing the pneumonia through the early use of antibiotics.

The anthrax attack in 2001 made headlines for weeks temporarily shutting down Congress and much of Washington, killing five people and causing severe illness in 17 others. The episode also brought attention and funding to public health programs. It was soon recognized that even large health departments with extensive responsibilities and expertise were not prepared to address bioterrorism and ensure availability of public health laboratories to diagnose anthrax-related illness and other potential agents of bioterrorism.

Preparation for bioterrorism also focuses on the unique characteristics of bioterrorism and the specific organisms that may be involved with it. The anthrax episode highlighted how terrorism, in general, and bioterrorism, in particular, differ from the types of emergencies and disasters that have become familiar. First, they may involve the military, as well as law enforcement. Second, they require knowledge of agents that are often very rare. Little expertise exists in either the public health or medical communities about agents such as anthrax, botulism, smallpox, and plague. In addition, bioterrorism may not be easily detected, allowing the agent to spread widely before it is noticed and action can be taken. Finally, there is the potential for multiple simultaneous threats at multiple locations. Thus, bioterrorism requires special preparation above and beyond the evolving preparedness system for emergencies and disasters. Public health agencies, including the CDC and local health departments, were on the front lines of the anthrax attack and will continue to be part of the first response to bioterrorism attacks if they occur in the future.

In recent years, public health agencies have been increasingly integrated into a National Incident Management System (NIMS), which is part of the Department of Homeland Security (DHS).[3] A central feature of the NIMS is an incident command system (ICS), widely used by police, fire, and emergency management agencies. The ICS attempts to establish uniform procedures and terminology, and an integrated communications system with established and practiced roles for each agency. The goal is to integrate these approaches into ongoing operations and not reserve them solely for emergency situations. The DHS has established a color-coded hierarchy of response levels with corresponding increasing public health agency responsibility at each of these levels. These levels are:

Green—low
Blue—guarded
Yellow—elevated
Orange—high
Red—severe threat

Public health agencies have specific roles to play at each level of the process. When levels are orange and red, public health agencies' responsibilities include: active surveillance for disease and disease agents; organization of systems for triaging patients to hospitals and other healthcare facilities; and key roles in accurate and timely communication of information on hazards to the public.

The DHS has developed what is called an **all-hazards approach**. An all-hazards approach to public health preparedness uses the same approach to preparing for many types of disasters, including use of surveillance systems, communications systems, evacuations, and an organized healthcare response. The all-hazards approach has been widely endorsed by public health agencies and organizations in part at least because it recognizes the need for basic public health infrastructure to respond, not only to the dramatic crisis or emergency, but to day-to-day needs as well.

Preparing for and responding to emergencies and disasters is key to addressing the expected and unexpected crises that we will inevitably face in the future. Preparing for the future also requires that we learn from the past. We will therefore examine approaches that look at history in order to plan for the future.

The first approach looks at past mistakes to derive principles we can use in planning for the future. The second looks at past trends and uses them to better understand the problems that we can expect to face in the future. Finally, we will take a look at the approach known as systems thinking that focuses on how to connect the components of the healthcare system and the public health system to make for a more effective and efficient overall health system.

WHAT CAN WE LEARN FROM THE MISTAKES OF THE PAST?

Some of the most important lessons for the future come from learning from past mistakes. Learning from hindsight is easier than having foresight, but looking back can help us learn from our past mistakes. Let us take a look at some examples.

Avoid Implementing Interventions When Preparation Is Enough

In 1976, public health authorities moved rapidly to vaccinate the entire U.S. population against what was called the swine flu. They feared that a handful of new influenza cases contracted from pigs resembled the influenza of 1918 that caused over 40 million deaths worldwide. Unfortunately, the swine flu vaccine was associated with an unexpected number of cases of Guillain-Barré syndrome, a rapidly progressive potentially life-threatening neurological condition. Despite the early termination of the swine flu campaign, the disease never spread from human to human. Today we recognize that person-to-person spread needs to be established and the ease of transmission measured in order to assess the epidemic potential of influenza and other potential threats.

Another episode of acting rather than preparing occurred after 9/11 and the subsequent bioterrorism scare. The federal government developed and rapidly implemented a campaign to vaccinate healthcare providers and other first responders using the original smallpox vaccine. The vaccine produced a large number of side effects, including life-threatening effects on the heart. The campaign was ended before it moved into full-scale implementation. In retrospect, it was recognized that the smallpox vaccine has long been known to cause severe side effects, especially in adults. Preparation and research is often better than large scale interventions. We have hopefully learned from incidences like these to extensively prepare and carefully act.

Interventions Routinely Used on Large Numbers of People Need to Be Especially Safe

In the 1960s and 1970s, the widespread use of an intrauterine device to prevent pregnancies known as the Dalkon Shield caused a large number of cases of fallopian tube infections, infertility, as well as pregnancies in the fallopian tubes called ectopic pregnancies. This led to the regulation of medical devices by the FDA.

Estrogen therapy was widely used in the late 20th century for women beginning menopause. The treatment seemed to make sense as a replacement for the declining level of estrogen that occurs at this time in a woman's life. It took the Women's Health Study, a large randomized clinical trial, to demonstrate the risks of postmenopausal estrogen on the heart, as well as the increased risk of breast cancer.

While we often cannot anticipate adverse effects of interventions, we need to have a system to detect and address side effects, especially when they are used on large numbers of people. Safety cannot be guaranteed by biological plausibility or even by long-term use.

Control of a Disease Is Often Possible; Elimination Is Rarely Realistic

As we have seen, elimination of a disease requires special conditions and a concerted global effort. Putting forth a campaign to eliminate a disease when these conditions are not present can do more harm than good. In the 1950s, the World Health Organization set out to eliminate malaria, only to have it rebound in recent years. More recently, the United States proclaimed an intention to eliminate tuberculosis, an equally unattainable goal, before eventually turning attention to controlling increasingly resistant strains. Based upon what we know, it is important not to talk about the "end of AIDS," which seems well beyond reality at least for the immediate future. In addition to learning from the mistakes of the past, there is much to learn from the trends of the past.

WHAT CAN WE LEARN FROM PAST TRENDS?

A number of trends in the pattern of disease have been described in recent years that have implications for what we can expect to happen throughout the 21st century. We will call these the demographic, epidemiological, and nutritional transitions.

The **demographic transition** describes the impact of falling childhood death rates and extended life spans on the size and the age distribution of populations.[4] During the first half of the 20th century, the death rates among the young fell dramatically in today's developed countries. Death rates continued their dramatic decline in most parts of the developing world during the second half of the 20th century.

Birth rates tend to remain high for years or decades after the decline in deaths. High birth rates paired with lower death rates lead to rapid growth in population size, as we have seen in much of the developing world. This trend continues today and is expected to go on in many parts of the world well into the 21st century. Figure 13-1 illustrates how the population of the Nigeria is expected to grow during the first half of the 21st century due to a high birth rate and a lowered death rate.

FIGURE 13-1 Population Pyramid Expected for Nigeria

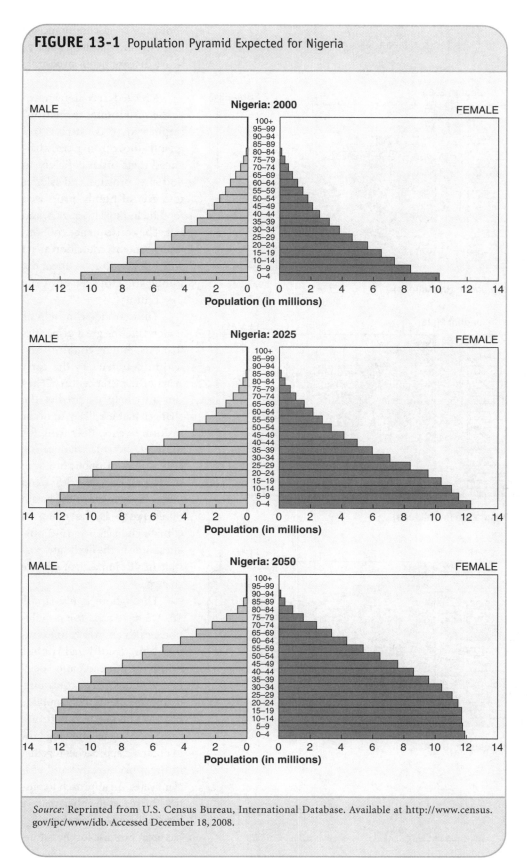

Source: Reprinted from U.S. Census Bureau, International Database. Available at http://www.census. gov/ipc/www/idb. Accessed December 18, 2008.

Despite the delay, a decline in birth rates reliably occurs following the decline in childhood deaths. This decline in births gradually leads to aging of the population. We are now seeing societies in much of Europe and Japan with growing elderly populations. Improved health care and extended life spans for the elderly has magnified this trend. Take a look at Figure 13-2, which shows what is expected to occur in the coming years in much of Europe and Japan. Japan is used as an example of the emergence of an inverted population pyramid with a smaller young population and a larger older population.

The large number of immigrants to the United States and their generally higher birth rates has slowed this process in the United States, but the basic trend of a growing elderly population continues. The U.S. baby boom, which occurred between 1946 and 1964, is expected to have major impacts on the numbers of elderly in coming years, as illustrated in Figure 13-3.

As we saw in Section III, a second transition has been called the **epidemiologic transition**,[5] or public health transition. The epidemiologic or public health transition implies that as social and economic development occurs, different types of diseases become prominent. Deaths in less-developed societies are often dominated by epidemic communicable diseases and diseases associated with malnutrition and childhood infections. As a country develops, communicable diseases often come under

FIGURE 13-2 Population Pyramid Expected for Japan

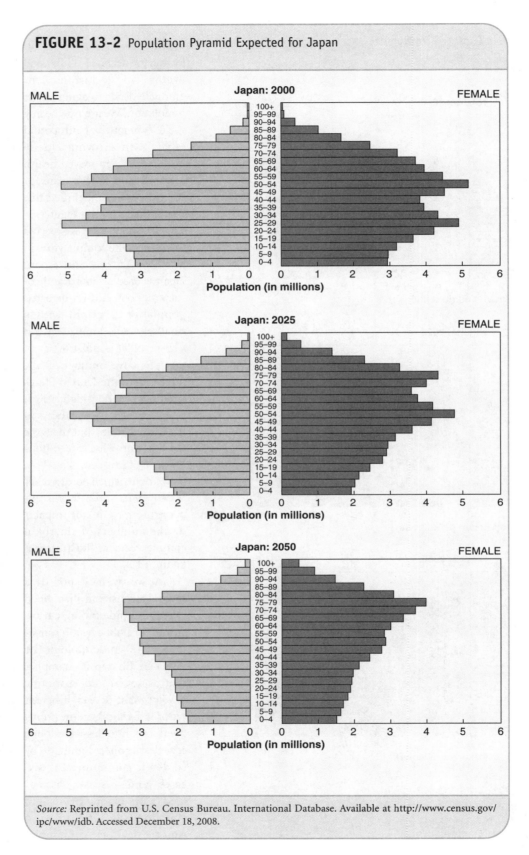

Source: Reprinted from U.S. Census Bureau. International Database. Available at http://www.census.gov/ipc/www/idb. Accessed December 18, 2008.

control and non-communicable and chronic diseases, such as heart disease often predominate.

A related transition known as the **nutritional transition**[6] implies that countries frequently move from poorly balanced diets often deficient in nutrients, proteins, and calories to a diet of highly-processed food including fats, sugars, and salt. The consequences of both under- and overnutrition affect and will continue to affect the public's health well into the 21st century.

These trends can help us understand the great disparities that exist among countries and within countries in the early years of the 21st century. They can also help us predict the changes that are likely to occur in future years. Preparing for these predictable changes is a critical goal for public health in the 21st century. One clear trend that is likely to affect the health of everyone is the effect of climate change. Box 13-3 outlines some of the likely and possible health impacts of climate change.[7, 8]

Throughout *Public Health 101* we have used the population health approach to examine how traditional public health, health care, and social interventions can all contribute to improvements in the public's health. The key to our future successes may be knowing how to put these approaches together in the most effective and efficient ways. An approach to putting the pieces together, that we have called systems thinking, has great promise for the future.

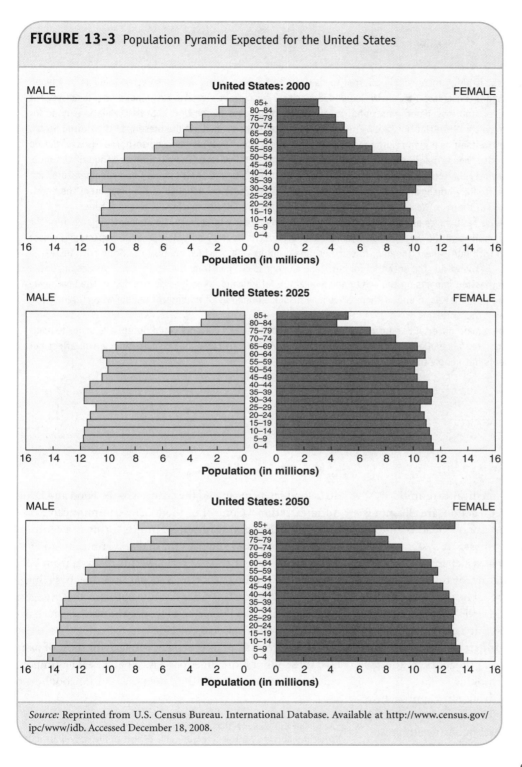

FIGURE 13-3 Population Pyramid Expected for the United States

Source: Reprinted from U.S. Census Bureau. International Database. Available at http://www.census.gov/ipc/www/idb. Accessed December 18, 2008.

WHAT IS SYSTEMS THINKING AND HOW CAN IT IMPROVE PUBLIC HEALTH EFFORTS?

Systems thinking is a comprehensive strategy for thinking about a problem as part of an interrelated network or sys-tem. In health, systems think-ing is increasingly used to integrate public health and healthcare systems into an in-tegrated health system. System thinking focuses on identify-ing **leverage points** or points in the system at which to in-tervene. It also looks at how to combine interventions to maximize their effectiveness and efficiency.[9]

The systems-thinking ap-proach contrasts with tra-ditional approaches that study problems by breaking them down into their separate elements. Systems thinking focuses on the connections between problems and the im-pacts of multiple interven-tions at key leverage or control points.

To begin to understand systems thinking, let us go back to where we began with a look at the problems of ciga-rette smoking and health. We will then look at an even more complex problem, the issue of food safety, and see how sys-tem-thinking approaches can help. We have seen that to-bacco control efforts have been responsible for a reduc-tion in tobacco use of approx-imately 50 percent compared to the 1950s. Nonetheless, to-bacco remains the number one cause of preventable death. Recently, the National Cancer Institute (NCI) and the Institute of Medicine (IOM) have looked at tobacco control efforts and concluded: "We are long past the time that tobacco use is purely a matter of individual choice and its control dependent on a strategy of one-person-at-a-time. Tax policy, school interventions, clean indoor air regulations, agricultural

BOX 13-3   Climate Change.

Global warming, or climate change as it is being increasingly referred to, is likely to have expected and unexpected impacts on human health. The most predictable changes are those associated with expanded territory for currently existing communicable diseases. For instance, cases of malaria, dengue fever, and insect-borne encephalitis are likely to increase in the United States. Malaria existed for many years in the country as far north as the Mid-Atlantic states. The mosquitoes that transmit malaria are present in the United States and the disease could readily reestablish itself as a major pathogen. Dengue, or "breakbone fever" is a mosquito-borne disease related to yellow fever. One strain of the disease, hemorrhagic dengue fever, has a high case-fatality rate. The geographic range of the mosquito that carries dengue fever is currently limited because frost kills both the adult insects and their larvae. Rising temperatures are expected to allow the disease to move steadily northward in future decades. Outbreaks of acute encephalitis (inflammation of the brain) transmitted by mosquitoes are already on the rise. We can expect to see more frequent and severe outbreaks in the future.

In addition, more frequent and intense heat waves are likely to occur, especially in currently temperate climates covering much of the United States. Deaths among the very young and the very old can be expected during heat waves. Additional possible impacts of climate change on health are those associated with hurricanes, flooding, forest fires, and drought—all of which are likely to occur with increased frequency and severity in specific areas of the world. The potential for hurricane damage is not just from the acute storm. As demonstrated by Hurricane Katrina, there can be long-lasting impacts on the safety and availability of housing, as well as destruction of the healthcare and public health infrastructure. Rising ocean levels in and of themselves may displace hundreds of millions of people who currently live in low-lying river delta areas throughout the world.

The exact impacts of climate change remain uncertain and controversial. Alterations in ocean currents could potentially lower temperatures in Europe and other highly-populated areas. Despite the great uncertainties ahead, it is clear that climate change will affect not only the lives of today's college students but people's lives for centuries to come.

---

initiatives, advertising campaigns, medical care initiatives, community mobilization, and political action, are all among the elements at work to reduce the use of tobacco among Americans." NCI and IOM go on to say: "A systems-level focus on tobacco control is a logical next step in understanding and managing the complex nature of tobacco use, as both an epidemiological and a personal health issue."[10] Box 13-4 outlines a number of key principles that distinguish systems thinking from a traditional one issue at a time **reductionist approach**. It also demonstrates how systems thinking leads to new and different approaches to address health problems, such as cigarette smoking.

Thinking in systems is a relatively new approach in public health though it has already become a "crosscutting competency" expected of master's level public health professionals who pursue certification.[11] Systems thinking is often useful for the most challenging public health issues. One such issue is food safety.

Food safety is not a new issue in public health; it has a long history. Early 20th-century public health efforts to ad-

dress food safety prompted the creation of the Food and Drug Administration.[a] Control of foodborne communicable diseases has been central to public health for over a century. Knowledge of causes and patterns of disease transmission has led to successful efforts to control specific diseases from botulism due to canning processes to hepatitis A due to shellfish. Despite these successes, it has become apparent that we have much to learn about the spread of foodborne disease, which increasingly crosses national borders.

Food affects all of us every day—in fact, for most of us at least three, if not more times per day. What we eat has important implications for nutrition, the potential for foodborne

---

[a] As we saw in Chapter 1, the case of Typhoid Mary came to symbolize public health efforts to control communicable disease in the early years of the 20th century. Typhoid Mary was a chronic carrier of typhoid who transmitted the disease as she moved from restaurant to restaurant serving food to a large number of unsuspecting customers. Typhoid Mary, despite being a chronic carrier, remained in good health. A widely-publicized legal action eventually resulted in her being quarantined on a New York City island to prevent her from continuing to spread typhoid.

BOX 13-4 Systems Thinking versus Reductionist Thinking and Cigarette Smoking.

The work of the National Cancer Institute and the Institute of Medicine on tobacco control encourages a systems-thinking approach. Systems thinking is more easily understood by contrasting it with the traditional approach, which has been called the **reductionist approach**. The following three concepts are key to understanding the differences between systems thinking and reductionist thinking:

1. *One intervention at a time versus multiple simultaneous interventions*

   A reductionist approach attempts to look at one factor or intervention at a time. An intervention, such as a smoking cessation program, might be investigated to determine whether it works when used alone. Rather than looking at one intervention at a time, systems thinking asks about the best combination of interventions. Systems thinking might identify smoking cessation programs, social marketing, and higher taxes as three important compatible interventions that need to be effectively and efficiently combined.

2. *Straight-line or linear projections versus measuring complex interactions*

   A reductionist approach usually assumes a straight-line or linear relationship implying that increased levels of an intervention, such as increasing taxes on tobacco, will produce a straight-line decrease in the levels of tobacco use. However, it is possible that small increases in taxes have little effect, while slightly larger increases have dramatic effects. In addition, reductionist approaches do not look at how the impact of one intervention may be affected by connecting it with other interventions, whereas systems thinking looks at these interactions. Thus, systems thinking would ask questions about how to most effectively utilize cigarette taxes by combining them with other approaches, such as using the taxes to support tobacco education programs, or reduce exposure to radon, asbestos, or other causes of lung cancer.

3. *One-point-in-time or static analysis versus a changing or dynamic analysis*

   Reductionist approaches look at the relationships at one point in time. That is, they use **static models** and do not take into account changes that often occur over time. For instance, they would not look at how changes over time in social attitudes may alter the effectiveness of tobacco cessation programs or set the stage for enforcement of public smoking regulations or increased tobacco taxes. Rather than seeing interventions as static or at one point in time, systems thinking develops **dynamic models** that look at the feedback process, the changes that occur over time, and bottlenecks that slow down change. For instance, systems thinking might identify a need to train large numbers of clinicians in smoking cessation methods so that they can address the demand for smoking cessation services created by social marketing, increased cigarette taxes, and better drug treatments.

disease, and has become an effective vehicle for implementing public health interventions.[b]

Today, our food comes from all parts of the world, many times going through multiple levels of processing to create prepared food, and is often stored for long periods of time before reaching our dinner plate. The World Health Organization estimates that approximately 1.8 million people die worldwide from foodborne disease each year.[12] In the United States, the CDC estimates that the number is approximately 5000 per year. However, hospitalizations are es-

timated at over 300,000 per year, making it a major cause of disability.[13 c]

The complexity of issues related to food and food safety has resulted in a complicated mix of local/state, federal and global agencies involvement. Table 13–1 outlines many of the agencies involved and suggests the need for a great deal of coordination to successfully achieve food safety.

Because of the inherent complexity of the problems of food safety and the large number of organizations involved at every level, systems-thinking approaches are key to food safety.

[b]Supplementation of food with vitamins and minerals has been an effective method for addressing specific disease. The addition of iodine to salt beginning in the 1920s is credited worldwide with a dramatic reduction in goiters (enlargements of the thyroid). Supplementation of milk with vitamin D greatly reduced the incidence of rickets, a deforming bone disease of children.

[c] Supplementation of bread with niacin dramatically reduced pellagra, a disease characterized by the 4 Ds: dermatitis, diarrhea, dementia, and death. Most recently, the addition of folic acid to a variety of products generally consumed by pregnant women is credited with a nearly 50 percent reduction in spina bifida, a birth defect in which the spinal column fails to fuse.

TABLE 13-1 Levels of Public Health Coordination Needed for Successful Food Safety

Level	Organizations involved	Roles
Global	The Food and Agriculture Organization of the United Nations (FAO)	The United Nations agency with overall responsibility for the food supply with special emphasis on ensuring an adequate supply of food worldwide
	The World Health Organization (WHO)	Not a regulatory agency, but establishes policy and makes recommendations regarding the safety of the world food supply through its Food Safety Department (FOS)
	The Codex Alimentarius Commission (CAC)	Initiated as a joint program of FAO and WHO that develops food standards, guidelines, and codes of practice. These now form the basis for the rules of global trade under the jurisdiction of the World Trade Organization (WTO)
Federal	The United States Food and Drug Administration (FDA)	Overall regulatory responsibility for food safety regulation in the United States
	The United States Department of Agriculture (USDA)	Regulatory responsibilities for meat, poultry, and eggs in the United States
	The United States Environmental Protection Agency (EPA)	Regulation of pesticide usage and the establishment of water quality standards
	The Centers for Disease Control and Prevention (CDC)	Not a regulatory agency, but responsible for ongoing surveillance, as well as acute investigations in collaboration with state and local health department
State/Local	State and local health departments	Restaurant inspections
Consumer	Consumer protection agencies	Education in safe food purchasing, preparation, and storage

Source: Awofeso N. What's new about the "New Public Health"? *American Journal of Public Health.* 2004;94(5): 705–709.

HOW CAN SYSTEMS-THINKING APPROACHES BE APPLIED TO FOOD SAFETY?

Two basic systems-thinking approaches to food safety have been put forward in recent years. In the first strategy the focus is on one type of food at a time. This process has been called the Hazard Analysis and Critical Control Point (HACCP) system.[14, 15] In a second systems-thinking approach, the food's detailed location and time of production down to the level of the farm or factory is identified on the label, allowing officials to trace the food back to where and when the problem occurred. Putting these two approaches together is now seen as

key to a successful systems approach. Let us take a look at these two approaches.

HACCP is a systems approach that looks for key leverage or control points to manage food safety issues. It is built upon a series of prerequisite conditions designed to first ensure basic environmental and operating conditions. These include: facilities that maintain sanitary conditions; proper equipment construction, installation, and maintenance; personal hygiene by employees, etc.

Once these basic conditions of food safety are accomplished, HACCP looks for options for interventions at multiple leverage or control points and institutes a series of safeguards at these specific points, as illustrated for ground beef in Box 13-5.

Knowing the type of food that causes an outbreak is not enough if we do not know where the food came from and cannot trace it back to the point of contamination. This became clear in an often fatal U.S. outbreak of salmonella from peppers coming from Mexico because there was delay in resolving the cause of the outbreak and tracing the product across national boundaries.[16] It is key to an effective and efficient systems approach to be able to rapidly trace the source of contamination to avoid shutting down whole industries to solve the problem caused by a single source. Efforts are underway to label foods to be able to identify and trace their origins. This tracking system can then draw upon the data collected as part of the HACCP system. Putting these two strategies together should allow public health officials to more quickly and reliably respond to foodborne disease that occurs often thousands of miles from the source of the food.

Protection against foodborne communicable disease is an ongoing daily public health challenge that is not about to go away. Systems thinking is now a well-established approach to control this rapidly changing and challenging problem.

BOX 13-5 Foodborne Communicable Diseases and Systems Thinking.

The systems approach known as Hazard Analysis of Critical Control Points (HACCP) attempts to understand, monitor, and quickly respond to breakdowns in the food safety system. This methodology, originally developed for the U.S. space program, requires that food be monitored from the field to the consumer. HACCP is increasingly being adopted for such products as seafood, meat, poultry, and fruit juices. HACCP includes the following seven steps:

- **Analyze hazards.** Potential hazards associated with a food and potential interventions to control those hazards are identified. The hazard could be biological, such as a microbe; chemical, such as a toxin; or physical, such as ground glass or metal fragments.
- **Identify critical control points.** These are points in a food's production—from its raw state through processing and shipping to consumption by the consumer—at which the potential hazard can be controlled or eliminated. Examples are: cooking, cooling, packaging, and metal detection.
- **Establish preventive measures with critical limits for each control point.** For a cooked food, for example, this might include setting the minimum cooking temperature and time required to ensure the elimination of any harmful microbes.
- **Establish procedures to monitor the critical control points.** Such procedures might include determining how and by whom cooking time and temperature should be monitored.
- **Establish corrective actions to be taken when monitoring shows that a critical limit has not been met.** For example, reprocessing or disposing of food if the minimum cooking temperature is not met.
- **Establish procedures to verify that the system is working properly.** For example, testing time- and temperature-recording devices to verify that a cooking unit is working properly.
- **Establish effective recordkeeping to document the HACCP system.** This would include records of hazards and their control methods, the monitoring of safety requirements, and actions taken to correct potential problems. Each of these principles must be backed by sound scientific knowledge—for example, published microbiological studies on time and temperature factors for controlling foodborne pathogens.

Meat safety issues reflect this approach. Toxin-producing strains of E. coli are widespread in beef products and have been responsible for a number of fatal outbreaks of foodborne illness. The threats to health have led to a more coordinated systems-thinking approach using the HACCP system. Ground beef, which combines meat often leftover from multiple animals, has been identified as a high-risk product or potential hazard. Key control points at which ground beef may be contaminated in the meatpacking process have been identified. Monitoring by testing includes a random testing process on all batches of ground beef. The process uses rapid testing of a sample of the finished ground beef and holding up distribution until the results are available.

These are among the efforts to identify control points, establish interventions at these leverage points, and implement corrective actions to address the potential hazards of contaminated ground beef. This systems approach has already reduced the frequency and severity of outbreaks of life-threatening disease from toxigenic E. coli.

In *Public Health 101*, we have examined the population health approach to public health. We have viewed population health as putting together individual, at-risk group, and population approaches to address public health problems using an evidence-based approach. We have seen that the key to successful population health approaches in the future requires a systems-thinking approach combining these types of strategies to maximize the efficiency and effectiveness of our health system.[d]

Seeing the big picture and finding the most effective and efficient combination of interventions using a systems-thinking approach is key to the future of public health. Perhaps at least as important to the future of public health is the active engagement of an educated citizenry that understands what is meant by public health and supports its methods and interventions.

HOW CAN AN EDUCATED CITIZENRY MAKE THE 21ST CENTURY DIFFERENT FOR THE PUBLIC'S HEALTH?

The history of American public health is a history of crisis and response. From the yellow fever and cholera epidemics of the colonial period that produced the first Boards of Health, to the food and drug safety scares that produced the Food and Drug Administration to the terrorism of 9/11 and anthrax, we have repeatedly responded rapidly to crises with new funding, new structures, and new energy. Once each of these emergencies passed from the public mind and the media focused elsewhere, it becomes more difficult to support the efforts and implement the programs envisioned in the aftermath of crisis. Public health approaches require sustained attention and big-picture thinking. It requires an educated citizenry.

In 2003, the IOM recommended that all undergraduates have access to education in public health. This recommendation was supported by the contention that "public health is an essential part of the training of citizens."[18] That is, education in public health is important not just for the future health professional, but for all those who will participate in decision making, including all those who vote in local, state, and national elections.

The IOM recommendations lay the groundwork for what has become the Educated Citizen and Public Health movement. This movement aims to develop an educated citizenry that understands public health issues and supports population health approaches for addressing them. *If you have read this book, you are part of the Educated Citizen and Public Health movement.*

---

[d] Systems thinking principles are increasingly being applied to public health using what is called a **syndemic orientation**.[17] A syndemic orientation focuses attention on how specific health problems interact as parts of larger systems. For instance, what are the consequences of the spread of AIDS and the simultaneous spread of tuberculosis? Large-scale public health problems, such as health disparities, may also be better understood by focusing not on one disease or condition at a time, but on the connections among diseases and their relationships to socioeconomic, organizational, and cultural issues.

Key Words

- All-hazards approach
- Demographic transition
- Epidemiologic transition
- Nutritional transition
- Leverage points
- Reductionist approach
- Static models
- Dynamic models
- Syndemic orientation

Discussion Question

Write your own mini-scenarios for what the world of public health will look like in the years 2015, 2025, 2035, 2055, and 2076.

REFERENCES

1. Reingold RL. Outbreak Investigations—A Perspective. Available at: http://www.cdc.gov/ncidod/EID/vol4no1/reingold.htm. Accessed April 3, 2009.

2. Hugh JM, Gerberding JL. Anthrax Bioterrorism: Lessons Learned and Future Directions. Available at: http://www.cdc.gov/ncidod/EID/vol8no10/02-0466.htm. Accessed April 3, 2009.

3. United States Federal Emergency Management Administration. National Incident Management System. Available at: http://www.fema.gov/emergency/nims/. Accessed April 3, 2009.

4. U.S. Census Bureau. International Database. Available at: http://www.census.gov/ipc/www/idb/pyramids.html. Accessed April 3, 2009.

5. Omran AR. The epidemiologic transition: a theory of the epidemiology of population change. *The Milbank Memorial Fund Quarterly.* 1971; 49(4): 509–538.

6. Skolnik R. *Essentials of Global Health.* Sudbury, MA: Jones and Bartlett Publishers; 2008.

7. Sierra Club. Global Warming Impacts: Health Effects. Available at: http://www.sierraclub.org/energy/health/. Accessed December 17, 2008.

8. Science Daily. Global Warming and Your Health. Available at: http://www.sciencedaily.com/releases/2006/10/061023192524.htm. Accessed April 3, 2009.

9. Meadows H. *Thinking in Systems: A Primer.* White River Junction, Vermont: Chelsea Green Publishing; 2008.

10. National Cancer Institute–United States Department of Health and Human Services. *Greater than the Sum: Systems Thinking in Tobacco Control—Executive Summary.* Washington, DC: U.S. Department of Health and Human Services–National Institutes of Health; 2007.

11. Association of Schools of Public Health. MPH Core Competency Development Project. Available at: http://www.asph.org/document.cfm?page=851. Accessed April 3, 2009.

12. World Health Organization. Food Safety. Available at: http://www.who.int/foodsafety/en/. Accessed April 3, 2009.

13. Centers for Disease Control and Prevention. Foodborne Illness. Available at: http://www.cdc.gov/ncidod/dbmd/diseaseinfo/foodborneinfections_g.htm. Accessed April 3, 2009.

14. Hoffmann S. Mending our food safety chain. *Resources.* 2007; 166: 11–15.

15. United States Food and Drug Administration. HACCP: A State-of-the-Art Approach to Food Safety. Available at: http://www.cfsan.fda.gov/~lrd/bghaccp.html. Accessed April 3, 2009.

16. Consumer Reports. Country-of-origin labeling: A shopper's guide. Available at: http://www.consumerreports.org/health/healthy-living/health-safety/country-of-origin-labeling-tool/overview/country-of-origin-labeling-tool-ov.htm. Accessed April 3, 2009.

17. Centers for Disease Control and Prevention. Syndemics Overview—What Principles Characterize a Syndemic Orientation? Available at: http://www.cdc.gov/SYNDEMICS/overview-principles.htm. Accessed April 3, 2009.

18. Gebbie K, Rosenstock L, Hernandez LM, eds. *Who Will Keep the Public Healthy? Educating Public Health Professionals for the 21st Century.* Washington, DC: National Academies Press; 2003: 144.

Section V:
Cases and Discussion Questions

Public Health Departments—Getting the Lead Out

A series of articles appears in your local newspaper investigating reports of elevated lead levels and reduced academic performance among students in a local grade school. The series ends with an editorial asking: "Where was the health department and what are they going to do now?"

The health department was aware of these reports and had sent a letter to each parent alerting them to the dangers of increased lead levels and letting them know of doctors and local clinics that could follow up and provide treatment through a health department-funded program. The mayor was not satisfied. He asked: "But isn't public health about prevention? How can we prevent this from happening again?" He asks the health department for a full report within a month.

The health department sets out to evaluate the range of potential sources of lead exposure in the community. They find the following contributing factors: a local factory releases fumes that contain lead; local playgrounds are still contaminated by lead from gasoline despite the fact that lead was removed from gasoline well over a decade ago; lead paint in older homes; possible exposure from lead used in water pipes; and lead from painted toys and glazes on homemade pottery. The health department's report to the mayor concluded that prevention of lead exposure requires not just the health department's role, but the cooperation of schools, parks, the environmental protection agency, the water system, the housing agency, as well as local industry and merchants. "We can't do it alone," the report concludes.

"Okay," says the mayor, "it sounds like this is a job for the whole city. I'm issuing an order requiring all city agencies to cooperate with the health department to find the sources of lead and develop a plan to reduce

them." Then, he turns to you, a new health department employee. "Work on this and write me a report by next month, but I want a press release out this afternoon."

1. How does this case reflect the role that the media and effective communications play in public health?
2. How does this case reflect the multiple collaborations that are needed to practice public health effectively?
3. How does this case reflect the relationship between public health agencies and clinicians?
4. How does this case illustrate the inherently political nature of public health?

Community-Oriented Primary Care (COPC)

A community-oriented primary care team was developed in a large Hispanic/Latino community defined by census tracks. The vast majority of the community is employed and over half of the working population receive minimum wage and have no health insurance. There are a large number of immigrants from Central America. Over 25 percent of the community is estimated to be undocumented aliens, most of whom live in crowded conditions. A high percentage of those over 18 are married with an average family size of 5—considerably larger than other communities in the same city. The population of the community is generally younger than surrounding more affluent communities. The vast majority of the community receives its health care at one community clinic.

The community's priority issues according to community residents include tuberculosis (TB), HIV/AIDS, a lack of recreational facilities for children, a lack of dental services, and a lack of Spanish-speaking healthcare professionals. The COPC team, consisting of health professionals, public health experts, a clinical administrator, and members of the community, identified tuberculosis for further study. They found CDC evidence-based guidelines that recommends the following:

- early and accurate detection, diagnosis, and reporting of TB cases leading to initiation and completion of treatment
- identification of contacts of patients with infectious TB and treatment of those at risk with an effective drug regimen

- identification of other persons with latent TB infection at risk for progression to TB disease and treatment of these persons with an effective drug regimen
- identification of settings in which a high risk exists for transmission of *Mycobacterium tuberculosis* and application of effective infection-control measures

To implement these recommendations, risk factors for tuberculosis were identified in the community including: crowded conditions, HIV infections, high numbers of recent immigrants from endemic areas, and poor follow-up of treatment.

The COPC team found data on the estimated prevalence of a positive skin test for TB, the prevalence of active TB, the percentage of HIV-positive patients among those with active TB, and the percentage of active TB patients who completed a full course of treatment. The team recommended interventions for those factors that are most amenable to change including intensive testing and follow-up of HIV-positive patients and special home health assistance to ensure completion of TB treatment.

The team recommended monitoring the percentage of HIV patients who were given tuberculosis skin tests and the percentage of TB patients who completed a full course of treatment. They also recommended measuring the prevalence of active TB before and after the interventions. Finally, they advised working closely with the local health department so that recommended TB follow-up practices are successfully performed. This included making sure that whenever active TB is diagnosed, all those in contact with the individual are offered TB skin testing and preventive treatments if they convert to positive.

1. Identify how the COPC team accomplished each of the six steps in the COPC process.
2. What factors would you consider in selecting a particular condition, such as tuberculosis, for special interventions efforts?
3. Identify one of the community's other priority issues and suggest interventions that you would use for addressing it and assessing, monitoring, and evaluating the impact of your intervention.
4. What are the strengths and limitations of the COPC approach?

Hurricane Karl and the Public Health Success in Old Orleans

Hurricane Karl, a Category 4 hurricane, made landfall last August 29th on the gold coast of the state of Good Fortune. The state was home to the town of Old Orleans, an historical community built below sea level and home to a large community from a range of socioeconomic backgrounds. Old Orleans has a model health department that seeks to provide the ten essential public health services.

Before Hurricane Karl made its impact on the community, preparation for hurricanes had been an ongoing activity of the health department, which worked closely with first responders to ensure safe evacuation and protection from fire and looting. The department also worked with the local TV and radio stations to advise citizens on the purchasing and storing of essential food, water, and first aid supplies. It organized a community-wide emergency care network to ensure that 911 calls were responded to as quickly as possible in the event of a hurricane and worked with local hospitals to ensure that a triage system was in place to allocate patients to available emergency facilities, while not overwhelming any one healthcare institution.

When Hurricane Karl did strike, the damage was more extensive than expected. Leaks in the public sewer system led to water contamination. A local chemical plant experienced a major chemical discharge. Almost 200 residents were stranded in their homes without adequate food. Nearly half of the homes experienced water damage and rapid growth of mold. Many older residents did not have access to their daily medications.

The local health department had prepared for disasters like Hurricane Karl. After testing the water for contamination, supplies of stockpiled bottled water were distributed to homes in the contaminated areas by the National Guard. The police department had purchased specially-equipped vehicles on the recommendation of the health department and were able, with the help of community organizations, to evacuate the stranded residents. The health department also sent out trained teams to diagnose the type and extent of hazards related to chemical contamination. With the help of the emergency radio system and cell phones, all individuals in the contaminated areas were notified and educated about methods for protecting themselves and their children.

Based on the emergency plan, the health department set up temporary healthcare sites and pharmacies staffed by nurses, physicians, and pharmacists who had been certified as emergency responders. The department also worked with representatives of the building industry to test water-exposed homes for mold and provided assistance to minimize the damage.

After the emergency, the health department joined with the local Schools of Public Health and Medicine to evaluate the response to Hurricane Karl and make recommendations for future emergencies. The data on infections, injuries, and deaths, as well as the use of services during the emergency was collected and published. A national network was set up as a result to coordinate efforts for future disasters and learn from the experience in dealing with Hurricane Karl.

1. Which of the ten essential services did the health department of Old Orleans fulfill?
2. What other efforts were needed to accomplish the ten essential public health services?
3. In addition to providing the ten essential public health services, to what extent are efforts required to deal with a disaster such as Hurricane Karl?
4. How does this case illustrate the complementary relationship between public health and medicine. What are the benefits of working together?

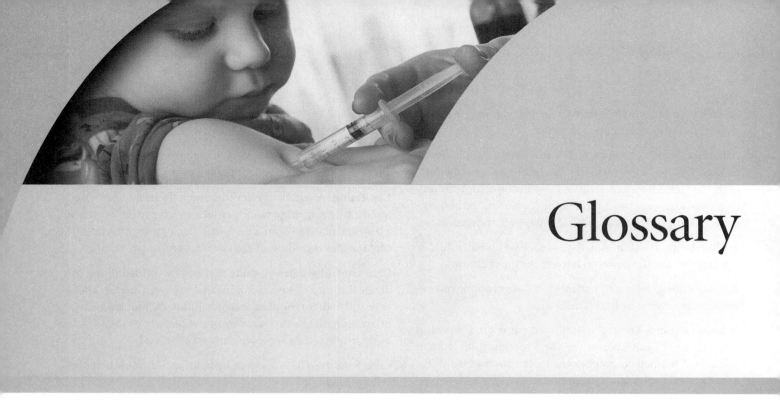

Glossary

Absolute risk–The actual chances or probability of developing the disease expressed as a probability such as 0.01 or a percentage such as 1%.

Academic Health Center–An organization that includes a medical school, one or more other health professions schools and an affiliated hospital.

Accreditation–A process applied to educational institutions, healthcare institutions, and proposed for governmental health departments to define and enforce required structures, processes, and outcomes.

Action phase–The fourth phase of the stages of change model in which the change in behavior takes place.

Actual causes of death–Modifiable factors that lead to major causes of mortality.

Administrative law–In the United States the type of law produced by executive agencies of federal, state, and local governments.

Age-adjustment–Taking into account age-distribution of a population when comparing population or when comparing the same population at two different points in time.

Age-distribution–The number of people in each age group in a population.

All hazard approach–An approach to public health preparedness that uses the same approach to preparing for many types of disasters including use of surveillance systems, communica-

tions systems, evacuations, and an organized healthcare response.

Antibody–A protein produced by the body in response to a foreign antigen which can bind to the antigen and facilitate its elimination.

Artifactual association–An association observed in the data that is actually the result of the method of data collection.

Artifactual difference or changes–Differences between population or changes in a population over time due to changes in interest in identifying the disease, change in ability to recognize the disease or changes in the definition of the disease.

Assessment–A core public health function that includes obtaining data that defines the health of the overall population and specific groups within the population including defining the nature of new and persisting health problems.

Association–The occurrence together of two factors, such as a risk factor and a disease, more often than expected by chance alone.

Assurance–A core public health function that includes governmental public health's oversight responsibility for ensuring that key components of an effective health system including health care and public health are in place even though the implementation will often be performed by others.

Asymptomatic–Without symptoms. When referring to screening for disease, it implies the absence of symptoms of the disease being sought.

At-risk population–The group of people who have a chance or probability of developing a disease.

Attributable risk percentage–The percentage of the disease or disability that can potentially be eliminated, among those with the factor being investigated, assuming a contributory cause and assuming the impact of the "cause" can be immediately and completely eliminated (*Synonym:* percent efficacy).

Authoritative decision–A decision made by an individual or a group that has the power to implement the decision.

Balance billing–Billing of patients for charges above and beyond those covered by health insurance.

Belmont Report–The commonly used name for a report of The National Commission for the Protection of Human Subjects of Biomedical and Behavioral Research which established key principles upon which the current approach to protection of human subjects is based.

Beneficence–An ethic principle which states that persons are treated in an ethical manner not only by respecting their decisions and protecting them from harm, but also by making efforts to secure their well-being.

Benefits–The positive outcomes that occur with or without an intervention.

BIG GEMS–A mneumonic which summarizes the determinants of disease including behavior, infection, genetics, geography, environment, medical care, and socioeconomic status.

Bioethics–Lies at the intersection of health law and policy and attempts to apply individual and group values and morals to controversial issues.

Biological plausibility–An ancillary or supportive criteria for contributory cause in which the disease can be explained by what is currently known about the biology of the risk factor and the disease.

Block grants–A system of federal funding to states and local jurisdictions that consolidates overall funding for a number of categories. They provide greater flexibility and allow the states to allocate funds to coordinate the delivery of services and to areas of greatest perceived need.

Branding–A marketing concepts for creating identification with a product or service that is also used in social marketing.

Built environment–The physical environment constructed by human beings.

Burden of Disease–Generically an analysis of the morbidity and mortality produced by disease. Often used to refer to the use of DALYs to estimate the burden of morbidity and mortality.

Cap–A limit on the total amount that the insurance will pay for a service per year, per benefit period, or per lifetime.

Capitation–A system of reimbursement for health care based upon a flat payment per time period for each person for whom a provider of care assumes responsibility for providing health-care services regardless of the services actually provided.

Case-control studies–A study that begins by identifying individuals with a disease and individual without a disease. Those with and without the disease are identified without knowledge of an individual's exposure or non-exposure to the factors being investigated (*Synonym:* retrospective study).

Case-Fatality–The chances of dying from a condition once it is diagnosed.

Case finding–As used in public health an effort to identify and locate contacts of individuals diagnosed with a disease and evaluate them for possible treatment.

Categorical funding–Providing funds for public health program based upon categories such as heart disease, tuberculosis, HIV/ AIDS, maternal and child health.

Cell mediated immunity–Immunological protection that is produced by t-lymphocytes and other white blood cells that combats intracellular pathogens and tumor cells.

Certainty effect–A risk-taking attitude in which the decision maker favors the status quo rather than a probability of obtaining a better or a worse outcome.

Certification–A nongovernmental process designed to ensure competence by individual health professionals based upon completion of educational requirement and performance on an examination or other evaluation procedure.

Cohort study–An investigation that begins by identifying a group that has a factor under investigation and a similar group that does not have the factor. The outcome in each group is then assessed (*Synonym:* prospective study).

Communicable disease–A disease due to an organism such as a bacteria or virus which is transmitted person-to-person or from animals or the physical environment to human by a variety of routes from air and water, to contaminated articles or fomites, to insect bites and animal bites. Here considered a subset of infectious disease.

Community Oriented Primary Care (COPC)–A structured six step process designed to move the delivery of health services from a focus on the individual to an additional focus on the needs of communities.

Community Oriented Public Health (COPH)–An effort on the part of governmental health agencies to reach out to the community and to the healthcare delivery system to address specific health issues.

Community rating–Insurance rates set the same for all eligible individuals and families based on the previous expenses in a defined community.

Concierge practice–A form of private practice of medicine that aims to provide personalized health care to those who can afford to pay for additional access and services out-of-pocket.

Confounding variable–A difference in the groups being compared that makes a difference in the outcome being measured.

Co-insurance–The percentage of the charges that the insured is responsible for paying.

Consistency–A supportive or ancillary criteria implying that the relationship has been observed in a wide range of populations and settings.

Constitutional law–In the United States a form of law based upon the United States constitution or the constitution of a state.

Contemplation phase–The second phase of the stages of change model in which an individual is actively thinking about the benefits and barriers to change.

Contributory cause–A definition of causation that is established when all three of the following have been established: (1) the existence of an association between the "cause" and the "effect" at the individual level; (2) the "cause" precedes the effect in time; and (3) altering the "cause" alters the probability of the "effect."

Co-payment–An amount that the insured is responsible for paying even when the service is covered by the insurance.

Core public health functions–Describes governmental public health functions that cannot be delegated and remain the responsibility of governmental public health. The Institute of Medicine has defined these functions as assessment, assurance, and policy development.

Cost effective–A measure of the cost of an intervention relative to its benefit. A cost effective intervention implies that any additional benefit is considered worth the cost. Cost effective can also imply that a large cost savings is worth a small reduction in net effectiveness.

Covered service–A service for which health insurance will provide payment if the individual is otherwise eligible.

Credentialing–A general term indicating a process of verifying that an individual has the desirable or required qualifications to practice a profession.

Customary, prevailing, and reasonable–These standards are used by many insurance plans to determine the amount that will be paid to the provider of services.

Data–Facts or the representation of facts as opposed to information.

Database–A collection of data organized in such a way that a computer program can select and compile the desired pieces of data.

Decision Analysis–A method of quantitative decision making that incorporates probabilities and utilities and the timing of events into the process of comparing options and making recommendations.

Decision Maker–A generic term that can be applied to a range of individuals and organizations that make health decisions including individuals, health professions and organizations ranging from non-profits to corporations to government agencies.

Deductible–The amount that an individual or family is responsible for paying before being eligible for insurance coverage.

Demographic transition–Describes the impact of falling childhood death rates and extended life spans on the size of populations and the age distribution of populations.

Determinants–Underlying factors that ultimately bring about disease.

Dietary supplements–A category within FDA law that includes vitamins, minerals, and many herbal remedies.

Diffusion of Innovation Theory–A theory that identifies stages of dissemination and types of adopters of new technology and other changes including behavioral change.

Disability Adjusted Life-Years (DALYs)–A population health status measure that incorporates measures of death and disability and allow for measurement of the impact of categories of diseases and risks factors.

Discounting–A process in which we place greater importance on events which are expected to occur in the immediate future than on events that are expected to occur in the distant future.

Distribution of Disease–How a disease is spread out in a population often using factors such as person, place, and time.

Dose-response relationship–A relationship which is present if changes in levels of an exposure are associated with changes in frequency of the outcome in a consistent direction.

Downstream factors–Factors affecting behavior that directly involve an individual and can potentially be altered by individual interventions such as an addiction to nicotine.

Dread effect–Perception of an increase in the probability of occurrence of an event due to its ease of visualability and its feared consequences.

Dynamic model–An approach to understanding a problem or system that looks at the components over a period of time.

Early adopters–Individuals categorized by Diffusion of Innovation theory as those who seek to experiment with innovative ideas.

Early majority adopters–Individuals categorized by Diffusion of Innovation theory as opinion leaders whose social status frequently influences others to adopt the behavior.

Ecological assessment–An assessment of the impact of an alteration of the physical environment on plants and animals.

Effectiveness–An intervention has been shown to increase the positive outcomes or benefits in the population or setting in which it will be used.

Efficacy–An intervention increased positive outcomes or benefits in the population on which it is investigated.

Eligible–An individual may need to meet certain criteria to be eligible for enrollment in a health insurance plan.

Employer Mandates–Employers are required to directly or indirectly provide comprehensive insurance coverage for all their employees.

Epidemiological transition–A concept indicating the change that has been historically observed as part of social and economic development from mortality and morbidity dominated by infections to morbidity and mortality dominated by what has been called non-communicable disease or degenerative and man-made diseases (*Synonym:* public health transition).

Epidemiological treatment–Treatment of contacts of an individual with a disease even in the absence of evidence of transmission of the disease.

Epidemiologists–An investigator who studies the occurrence and control of disease or other health conditions or events in defined populations.

Essential public heath services–The ten services that have come to define the responsibilities of the combined local, state, and federal governmental public health system.

Estimation–A statistical term implying a measurement of the strength of an association or the size of a difference.

Evidence–Reliable quantitative or qualitative information or data upon which a decision can be based.

Experience rating–Health insurance rates set on the basis of a group's past history of healthcare expenses (*Synonym:* Medical underwriting).

False negative–Individuals who have a negative result on a screening test but turn out to have the disease.

False positive–Individuals who have a positive result on a screening test but turn out not to have the disease.

Fee-for-service–A system of reimbursement for health services provided based on charges for health services actually provided to patients.

Group association–Two factors such as a characteristic and a disease occur together more often than expected by chance alone in the same group or population. Does not require that the investigator have data on the characteristics of the individuals that make up the group or population (*Synonym:* ecological association).

Harm–The negative outcomes that may occur with or without an intervention (see side effect).

Hazard–A measure of the inherent capability of a substance to produce harm.

Health Adjusted Life Expectancy (HALE's)–A population health status measure that combines life expectancy with a measure of the population's overall quality of health.

Healthcare delivery system–A linkage of institutions and healthcare professional that together take on the responsibility of delivering coordinated care.

Healthcare system–A healthcare delivery system plus the financial system that pays for the delivery of health care.

Health Communications–Method for conveying, interpreting, and utilizing health information as the basis for decision making.

Health Informatics–Methods for obtaining and compiling health information.

Health Related Quality of Life (HRQOL)–A health status measure that reflect the number of days of unhealthy days due to physical plus mental impairment. HRQOL provides an overall quality of health measure but it does not incorporate the impact of death.

Health system–The healthcare system plus the public health system.

Herd immunity–Protection of an entire population from a communicable disease by obtaining individual immunity through vaccination or natural infections by a large percentage of the population (*Synonym:* population immunity).

Heuristics–Rules of thumb for decision making that often allow more rapid decision making based on a limited amount of information.

Home rule–Authority granted to local jurisdictions such as cities or countries by state constitutions or state legislative actions.

Immunization–The strengthening of the immune system to prevent or control disease through exposure to antigens or administration of antibodies.

Inactivated vaccine–Injection of a nonliving organism or antigens from an organism designed to develop antibodies to protect an individual from the disease (*Synonym:* dead vaccine).

Incidence–Rates which measure the chances of occurrence of a disease or other condition over a period of time usually one year.

Incremental cost effectiveness–A measurement of the additional cost relative to the additional net-effectiveness (see net-effectiveness).

Individual mandates–Individuals are required to purchase individual health insurance policies which include at least standardized minimum coverage.

Infant mortality rate–A population health status measure that estimates the rate of death in the first year of life.

Infectious disease–A disease caused by an organism such as a bacteria or virus. Here used to include communicable diseases as well as other infections that are not communicable.

Infectivity–The ability of a pathogen to enter and multiply in a susceptible host.

Inference–A statistical term used to imply the drawing of conclusions about a population based upon data from a sample using statistical significance testing.

Inform of decision–A decision making approach in which a clinician is merely expected to inform the patient of what is planned.

Information–As used here, the compiling or presenting of data for a range of uses.

Informed consent–A decision making approach in which a clinician is expected to provide information and obtain agreement to proceed from the patient.

Inpatient facility–A healthcare facility in the United States in which an individual may remain for more than 24 hours. Examples include hospitals and nursing homes.

Institutional Review Board (IRB)–An institution-based group that is mandated by federal regulations to review human research conducted at the institution and determine whether it meets federally defined research standards.

Interaction analysis–An approach to environmental health assessment that looks at the consequences of two or more exposures.

Interventions–The full range of strategies designed to protect health and prevent disease, disability, and death.

Judicial law–Law made by courts when applying statutory or administrative law to specific cases (*Synonym:* case law, common law).

Justice–An ethical principle based on a sense of fairness in distribution of what is deserved.

Koch's postulates–Four postulates that together definitely establish a cause and effect for a communicable disease: the organism must be shown to be present in every case of the disease; the organism must not be found in cases of other diseases; once isolated the organism must be capable of replicating the disease in an experimental animal; and the organism must be recoverable from the animal (see Modern Koch's postulates).

Late adopters–Those identified by Diffusion of Innovation theory as in need of support and encouragement to make adoption as easy as possible (*Synonym:* laggard).

Lead time bias–The situation in screening for disease in which early detection does not alter outcome but only increases the interval, between detection of the disease and occurrence of the outcome such as death.

Legislative law–In the United States the type of law that includes statutes passed by legislative bodies at the federal, state, and local levels.

Leverage points–Points or locations in a system in which interventions can have substantial impacts (*Synonym:* control points).

License–A legal document granted by a governmental authority that provide permission to engage in an activity such as the practice of a health profession.

Life Expectancy–A population health status measure that summarizes the impact of death in an entire population utilizing the probability of death at each age of life in a particular year in a particular population.

Live vaccines–Use of a living organism in a vaccine. Living organism included in vaccines are expected to be attenuated or altered to greatly reduce the chances that they will themselves produce disease (*Synonym:* attenuated vaccine).

Long shot effect–A decision making attitude in which a decision maker perceives the status quo as intolerable and is willing to take an action with only a small chance of success and a large chance of making the situation worse.

Mainstream factors–Factors affecting behavior that result from the relationship of an individual with a larger group or population such as peer pressure to smoke or the level of taxation on cigarettes.

Maintenance–The fifth phase of the stages of change model in which the new behavior become a permanent part of an individual's lifestyle.

Market justice–The philosophy that market forces should be relied upon to organize the delivery of healthcare services.

Medicaid–A federal-state program which covers groups defined as categorically needed as well as groups that may be covered at the discretion of the state including those defined as medically needy such as those in need of nursing home care.

Medical Home–A term describing a concept of primary care that includes a team approach as part of a larger healthcare system.

Medical loss ratio–The ratio of benefits payments paid to premiums collected, indicating the proportion of the premiums spent on medical services.

Medical malpractice–A body of state civil law designed to hold practitioners accountable to patients for the quality of health care.

Medicare–A federal health insurance system that covers most individuals 65 and older as well as the disabled and those with end-stage renal disease.

Medigap–A supplemental health insurance linked to Medicare designed to cover all or most of the charges that are not covered by Medicare including the 20% co-payment required for many outpatient services.

Modern Koch's postulates–A set of criteria for establishing that an organism is a contributory cause of a disease requiring evidence of an epidemiological association, isolation, and transmissions (see Koch's postulates).

Morbidity–A public health term to describe the frequency of impairments or disability produced by a disease or other condition.

Mortality–A public health term to describe the frequency of deaths produced by a disease or other condition.

Multiple risk factor reduction–Simultaneous efforts to reduce more than one risk factor.

Multiplicative interaction–A type of interaction between two or more exposures such that the overall risk when two or more exposures are present is best estimated by multiplying the relative risk of each of the exposures.

Natural experiment–A change that occurs in one particular population but not another similar population without the intervention of an investigator.

Necessary cause–If the "cause" is not present the disease or "effect" will not develop.

Negative constitution–The principle that United States constitution allows but does not require government to act to protect public health or to provide healthcare services.

Negligence law–A body of law designed to protect individuals from harm.

Net effectiveness–A measure of the benefits minus the harms of an intervention (*Synonym:* Net benefit).

No-duty principle–The principle of United States law that healthcare providers, either individuals or institutions, do not have an obligation to provide health services.

Nutritional transition–Countries frequently move from poorly balanced diets often deficient in nutrients and calories to a diet of highly processed food including fats, sugars, and salt.

Odds ratio–A measure of the strength of the relationship that is often a good approximation of the relative risk. This ratio is calculated as the odds of having the risk factor if the disease is present divided by the odds of having the risk factor if the disease is absent.

Outcome measures–Measures of quality that imply a focus on the result of health care ranging from rates of infection to readmissions with complications.

Out-of-pocket expenses–Payments for health services not covered by insurance that are the responsibility of the individual receiving the services.

Outpatient facility–A healthcare facility in the United States in which patients can remain for less than 24 hours. These facilities include the offices of clinicians, general and specialty clinics, emergency departments and a range of new types of community-based diagnostic and treatment facilities.

Passive immunization–Administration of antibodies to provide short term protection against a disease.

P.E.R.I. Process–A mnemonic which summarizes the evidence-based public health process including problem description, etiology, recommendations based upon evidence, and implementation.

Phenotypic expression–The clinical presentation of a disease which may be quite variable despite the same genetic composition or genotype.

Point of Service Plans (POS)–A type of health plan that is a modification of staff model HMOs that allow enrollees to obtain care outside the HMO but require that the patient pay for a portion of the cost of the care received.

Police powers–Authority of governmental public health based on the power of state government to pass legislation and implement actions to protect the common good.

Policy development–A core public health function that includes developing evidence-based recommendations and other analyses of options such as health policy analysis to guide implementation including efforts to educate and mobilize community partnerships to implement these policies.

Population comparisons–A type of investigation in which groups are compared without having information on the individuals within the group (*Synonym:* ecological study).

Population health approach–As used here, a term used to describe an evidence-based approach to problem solving that considers a range of possible interventions including health care, traditional public health and social interventions (*Synonyms:* ecological approach, socio-ecological approach).

Population health status measures–Quantitative summary measures of the health of a large population such as life-expectancy, HALEs, and DALYs.

Portability–The ability to continue employment-based health insurance after leaving employment usually by paying the full cost of the insurance. A federal law known as COBRA generally ensures employees of 18 months of portability.

Potential risk factors–Factors that are thought to be associated with an increased probability of disease.

Precontemplation phase–The first phase of the stages of change model in which an individual has not yet considered changing their behavior.

Prediction rule–A quantitative formulae designed to increase the ability to predict the outcome of an condition and thereby guide the use of interventions.

Preferred Provider Plans (PPOs)–An insurance system that works with a limited number of clinicians. These providers agree to a set of conditions that usually includes reduced payments and other conditions. Patients may choose to use other clinicians but they often need to more pay more out-of-pocket.

Preparation phase–The third phase of the stages of change model in which the individual is developing a plan of action.

Preponderance of the evidence–A legal term implying that a trial is decided based upon the conclusion that the evidence is more supportive of the plaintive than the defendant or visa versa.

Prevalence–A measurement of the number of individuals who have a disease at a particular point in time divided by the number of individuals who could potentially have the disease.

Primary care–Traditionally refers to the first contact providers of care who are prepared to handle the great majority of common problems for which patients seek care.

Primary intervention–An intervention that occurs before the onset of the disease.

Procedural due process–A form of due process that prohibits governments from denying individuals a right in an arbitrary or unfair way.

Process measures–Measurement of quality that focus on the procedures and formal processes that go in delivering care from procedures to ensure credentialing of health professionals to procedures to ensure timely response to complaints.

Proportion–A fraction in which the numerator is made up of observations that are also included in the denominator.

Protective factor–A factor which is associated with a reduced probability of disease.

Provider–A term used to include a wide range of health professionals that provide health services.

Proximate cause–A legal concept of causation which asks whether the injury or other event would have occurred if the negligent act had not occurred.

Public health assessment–A formal assessment that incorporates risk assessment but also includes data on the actual exposure of a population to a hazard.

Public health surveillance–Collection of health data as the basis for monitoring and understanding health problems, generating hypotheses about etiology, and evaluating the success of interventions (*Synonym:* Surveillance).

Quality Adjusted Life Year (QALY)–A measurement that asks about the number of life-years saved by an intervention rather than the number of lives.

Quarantine–The compulsory physical separation of those with a disease or at high risk of developing a disease from the rest of the population.

Randomization–As part of a randomized clinical trial, assignment of participants to study and control groups using a chance process in which the participants are assigned to a particular group with a known probability (*Synonym:* Random assignment).

Randomized clinical trial–An investigation in which individuals are assigned to study or control groups using a process of randomization. (*Synonym:* experimental study).

Range of normal–The range of values on a test that is established by performing the test on those who are believed to be free of a disease. (*Synonym:* reference interval).

Rates–Used here as a generic term to describe measurements that have a numerator and a denominator.

Recommendations–Statements based upon evidence indicating that actions such as cigarette cessation will improve outcomes such a reducing lung cancer.

Reductionist approach–An approach to problem solving that looks at each of the components of a problem one at a time.

Relative risk–A ratio of the probability of the outcome if a factor known as a risk factor is present compared to the probability of the outcome if the factor is not present.

Respect for persons–An ethical principle that incorporates two ethical convictions: first, individuals should be treated as autonomous agents, and second, that persons with diminished autonomy are entitled to protection.

Revenue sharing–A system of allocating federal funding to states and local jurisdictions according to a specific formula with few restrictions on its use.

Reverse causality–The situation in which the apparent "cause" is actually the "effect."

Rights–Protections afforded individuals on the basis of the United States constitution, a state constitution, or legislative actions.

Ring vaccination–As used in the smallpox eradication program, immediate vaccination of populations in surrounding geographic areas after identification of a case of disease.

Risk assessment–A process used in environmental health to formally assess the potential for harm due to a hazard taking into account factors such as the likelihood, timing, and duration of exposure.

Risk avoider–A decision maker who consistently favors avoiding an action even when a decision analysis utilizing probabilities, utilities, and timing argues for the action.

Risk indicator–A characteristic such as gender or age that is associated with an outcome but is not considered a contributory cause (*Synonym:* risk marker).

Risk factor–A characteristics of individuals or an exposure that increases the probability of developing a disease. It does not imply that a contributory cause has been established.

Risk taker–A decision maker who consistently favors taking an action even when a decision analysis utilizing probabilities, utilitizes, and timing argues against the decision.

Risk taking attitudes–A decision making attitude in which an individual or group consistently favors taking action or avoiding action that differ from the recommendations of a decision analysis utilizing probabilities, utilities, and the timing of events.

Safety net–The provision of services for those who cannot afford to purchase the services.

Sample–A small subset drawn from a larger group or population.

Score–In the context of evidence-based recommendations, a measurement of the quality of the evidence and a measurement of the magnitude of the impact.

Screening–As used here, testing individuals who are asymptomatic for a particular disease as part of a strategy to diagnose a disease or identify a risk factor.

Secondary care–Refers to specialty care provided by clinicians who focus on one or a small number of organ systems or on a specific type of service such as obstetrics or anesthesiology.

Secondary intervention–Early detection of disease or risk factors and intervention during an asymptomatic phase.

Sensitivity–A measurement of how well a test performs in the presence of disease.

Sequential testing–A screening strategy that uses one test followed by one or more additional tests if the first test is positive (*Synonym:* two-stage testing).

Shared decision making–A decision making approach in which a clinician is expected to directly or indirectly provide information and options for intervention to a patient and then rely on the patient to synthesize the information and make their own decision.

Side effect–A negative outcome that may occur from an intervention.

Single Payer–A single source of payment for all healthcare services usually envisioned as government at the state or federal level as the payer for all basic healthcare services.

Simultaneous testing–A screening strategy that uses two tests initially with follow-up testing if either test is positive (*Synonym:* parallel testing).

Skimming–Enrolling predominating healthy individuals into a health plan to reduce the costs to the plan.

Social justice–A philosophy that aims to provide fair treatment and a fair share of the reward of society to individuals and groups.

Social marketing–The use of marketing theory, skills, and practice to achieve social change, e.g., in health promotion.

Socio-economic status–In the United States a measurement using scales reflecting education, income, and professional status.

Specificity–A measure of how well a test performs in the absent of disease. Equals 1 minus the false negative rate.

Stages of Change model–A model of behavioral change that hypothesizes five steps in the process of behavioral change including pre-contemplation, contemplation, preparation, action, and maintenance.

Standard population–The age distribution of a population that is often used as the basis for comparison with other populations. The age distribution of the United States population in the year 2000 is generally used.

State Child Health Insurance Program (SCHIP)–A federally funded health insurance program that provides funds to the states to use to expand or facilitate the operation of Medicaid or other uses to serve the health needs of lower income children.

Static model–An approach to understanding a problem or system that looks at the components at one particular point in time.

Statistical significance test–A method used to draw conclusions or inferences about populations from data on sample(s) of the population.

Strength of the relationship–A supportive or ancillary criteria implying that a measurement of the strength of an association such as a relative risk or odds ratio is large or substantial.

Structural measures–Measure of quality of health care focused on the physical and organizational infrastructure in which care is delivered.

Substantive due process–A type of due process in which state and federal governments must justify the grounds for depriving an individual of life, liberty, and property.

Sufficient cause–If the "cause" is present the disease or "effect" will occur.

Supportive criteria–Criteria that may be used to argue for a cause and effect relationship when the definitive requirements have not been fulfilled (*Synonym:* ancillary criteria).

Surrogate outcome–A measurement of outcome that looks at short term results such as changes in laboratory tests that may not reflect longer term or clinical important outcomes.

Syndemic–A systems thinking approach that focuses attention on how health problems interact as part of larger systems.

System error–Problems resulting from deficiencies in the system for delivering health care or other services.

Systems analysis–An approach to environmental exposures as well as other public health problems that examines the interconnections between exposures or components of larger networks.

Tertiary care–A type of health care often defined in terms of the type of institution in which it is delivered, often academic or specialized health center. This type of care may also be defined in term of the type of problem that is addressed such as trauma centers, burn centers, or neonatal intensive care.

Tertiary intervention–An intervention that occurs after the initial occurrence of symptoms but before irreversible disability occurs.

True rate–A measurement that has a numerator which is a subset of the denominator and a unit of time, such as a day or a year, over which the number of events in the numerator is measured.

Uncontrollability effect–Perception of increased probability of occurance of an event due to the perceived inability of an individual to control or prevent the event from occurring.

Under-5 Mortality–A population health status measure that estimates the probability of dying during the first 5 years of life.

Undergraduate medical education–Refers to the four years of medical school leading to a MD or DO degree despite the fact that an undergraduate or bachelors degree is generally required for admission.

Unfamiliarity effect–Perception of increased probability of an event due to an individual's absence of prior experience with the event.

Universal coverage–Provision of at least basic or medically necessary health insurance for an entire population.

Upstream factors–Factors affecting behavior that are grounded in social structures and policies, such as government-sponsored programs that encourage tobacco production.

Utility scale–A scale that goes from 0 to 1 with zero reflecting immediate death and 1 reflecting full health. This scale is used to measure the value or important that an individual or a group places on a particular outcome.

Victim blaming–Placing the responsibility or blame for a bad outcome on the individual who experiences the bad outcome due to their behavior.

Viral load–A measurement of the quantity of a virus such as HIV which is present in the blood.

Index

technology used to improve quality of care, 149–150
types of, 142
healthcare safety net, 182
healthcare systems
Commonwealth Fund's Commission on, 166
comparing U.S. to other developed countries, 163–164, 166
controlling costs of health care in U.S., 164–167
describing Canadian and U.K. systems, 161–162, 164–165
describing U.S. systems, 161–163
employment-based insurance programs, 158–160
extent/consequences of uninsured and underinsured, 160–162
government-supported insurance programs, 156–158
vs. health systems and healthcare delivery systems, 146
how much is spent on health care in U.S., 156
overview of, 128, 155–156
partnerships between, 188
public health and, 4
scoring, 162–163
health-related quality of life (HRQOL), 44
heart disease
preventative practices, 3
screening tests for, 91
herd immunity
smallpox and, 104
types of immunization, 102
HHS (Health and Human Services), 183
high-risk approach, to public health, 10
highway safety, 4, 96
HIV/AIDS
case finding applied to, 103
contributory causes of, 11
options for controlling, 105–107
outbreak investigations, 194
as societal health concern, 9
TB and, 101
treatment as means of reducing risk of transmission, 103
HMOs (Health Maintenance Organizations), 158–159
home rule authority, 181–182
hospice movement, 143
hospitals, 142–143
The House of God, 142
HRQOL (health-related quality of life), 44
HRSA (Health Services and Resources Administration), 183–184
Hurley v. Eddingfiled, 73
hygiene movement, 6, 8
hypotheses, generating, 20

I
ICD (International Classification of Diseases), 19
identical twin case study, 79
IHS (Indian Health Service)
healthcare systems, 157
as key federal health agency, 184
immunizations, for communicable diseases, 102. *see also* vaccines
implementation
framework of options for, 31
of interventions, 30–32
in P.E.R.I. process, 17
post-implementation procedures, 33
improving-the-average approach, to public health, 10
inactivated (dead) vaccines, 102
incentives
behavioral change and, 60
federal authority exerted via, 69
for reducing cost of health care, 166
incidence rates, 19
incremental cost-effectiveness ratio, 94
Indian Health Service (IHS)
healthcare systems, 157
as key federal health agency, 184
individual mandate approach, to insuring the uninsured/underinsured, 162
infant mortality rates, 42–43
infections. *see also* communicable diseases
as determinant of disease, 12–13
diseases due to, 99
infectious diseases vs. communicable diseases, 99
influenza, 107–108
inform of decisions, clinical decision making approaches, 49, 51
informed consent
Belmont Report and, 75
clinical decision making approaches, 49–51
informed purchaser, competition as means of controlling healthcare costs, 167
inpatient facilities, 142–143
Institute of Medicine (IOM)
core functions, 181
Educated Citizen and Public Health movement, 204
electronic record keeping and, 147–149
To Error is Human report, 151
National Vaccine Plan, 189
systems thinking used by, 199
Institutional Review Boards (IRBs), 75–76
insurance programs